Complete Denture Prosthodontics

Complete Denture Prosthodontics

Sujit Kumar Das BDS MDS (Cal)
Formerly
Principal, Professor and Head
Department of Prosthodontics and Dental Materials
Kalinga Institute of Dental Sciences, KIIT University
Bhubaneswar, Odisha, India
Professor and Head
Department of Prosthodontics and Dental Materials
Dr R Ahmed Dental College and Hospital
Kolkata, West Bengal, India

JAYPEE The Health Sciences Publisher
New Delhi | London | Philadelphia | Panama

Jaypee Brothers Medical Publishers (P) Ltd

Headquarters

Jaypee Brothers Medical Publishers (P) Ltd
4838/24, Ansari Road, Daryaganj
New Delhi 110 002, India
Phone: +91-11-43574357
Fax: +91-11-43574314
Email: jaypee@jaypeebrothers.com

Overseas Offices

J.P. Medical Ltd
83, Victoria Street, London
SW1H 0HW (UK)
Phone: +44 20 3170 8910
Fax: +44 (0)20 3008 6180
Email: info@jpmedpub.com

Jaypee-Highlights Medical Publishers Inc
City of Knowledge, Bld. 237, Clayton
Panama City, Panama
Phone: +1 507-301-0496
Fax: +1 507-301-0499
Email: cservice@jphmedical.com

Jaypee Medical Inc
325 Chestnut Street
Suite 412, Philadelphia, PA 19106, USA
Phone: +1 267-519-9789
Email: jpmed.us@gmail.com

Jaypee Brothers Medical Publishers (P) Ltd
17/1-B Babar Road, Block-B, Shaymali
Mohammadpur, Dhaka-1207
Bangladesh
Mobile: +08801912003485
Email: jaypeedhaka@gmail.com

Jaypee Brothers Medical Publishers (P) Ltd
Bhotahity, Kathmandu
Nepal
Phone: +977-9741283608
Email: kathmandu@jaypeebrothers.com

Website: www.jaypeebrothers.com

Website: www.jaypeedigital.com

Inquiries for bulk sales may be solicited at: jaypee@jaypeebrothers.com

Complete Denture Prosthodontics

First Edition: **2016**

ISBN 978-93-5152-621-6

Printed at Sanat Printers

Dedicated to

My parents
and
My beloved wife Aparna

PREFACE

During my career in dental education, I have felt the need for a simple yet comprehensive textbook on *Complete Denture Prosthodontics* that would serve as an introductory text for the dental students and be a suitable refresher source for the general practitioners and the postgraduate students.

The concepts presented in this book have been developed over time under the influence of my teachers and in close cooperation with my coworkers and postgraduate students. I have had the good fortune of working with two great prosthodontists—Dr SP Mayer and Dr PK Basu at Dr R Ahmed Dental College and Hospital, Kolkata, West Bengal, India. They have the great influence on me and my respected gratitude toward these giants is never ending.

I hope this book will be of immense help to the students and clinicians alike. It is well understood that a text is not a substitute of a teacher and guide, whose presence will always be felt in every step of learning and execution.

Sujit Kumar Das

ACKNOWLEDGMENTS

I think teachers continue to learn as long as they have students. So, my thanks go to all my students, especially my postgraduate students. My thanks to my friends and coworkers who inspired me, namely Dr B Bera, Dr SK Sen, Dr A Banerjee, Dr PK Paul, Dr B Sengupta, Dr S Mukherjee, Dr D Dutta, Dr Tapas Gupta and Dr Sampa Roy.

My thanks are due to M/s Whip Mix Corporation, Loisville, USA, for their permission of using many photographs from MS PowerPoint version 12.04.

My thanks to the Department of Health and Family Welfare, Government of West Bengal, for permission of the literature works done during my service as the Professor and Head, Department of Prosthodontics, Dr R Ahmed Dental College and Hospital, Kolkata.

My thanks are due to Mr Subrato Sarkar, the photographer for his excellent work.

My thanks are also due to Dr A Samanta, and Mr P Parida, Kalinga Institute of Dental Sciences, Kalinga Institute of Industrial Technology (KIIT) University, Bhubaneswar, Odisha, India.

I take this opportunity to thank my sons Sarbadarshi and Avishek, and my daughter-in-law Sarmistha.

My special acknowledgment to Shri Jitendar P Vij (Group Chairman), Mr Ankit Vij (Group President), Mr Tarun Duneja (Director–Publishing), and the editorial team of M/s Jaypee Brothers Medical Publishers (P) Ltd, New Delhi, India, for publishing the book.

CONTENTS

1. Introduction and Scope **1**
Definition of Terms 1
Branches of Prosthodontics 1
Types of Prosthesis 2
Objectives of Complete Denture Prosthesis 2
History of Complete Dentures 3
Clinical and Laboratory Procedures of Complete Denture Prosthesis 4
Treatment Options for Edentulous Patients 5
Scope of Complete Dentures 5

2. Applied Anatomy **8**
Applied Anatomy of Important Oral Structures 8
Mucosa 8
Bones 10
Surrounding Muscles 14
Salivary Glands and Saliva 19

3. Examination, Diagnosis, Treatment Planning and Prognosis **29**
Definition of Diagnosis 29
Treatment Planning 29
Diagnostic Form 30
Explanation of Diagnostic Form 33
Prognosis 45

4. Retention, Stability and Support of Complete Dentures **49**
Retention 49
Definition 49
Factors Affecting Complete Denture Retention 49
Stability 54
Support 57

5. Principles and Techniques of Impression Making **60**
Impression 60
Complete Denture Impression 60
Anatomic Landmarks 62
Denture-bearing Areas 63
Theories of Impression Making 69
Impression Techniques 69
According to Degree of Compression 69
Mucocompressive Impression Technique 71
According to the Position of the Mouth 74

According to the Type of Impression Tray 75
Principles of Impression Making 75
Clinical Procedures of Impression Making 76
Preliminary Impressions 76
Final Impressions 85
Custom/Special Tray 85

6. Preparation of Casts, Special Trays, Denture Bases and Occlusal Rims............................ 92
Model 92
Cast 92
Laboratory Preparation 93
Boxing and Pouring of Master Casts 97
Record Bases and Occlusion Rims 100

7. Articulators and Facebows.. 107
Articulators 107
Facebows 113

8. Jaw Relations and Methods of Registration... 119
Jaw Relationship 119
Jaw Relationship Record 119
Importance of Maxillomandibular Relations 119
Vertical Dimension 120
Effects of Excessive Occlusal Vertical Dimension 121
Effects of Reduced Occlusal Vertical Dimension 122
Methods of Determining Vertical Dimension of Occlusion 122
Significance or Importance of Centric Relation 126
Difficulties in Recording Centric Relation 126
Contraindications of Gothic Arch Tracing Method 129
Clinical and Laboratory Procedures 130
Preliminary Vertical Dimension of Occlusion 130
Recording the Centric Relation 136

9. Artificial Tooth Selection and Arrangement 139
Anterior Tooth Selection, Arrangement and Esthetics 139
Objectives 139
Methods of Selection of Teeth 139
Number System of Artificial Teeth 146
Preliminary Arrangement of Artificial Teeth for Trial 148
Inclinations 151
Selection and Arrangement of Posterior Teeth 154
Selection of Posterior Teeth 154
General Principle of Arrangement of Posterior Teeth
Factors for Arrangement of Posterior Teeth 156
Laboratory Procedures (Arrangement of Teeth) 157
Arrangement of Teeth in Class I Relation 160
Selection and Arrangement of Teeth in Atypical Ridge Relations 163

Arrangement of Teeth in Angle's Class II, Division 1 163
Arrangement of Teeth in Angle's Class II, Division 2 163
Arrangement of Teeth in Angle's Class III 164
Arrangement of Teeth of Patient with Old Denture 164

10. Occlusion and Articulation in Complete Dentures 166
Nomenclature and Terminology of Occlusion 166
Balanced Articulation 168
Arrangement of Anatomic (Cusp) Teeth to Balanced Articulation 172
Arrangement of Nonanatomic (Cuspless) Teeth to Balanced Articulation 173

11. Try-in of Complete Dentures 177
Definition 177
Objectives 177
Instruments and Materials 177
Trial Denture Procedures 177
Postdam/Post-palatal Seal 181

12. Laboratory Procedures—Final Arrangement of Teeth, Waxing, Processing and Finishing of Dentures 185
Final Arrangement of Teeth 185
Wax Contouring (Waxing) of Complete Dentures 187
Conventional Method 188
Processing Complete Dentures 191

13. Correction of Occlusal Discrepancies 199
Causes of Occlusal Discrepancies 199

14. Delivery and Adjustments of Complete Dentures 205
Objectives 205
Instruments and Materials 205
Preparation for Insertion 206
Insertion Procedure 206
Check Record 208
Complains of Dentures 213

15. Sequelae of Wearing Complete Dentures 215
Effects of Complete Dentures on Oral Tissues 215
Residual Ridge Reduction (RRR) 216
Denture Stomatitis 217
Angular Cheilitis 217
Flabby Ridge 217
Burning Mouth Syndrome 217
Gagging 218
Control of Sequelae of Wearing Complete Dentures 218

16. Repair, Rebasing and Relining 220

Repair 220
Relining 225
Rebasing 227

17. Immediate Complete Dentures 228

Definition 228
Types of Immediate Denture 228
Requirements of Immediate Dentures 229
Advantages of Immediate Dentures 229
Disadvantages of Immediate Dentures 230
Indications 230
Contraindications 230
Treatment Planning for Immediate Dentures 230
Immediate Denture Techniques 231

18. Dental Implants 235

Dental Implants 235
Implants Treatment Course 239
Types of Implants Restoration for Edentulous Patients 242
Clinical Success for Endosseous Implant 243
Biomechanical Factors in Long-term Implant Success 243
Criteria for Implant Success 243
Complications of Implants 244

19. Overdentures 245

Definitions 245
Overlay Denture 245
Goals of Overdentures 245
Indications 245
Contraindications 246
Advantages of Overdenture 246
Disadvantages of Overdenture 246
Types of Overdentures 246
Techniques of Overdenture 247
Treatment Procedure for Overdenture 247

20. Single Complete Denture 250

Definition 250
Indications 250
Contraindications 250
Problems of Single Complete Denture 250
Fees for Single Complete Denture 251
Diagnosis and Treatment Planning 251
Tooth Modification 251
Methods Used to Obtain Balanced Occlusion 252
Occlusal Materials for the Single Complete Denture 253
Clinical Procedures for Single Complete Denture Opposing Natural Teeth 253

21. Maxillofacial Prosthetics **255**

Definition 255
Objectives 255
Classification of Maxillofacial Defects 255
Types of Surgical Defects in Maxilla 255
Types of Surgical Defects in Mandible 255
Types of Maxillofacial Prosthesis 256
Cleft Palate 257
Maxillary Prosthesis 258
Clinical and Laboratory Step by Step Procedures of Fabrication of Complete Denture with Obturator 260
Treatment Prosthesis 264
Mandibular Training Flange 265
Splints 265
Stents 267
Carrier 267
Mouth Protectors 267

Index *269*

Chapter 1

Introduction and Scope

DEFINITION OF TERMS

There are some special words and phrases that dentists use to communicate with one another. Thus a need for terminology was felt. A glossary of prosthodontics terms published in 1956 to standardize terms and other meanings. Since then these accepted terms under the name of *Glossary of Prosthodontic Terms* were published every four years in the Journal of Prosthetic Dentistry. The revised eighth edition of the glossary is now available. Some terms are defined here and additional terms used later in the text will be defined as they are used.

Prosthesis: Prosthesis may be defined as an appliance which replaces lost or congenitally missing tissue restoring both the function and the appearance of the tissue it replaces or one of these. Prosthesis, denture, denture prosthesis and restoration may be used synonymously.

Prosthetics: It is art and science of designing and fitting artificial substitutes to replace lost or missing tissues.

Prosthodontics/Prosthetic dentistry/Dental prosthetics: The branch of dentistry pertaining to the restoration and maintenance of oral function, comfort, appearance, and health of the patient by the restoration of the natural teeth and/or the replacement of missing teeth and contiguous oral and maxillofacial tissues with artificial substitutes (GPT-8).

BRANCHES OF PROSTHODONTICS

Prosthodontics has several branches as follows:

1. Removable prosthodontics
   a. Complete denture prosthodontics
   b. Partial denture prosthodontics
2. Fixed prosthodontics
3. Maxillofacial prosthodontics
4. Implant prosthodontics

Removable prosthodontics: The branch of prosthodontics concerned with the replacement of teeth and contiguous structures for edentulous or partially edentulous patients by artificial substitutes that are removable from the mouth.

Fixed prosthodontics: The branch of prosthodontics concerned with the replacement and/or restoration of teeth or both, by artificial substitutes that are not readily removable from the mouth.

Maxillofacial prosthetics: The branch of prosthodontics concerned with the restoration and/or replacement of the stomatognathic and associated facial structures with prosthesis that may or may not be removed on a regular or elective basis.

Implant prosthodontics: The phase of prosthodontics concerning the replacement of missing teeth and/or associated structures by restorations that are attached to dental implants.

Complete denture prosthodontics: The replacement of the natural teeth in the arch and their associated parts by artificial substitutes (GPT-8).

Removable partial denture prosthodontics: The science and techniques of designing and constructing partial denture (GPT-4).

TYPES OF PROSTHESIS

Denture: An artificial substitute for missing natural teeth and adjacent tissues (GPT-8). A denture may be partial or complete.

Partial denture: A dental prosthesis that restores one or more but not all of the natural teeth and/or associated parts and that is supported in part by natural teeth, dental implant supported crowns, abutments, or other fixed partial dentures and/or the mucosa.

Based on patient's capability to remove or not to remove the prosthesis, a partial denture may be fixed or removable.

Fixed partial denture: A partial denture that is luted or otherwise securely retained to natural teeth, tooth root and/or dental implant abutments that furnish the primary support for the prosthesis. They are of two types: (a) screw retained fixed partial denture, (b) cement retained fixed partial denture (GPT-8).

Removable partial denture: Any prosthesis that replaces some teeth in a partially dentate arch. It can be removed from the mouth and replaced at will (GPT-8).

Complete denture: A removable dental prosthesis that replaces the entire dentition and associated structures of maxillae and mandible (GPT-8).

INTRODUCTION

The loss of all teeth results in edentulous state for any person. He also loses some of the ability to perform important functions—chewing, speaking, facial expression and his appearance is impaired. The loss of teeth is also accompanied by the loss of bony support due to resorption. The complete denture not only replaces the loss of teeth, supporting bone and soft tissues but also restores the impaired functions and appearance.

OBJECTIVES OF COMPLETE DENTURE PROSTHESIS

The desired objectives in complete denture prosthesis are as follows:

1. *Esthetics*: The restoration of the facial dimension and lost contour with normal appearance.
2. *Mastication*: The restoration of the function of mastication for adequate nutrition.
3. *Phonetics*: The restoration of speech due to loss of teeth. The complete dentures help the patient to speak as distinctly as breathing factors will permit.
4. The complete dentures will provide the patient with oral comfort and improve the sense of wellbeing.
5. *Preservation of oral structures*: The patient should be informed about the changes to be expected in the supporting tissues and convinced him of the need for regular check-ups and further treatment.

Esthetics

The main part of the face to suffer change by the loss of the teeth and consequent resorption of the alveolar process is the lower third. The lips lose their normal pose and exhibit an unnatural expression. The wrinkle of face and aged appearance sets in. The prosthodontics should correct, and as far as possible restore the normal appearance. It requires an artistic sense to develop the correct facial contour in order to restore harmony in each individual type of expression. The color of artificial teeth must be harmonious with the color of the eyes, hair and patient's complexion. The form, size and arrangement of the teeth and their treatment by grinding to simulate wear appropriate to the age of the patient must also be done.

Phonetics

The third objective is the correction of speech defects resulted from absence of natural teeth or from improper arrangements of teeth. The best result is most often obtained by placing the teeth, as nearly as possible in position occupied by the natural teeth. These can be done by using the proper form of teeth selection and adjusting the bulk of base material, as well as the reproduction of the rugae of the palate.

Mastication

When the function of mastication is impaired, the digestive organs fail to properly digest the food which results in poor health and a curtailment of the span of life. The substitutes for the natural teeth should be provided that function as far as practicable.

The achievement of these objectives will, of course, be limited by the physiologic and psychologic condition of the patient. Unless he/she is physically and mentally able to adapt to an oral prosthesis, no one can improve these objectives on him/her. Paramount to success is the patient's cooperation, both subconscious and conscious.

HISTORY OF COMPLETE DENTURES

The practice of prosthodontics has been improved in more recent times by the following men:

1. *Lorenz Heister (1683–1758)*: Surgeon of Frankfort, was the first to make a removable prosthesis made of ivory of hippopotamus tusk.
2. *Fan Chard (1678–1761)*: Used human teeth and teeth of hippopotamus tusk, ivory or ox bone to make upper and lower complete dentures.
3. *Pierre Fouchard (1728)*: Described a process of attaching carved ivory tooth on a strip of gold.
4. *Philip Pfaff (1756)*: The dentist of Frederick the great of Prussia, was the first to make impression by asking the edentulous patient to bite into a softened ball of bees wax, thus obtaining simultaneously impressions of both the jaws. He poured the casts into plaster, keyed them and fabricated the prosthesis on it. It recorded close mouth impressions along with jaw relations.
5. *Duchateau and Dubois de Chemant (1774)*: Made a complete denture from fused porcelain.
6. *William Rae (1782)*: Described a technique of impression taking in wax and pouring the cast of plaster of Paris.
7. *Garriot (1805)*: A Frenchman, discovered metallic hinge articulator.
8. *G Fouzi of Italy (1808)*: Made individual poreclain tooth with steel pin.
9. *James Cameron and Denial Evans (1840)*: Developed hinge articulators and took patient for it.
10. *Claudius Ash of England (1837)*: Prepared porcelain tube teeth.
11. *Thomas W Evans (1854)*: First used vulcanite for dentures in United Kingdom followed by Goodyear in 1855 in USA.
12. *W GA Bone Will (1933–1899)*: Invented the first anatomical articulator to simulate the movement of the jaws. In 1858, he described the 'Bonewill triangle' and balanced complete dentures at three points in forward and lateral movements.
13. In 1887, *Hanes* designed a face bow for orientation of cast on articulator.
14. In 1896, *WE Walker* showed that dentures set on Bonewill's articulators are not exhibiting balanced occlusion in patient's mouth. He developed first adjustable articulator with adjustable condylar guides.
15. In 1899, *Snow* improved the face bow.
16. In 1907, Bakelite was discovered and in 1924 *Gorge W Stryker* constructed a full denture of Bakelite.
17. *Alfred Gysi* in 1913 designed anatomic tooth form known as 'Trubyte'.
18. *Monson* in 1918 presented the maxillo mandibular instrument based on the spherical theory of occlusion.

19. *Hanau* in 1927 designed articulator and came up with the theory of *'Balanced articulation'*.
20. The shortage of rubber vulcanite in world war time led to the discovery of acrylic resin in 1935.
21. In 1936, moulding of colored glass into dentures and swaged stainless steel was done as denture base materials were used as denture base material in combination with acrylic resin.

Indications of Complete Dentures

1. Presence of acceptable edentulous ridge or ridges with sufficient vertical space to accommodate the dentures or dentures without affecting any major change in the patients vertical dimension after the postextraction tissue changes occurred.
2. Serious loss of masticatory function or impairment of esthetics, speech, and psychologic wellbeing.
3. Treatment of patients where remaining teeth cannot be retained owing to extensive carious destruction or periodontal bone loss.

Contraindications of Complete Dentures

There is no absolute contraindication of complete denture prosthesis but it is difficult to fabricate complete denture in the following situations:

1. An edentulous patient who has not worn dentures in many years if ever.
2. Unmanageable mechanical problems associated with major lack of vertical interarch space.
3. Maxillary mandibular arch size or relation discrepancies.
4. Patient with no salivary function as a result of radiation or drug therapy.
5. Altered systemic health, e.g. uncontrolled diabetes, Parkinson's disease, epilepsy, etc.
6. Severe or total loss of alveolar ridge.
7. Allergy to acrylic resin.
8. Patient with severe or total paralysis of motor nerves of tongue, cheeks, lips, or floor of the mouth.
9. Excessive loss of maxilla or mandible as a result of radical surgery.
10. Unmanageable gag reflex.
11. Large maxillary or mandibular tori.

CLINICAL AND LABORATORY PROCEDURES OF COMPLETE DENTURE PROSTHESIS

First Appointment

1. History, examination, diagnosis, treatment planning, prognosis and patient education.
2. Preliminary impressions corrected and tested.

Laboratory Preparations for the Second Appointment

3. Pouring diagnostic casts, custom tray fabrication.

Second Appointment

4. Final impressions.

Laboratory Preparations for the Third Appointment

5. Boxing, cast pouring, occlusal rims on base plate.

Third Appointment

6. Recording of jaw relations.
7. Selection and arrangement of artificial teeth.

Fourth Appointment

8. Try-in.

Laboratory Preparation for the Fifth Appointment

9. Waxing, flasking, curing, polishing and finishing.

Fifth Appointment

10. Insertion and instructions to the patient.

Sixth Appointment

11. 24 hours postinsertion check-up for adjustments.
12. Recall for check-up periodically.

TREATMENT OPTIONS FOR EDENTULOUS PATIENTS

1. Edentulous in one or both arches with no prior denture experience
   a. Complete dentures or
   b. Implant-supported overdentures or
   c. Implant-supported fixed prosthesis.
2. Edentulous in both arches with an adaptive complete denture experience
   a. Complete dentures or
   b. Implant-supported overdentures or
   c. Implant-supported fixed prosthesis.
3. Edentulous in one or both arches with current maladaptive denture experience
   a. Implant-supported overdentures or
   b. Implant-supported fixed prosthesis.

SCOPE OF COMPLETE DENTURES

To discuss about the scope of complete denture let us discuss about the current statistics of magnitude of edentulism.

Due to improvement of medical science, antibiotics, vaccines the average life expectancy of people has been increasing rapidly over the last 50 years. So, the number of aged patients has been increasing.

The life expectancy during roman times was 25 years.

- In the middle age it was 30 years only.
- In 1775–34 years
- In 1850–42 years
- In 1900–50 years
- In 1920–56 years
- In 1940–64 years
- In 1970–70 years (Fig. 1.1)
- In recent years it is more than 70 years.

The decrease in child and young age mortality rate and decrease in number of stillborn child has given its substractive effect on overall mortality rate.

This causes the growing number of elders in our society. As complete edentulous cases are mostly of older age group, there is increasing demand of complete denture restoration.

On the other hand in recent years introduction of fluoridation and prevention of tooth degenerative diseases like periodontal diseases, caries has declined the number of tooth loss. So, decrease of complete edentulous cases with respect to population causing slight decline in percentage of complete denture cases.

In spite of advancement of dental sciences until knowledge of the cause and perfect treatment of caries and periodontitis is known, the necessity of complete denture prosthesis will remain unabated. Krajicek (1977) has estimated that there will be increase of edentulous persons from 23 to 28 lac in United State from 1977 to 2000.

A study conducted in USA by Douglass et al in 2002 showed that there is 10% decline in total edentulism in every decade. The 10% decline in edentulism each decade for last 30 years will

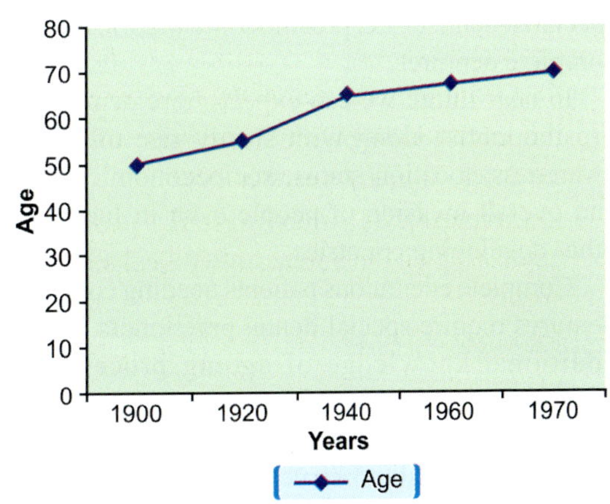

Fig. 1.1: Graphical representation of rise of life-expectancy from the year 1900 to 1970

be offset say the increase in population of 56 years of age by 79% in 2020 (Fig. 1.2). So, the speculation that "complete edentulism and need for complete denture has been declined markedly or will decline markedly in near future" was proved wrong. Probably no dramatic changes in the needs of complete denture prosthesis will be in our population in near future.

There may be a gradual reduction in the percentages of complete edentulous patient among the population but that is lower than the percentage of rise of life expectancy of the population. So, ultimately there is increase in the total number of edentulous person, i.e. increased demand of complete dentures.

Hickey (1985) has estimated that the number of edentulous patient seeking initial treatment and/or periodic maintenance case was 9.0 million in 1980 and became 10.4 million in 2000.

In India, continuous rise in total population along with the increase in their life expectancy gives a higher percentage of increment of old age group population so, increase in edentulous cases. Affordability and awareness of being restored by complete denture during edentulous state may not be markedly pronounced in poor socioeconomic and higher socioeconomic groups of people in India.

Increased demand of complete denture also increases the demand/need of particular trained or specialist dentists, i.e. prosthodontist fabrication of complete dentures.

In near future we can expect more demand of prosthodontist along with steady rise of public awareness, location status, socioeconomic status and overall invasion of people even in India and other developing countries.

Complete edentulous patients needing complete dentures require special dental practioners having additional knowledge of ageing process and awareness of differences need and response expected at older age levels.

Prosthodontists to serve the complete denture patients need to be very much concerned with

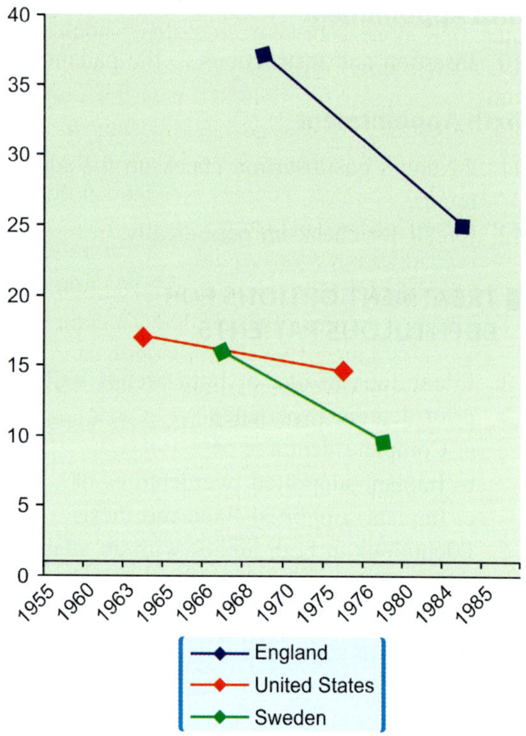

Fig. 1.2: Decrease in edentulous persons in each decade in three developed countries

geriatric management along with complete denture construction. Prosthodontists should have perfect knowledge about solution of complexities associated with complete dentures. Edentulous patients require competent, compassionate professional dental treatment even though providing such treatment is difficult and time-consuming. The understanding of people, their problems and their attitude is necessary for successful practice of prosthodontists and successful restoration of cases of complete dentures. Limitation of knowledge in genetics, periodontology, limitations of knowledge in psychology and dental materials and technology have made it difficult job for prosthodontists to fabricate complete satisfactory complete denture prosthesis. Keeping in mind the varied scope and increasing demand of complete dentures in future, a prosthodontist may work as a part of health team rather than alone. Moreover, the patient should also be educated about the periodic examination after the complete denture treatment and need for relining when necessary by change in supporting tissues. A complete and thorough knowledge of the age-related TMJ changes, support mechanism during masticatory load and in resting state on mucosa and bones of ridges is very essential.

In India number of dentist per 100,000 was 3 in a study by Zillen et al in 2000. To cope with the mounting demand for prosthodontic care, it is necessary to improve the quality of instruction and efficient use of adequate patient contact hours.

CONCLUSION

The increasing need for complete denture treatment has been met with 'denturist' some American states and some countries like Canada. The denturist is a nondentist licensed to provide complete dentures directly to the public. But to provide classic complete denture service for some elderly patients, a properly trained and experienced prosthodontist is still in need. It is, therefore, obvious that an abbreviated technique for a complete denture is necessary that yields an acceptable complete denture for the edentulous patient.

BIBLIOGRAPHY

1. Atwood DA. Practice of prosthodontists. J Prosthet Dent. 1969;21:393.
2. Douglas CW, Shih A, Ostry I. Will there be a need for complete dentures in the United States in 2020? J Prosthet Dent. 2002;87:58.
3. Hickey JC, Oral health status in the United States—Tooth loss and edentulism. J Dent Educ. 1985;49: 377-78.
4. Krajicek DD. The future of complete prosthodontics. J Prosthet Dent. 1977;37:126.
5. Love WB. Prosthodontics past, present and future. J Prosthet Dent. 1976;36:261.
6. Lytle RB, Atwood DA, Beck HO. Minimum standards of adequate prosthodontic service. J Prosthet Dent. 1968;19:108.
7. Overton RG, Bramblett RM. Prosthodontic service, a study of need and availability in the United States. J Prosthet Dent. 1972;21:329.
8. Payne SH. The future of prosthodontics. J Prosthet Dent. 1976;35:3.
9. Shary JJ. Curriculum curtailment in prosthodontic education. J Prosthet Dent. 1976;35:469.
10. Zillen PA, Mindak M. World dental demographics. Int Dent J. 2000;50:194-97.

Chapter 2

Applied Anatomy

INTRODUCTION

The complete dentures are fabricated for use in the oral environment. So, for successful complete denture treatment, the knowledge of anatomy and physiology is essential. Without a thorough knowledge of these basic sciences, denture fabrication becomes only a mechanistic approach. A combined knowledge of biological sciences and mechanics will be the biomechanical approach of present day. The anatomical structures of the oral cavity consist of denture-bearing soft tissues, underlying bone, surrounding muscles, tongue, salivary glands and saliva. All of them influence the construction of complete dentures. The knowledge of the temporomandibular joint and mandibular movements is also important because jaw relation and building up of occlusion is an important part of complete dentures fabrication.

APPLIED ANATOMY OF IMPORTANT ORAL STRUCTURES

It can be discussed under two following heads:

a. Applied anatomy of impression procedures: Tissues of denture-bearing area and its environment.
b. Applied anatomy for jaw relation records: Tissues of the temporomandibular joints and muscles performing mandibular movements and various movements of mandible.

Applied anatomy in impression procedures—Tissues of denture-bearing area and its environment: The oral tissues of denture-bearing area which come in contact with the complete upper and lower dentures are:

1. Mucosa
2. Bone
3. Tongue
4. Surrounding muscles
5. Salivary glands and saliva.

MUCOSA

The oral mucosa covers the hard and soft palate, the upper and lower alveolar ridges, sulcus and inner side of the lips and cheeks. It is related to bone only or supported by connective tissues and muscle. The oral mucosa is composed of two layers—the mucosa and the submucosa. The mucosa is further divided two layers—the external epithelium and an inner layer of thick and dense connective tissue, the lamina propria with a basement membrane in between them (Fig. 2.1). The mucous membrane is attached to the bone by the periosteum. There are several types of mucosa due to difference in function.

Types of Mucosa (Fig. 2.2 and Flow chart 2.1)

The mucosa can be classified as: (a) masticatory, (b) lining, and (c) specialized.

Masticatory Mucosa

The mucosa is present on the ridge and the hard palate.

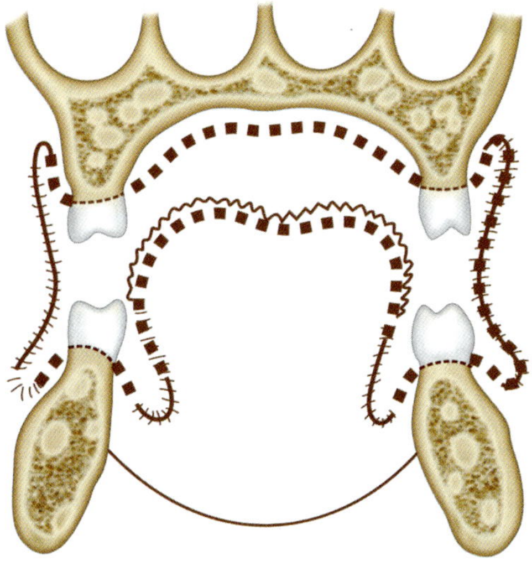

Fig. 2.1: Types of oral mucosa

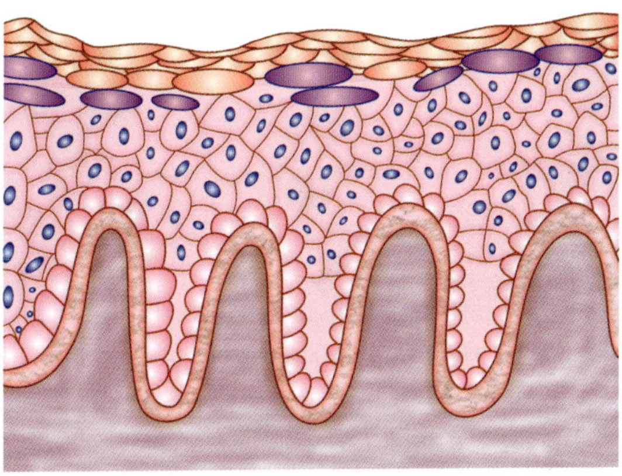

Fig. 2.2: Diagrammatic representation of keratinized mucosa

Flow chart 2.1: Type of mucosa

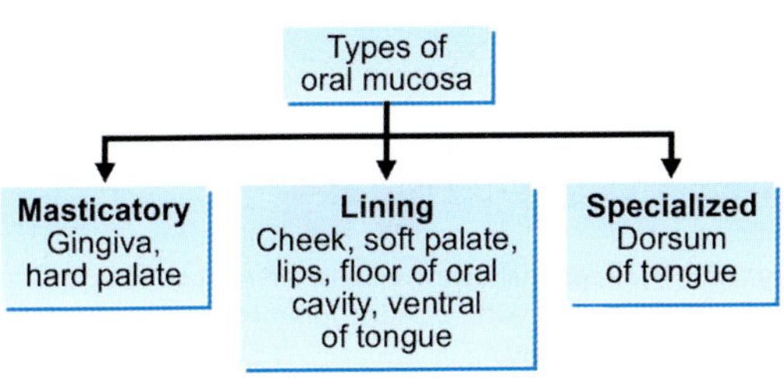

Lining Mucosa

This mucosa is seen lining the lips, inside the cheeks, vestibular sulcus, soft palate, floor of the mouth and undersurface of tongue. It has a thin and nonkeratinized layer of epithelium. It is ideal for forming and maintaining the peripheral seal.

Specialized Mucosa

It is found only on the dorsum of tongue and firmly attached to the muscles of the tongue. It is partially keratinized and resists pressure. It consists of papillae.

Oral Epithelium

It is made up of stratified squamous type. There are several layers of epithelium. The deepest layer lies on the basement membrane and is called basal cell layer. It consists of single layer of cuboid cells. This layer shows mitosis division and contains melanocytes with melanin pigment. Superficial to this layer there are several layers of polyhedral cell known as prickle cell. Superior to this layer there are one or two layers of granular cells containing basophilic granules. This layer is seen only in the masticatory mucosa and absent in lining mucosa. The cells of basal layer divide and form prickle cells which, in turn, change gradually into granular cells and then to surface layer. The rate at which the basal cell divides is the same as the rate of shedding of surface layer (Fig. 2.1).

Submucosa: The submucosa contains connective tissue, varying from dense to loose and varying in thickness. The submucosa may contain salivary glandular tissue, adipose tissue, and skeletal muscle fibers. In the sulcus of both the jaws, submucosa forms a soft cushion between the mucosa and the muscles below. The thick, loosely attached submucosa is ideal for a peripheral seal. A layer of submucosa containing minor salivary glands, adipose tissue, and arteries, veins and nerve fibers is present in the maxilla between the crest of the ridge and center of the palate.

Lamina Propria

It is a dense layer of connective tissue present beneath the basement membrane of the mucosa. It contains blood vessels, lymphatic, elastic fibers which extend into the epithelium. It is bound to the underlying bone in gingival hard palate and to muscles of cheeks, soft palate and tongue.

Mucoperiosteum

At the crest of the edentulous ridges and the center of the palate there is present no submucosa, the mucosa is firmly attached to the periosteum to form mucoperiosteum. It cannot tolerate stress. It is considered as a 'relief' area. The spacers and escape holes are mandatory in this area.

Clinical Significance

The loose submucosa in the vestibule has wide variations in position which may cause under-extension or overextension of denture borders during impression taking. The resiliency and like effects of mucosa are termed by Hanau as "realeff".

The following procedures are practiced to take the advantages of the resilient property of the mucosa:

a. The dentures in current use should be removed for tissue recovery before impression making. The period is 24 hours for young patient and several days for a geriatric patient.
b. A free flowing low viscous impression material should be used.
c. Impression material should have sufficient space to record the tissues undistorted by providing escape holes particularly in special trays for maxillary impression.
d. The impression after completion should not be removed and inserted more than necessary.
e. The border moulding should be completed before proceeding for the final wash impression.
f. Surgical removal of excessive thick tissues should be considered.

BONES

Gross Anatomy of Maxilla (Figs 2.3A and B)

The maxillary denture derives its support from the two maxillary and the two palatine bones. The basal seat is formed by the alveolar and palatine bones.

The *alveolar process* comes out of the lower part of the maxilla, is known as residual ridge after tooth loss. The residual ridge consists of two plates of compact bone surrounding a mass of cancellous bone. The labial and palatal cortical plates unite behind to form the maxillary tuberosity.

The *zygomaticoalveolar crest* starts from zygomatic process to alveolar process. It acts like buccal shelf area of mandible.

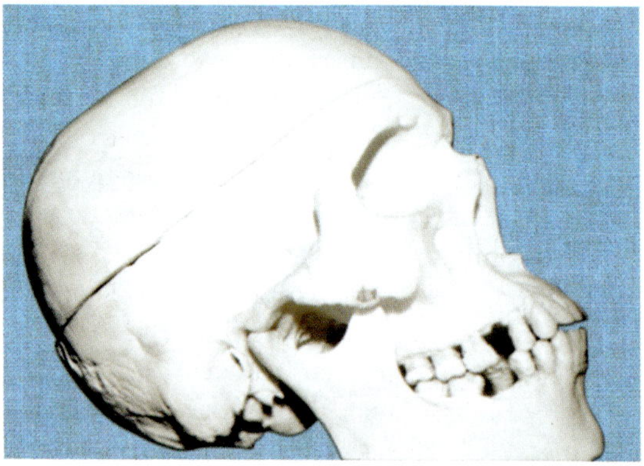

Fig. 2.3A: Gross anatomy of maxilla

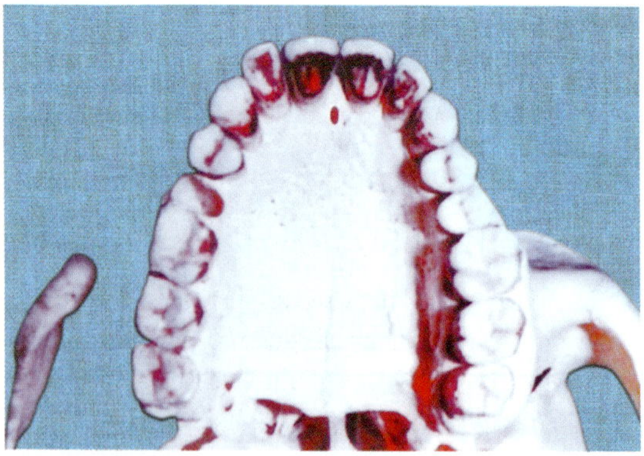

Fig. 2.3B: Hard palate showing incisive foramen, palatine process, midpalatal suture, greater palatine foramen, palatine processes and pterygoid hamulus

The *palatine processes* of the maxillary bones arise as horizontal plates which unite at midline by midpalatal suture. A bone growth called torus palatinus is seen in this area in 20–25% of population.

The palatine bones: The horizontal plates of the palatine bones articulate with the posterior horizontal processes of maxillae. The posterior margins of the hard palate serve as anterior attachment for the aponeurosis of the soft palate.

The *incisive fossa* is located in the midline of the palate, posterior to the maxillary central incisors or in edentulous mouth at palatal alveolar plate. The nasopalatine nerves and vessels pass through this. The opening is protected by soft tissue but relief of the denture base is required as the nerves and vessels are at right angle to the opening. The greater palatine foramina are located mandible to the third molars near the junction of the maxillary and palatine bones. The anterior palatine nerves and vessels pass through this opening. The openings are protected sufficiently by soft tissue so that no relief of the denture base is required.

The *pterygoid hamulus* is a thin, curved process at the end of the medial pterygoid plate of the sphenoid bone. The area between the pterygoid hamulus and the maxillary tuberosity is called hamular notch. The compressible tissue within the notch is utilized for posterior palatine seal.

Clinical Significance

1. Compact bone resists shearing stresses better whereas the alveolar bone withstand compressive stresses better. Compact bone covered by dense connective tissue at the crest of the maxillary ridge is considered to be the primary stress-bearing area. The slopes of the residual maxillary ridge may act as primary stress- bearing area if the crest is not suitable when covered by thick displaceable tissue that cannot be removed surgically due to patient state of general health.
2. *Size of ridge*: The size of the ridges is important for developing good retention. Within limits the larger the size of the ridges the greater will be the retention. A well-developed but not abnormally large ridges give resistance to denture movement both laterally and anteroposteriorly. Very large bulbous ridges require surgical removal whereas a small grossly resorbed ridge will provide poor retention. Excessive height creates insufficient space for setting.
3. *Form of ridge*: The forms of ridges when viewed in coronal section are classified into square, ovoid and tapering. The square and ovoid arches are favorable because the square ridges have more stability. The tapering arch shows less retentive quality (Figs 2.4A to C).
4. *Form of palatal vault*: The form of palatal vault influences denture stability and retention. The palatal vault of medium depth is the most favorable. A flat vault cannot resist movement of the maxillary denture. A high V-shaped palate is usually unfavorable for adequate retention (Figs 2.5A to C).
5. The posterior palatal seal should follow the contour of the posterior border of the hard palate from hamular notch to hamular notch but not in a straight line.
6. In the maxillary torus judicious relief should be given or if large surgical removal will be required.

Gross Anatomy of the Mandible (Fig. 2.6)

The mandibular denture is supported by one bone, the mandible. It consists of a body and the ramus. The superior surface of the body of edentulous mandible is narrow with an overlying soft tissue forming the residual ridge. The posterior part of the body curves upwards to form the ramus. The ramus divides into two processes, the condyloid and the coronoid. The condyle is the articular surface. The external oblique line is the inferior anterior continuation of the ramus laterally.

The *buccal shelf* lies between the external oblique ridge and the slope of the residual ridge. The bone of the buccal shelf is very dense because

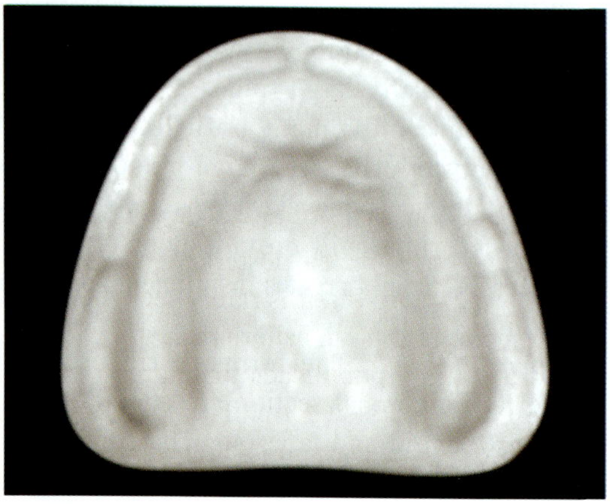

Fig. 2.4A: Square arch form of ridge

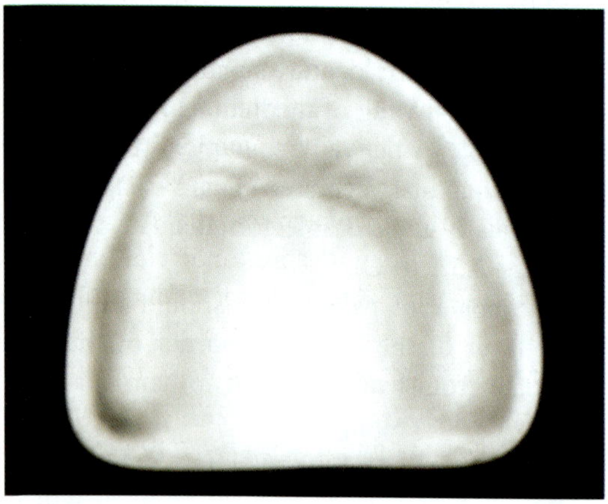

Fig. 2.4B: Ovoid arch form of ridge

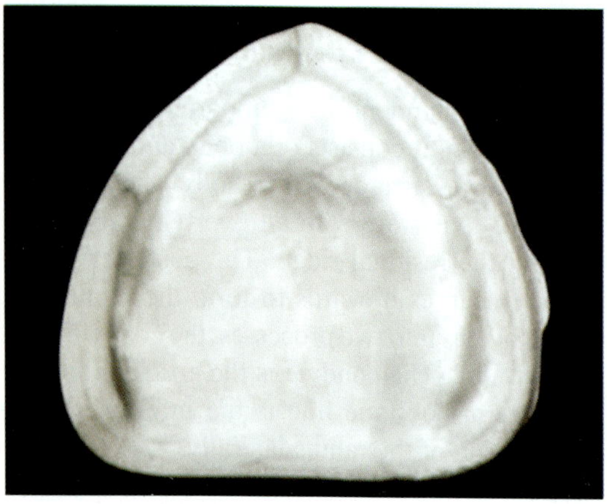

Fig. 2.4C: Tapering arch form of ridge

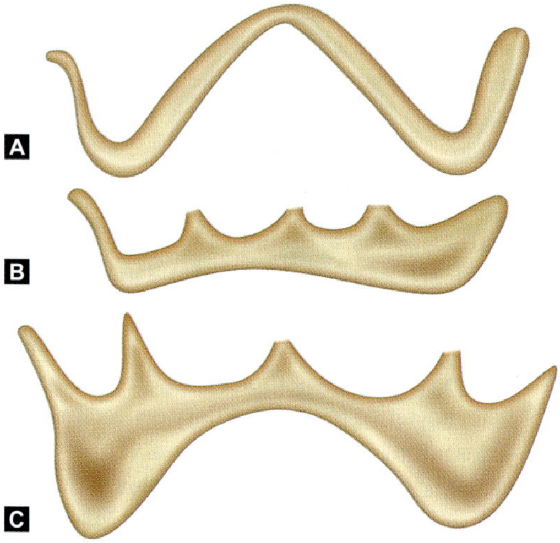

Figs 2.5A to C: Form of palatal vault: (A) High V-shaped; (B) Flat palate; (C) Medium vault

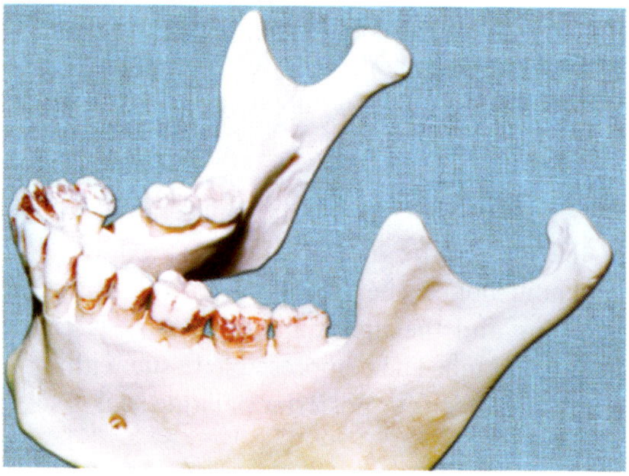

Fig. 2.6: Anatomy of the mandible showing condyle, coronoid processes and external oblique line

the forces of elevator muscles are directed to this area and the trabecular pattern of the bone is such to resist these forces.

The *mylohyoid ridge* is an irregular bony crest on the lingual side of the mandible. It extends from the third molar region to the mental spines near the lower border of the mandible. It may present severe undercut.

The *genial tubercles* (mental spines) are located on the lingual side of the body of the mandible in the midline near the border.

The *mental foramen* is located on the buccal aspect of the body of the mandible in the premolar area.

The *lingual tuberosity* lies as an irregular bony prominence on the distal end of the mylohyoid line.

The size, form and relationship of the alveolar ridge for the retention, stability, support and preservation are primarily important in complete denture fabrication.

Clinical Significance

1. The thickness of the distobuccal flange of the maxillary denture is determined by the coronoid process when the mandible is protruded or in lateral excursions.
2. The external oblique line is the anatomic guideline for lateral border of the buccal flange in most cases.
3. The buccal shelf is designed as the primary stress-bearing area in the mandibular arch because of its compact bony foundation which is at right angle to the occlusal plane.
4. The lingual flanges of the mandibular denture should extend inferior to, but not lateral to the mylohyoid ridge. Flange extended laterally, under the mylohyoid ridge would traumatize the very thin mucosa covering the ridge and causes discomfort and ulceration. If the bony crest is so prominent and sharp, surgical removal is required.
5. In case of extreme loss of residual ridge, the mental foramen occupies a more superior position and the denture base must be relieved over the foramen to keep the denture base free from irritating the mental nerve and vessels.
6. The mental spines are more superior in position than the crest of the existing ridge, surgical procedures are indicated.

   About 70% of denture patient can be treated successfully without much difficulty. A large number of patients of this group have significantly resorbed mandibular ridges, yet they wear mandibular denture without problem. The ridge augmentation by surgical measures is not necessary for good prognosis of denture.

Ridge relations: In case of a normal jaw relation, the upper ridge anteriorly will lay slightly oversized than the lower ridge but posterior a little narrower than the lower. Then the teeth can be set with normal over jet anteriorly and the posterior teeth can be set in normal relation. But it is rarely seen due to the difference in resorption pattern in the two jaws. In maxilla, the resorption leads to an arch narrower than its pre-extraction form. The position of the incisive papilla changes in relation to the anterior ridge. The reduction in the circumference of the maxillary arch is due to oblique placement of the teeth in alveolar ridge. The alveolar ridge is itself inclined laterally and anteriorly.

In the mandible, the opposite thing occurs particularly in the posterior areas. Thus, the circumference of the lower arch tends to widen in edentulous patients (Fig. 2.7). This difference in resorption patten between maxilla and mandible often wrongly diagnosed as malrelation of the alveolar ridges, and the posterior teeth are arranged in reverse relationship mediolaterally and anterior teeth are arranged with incisal edge to incisal edge. Anatomic landmarks aid in relocating the original center of the mandibular ridge, e.g. retromolar pads, retromolar papilla, etc.

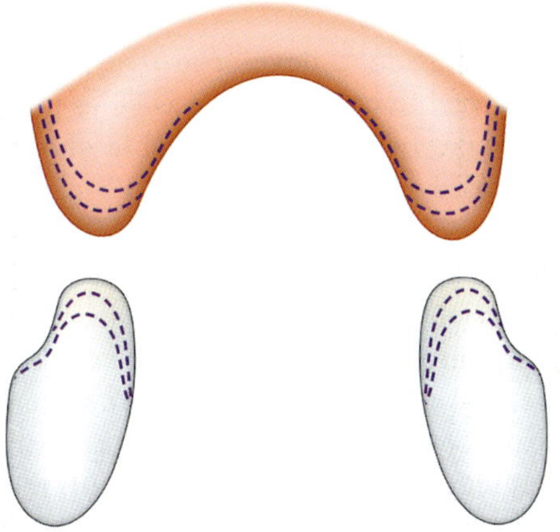

Fig. 2.7: The crests of residual ridges do not remain in their relative relations as resorption progresses

Residual Ridge Resorption (RRR)

It is universally agreed that any type of pressure from dentures causes ridge resorption due to an interruption of blood supply. The residual ridge has two sources of blood supply: (1) the alveolar arteries; and (2) the periosteal vessels. The periosteal vessels due to their comparatively superficial location are prone to interruption from pressure whereas the alveolar arteries due to their deep location are protected and continue supply blood containing nutrition to the bone despite the pressure of the prosthesis. At present there is no therapeutic solution for this problem.

Clinical Significance

The pressure on the residual ridges may be reduced in several ways as follows:

1. The prosthesis should be removed for at least 8 hours per day for tissue rest.
2. Impression should be recorded with the tissues at rest.
3. Extension of the denture base for maximum coverage within tissue limit.
4. The number of teeth on denture should be decreased.
5. Reducing stresses to the very delicate anterior ridges by removing anterior tooth contact in centric relation position and chewing with posterior teeth.
6. An occlusion is developed that eliminates horizontal forces and torque as far as possible.
7. The size of the occlusal table should be decreased.
8. Where systemic disease affects bone, the patient should be placed on a controlled recall at six-month intervals. At the recall visit, the following procedures should be done: (a) retaking of medical and dental history, (b) systematic evaluation of the prosthesis, (c) adjustments and remounting and adjustments, (d) relining and rebasing as necessary, (e) adhere to the patient instructions.

SURROUNDING MUSCLES

The muscles of mastication, facial expression, tongue, pharynx, muscles of soft palate and mandibular depression influence directly and indirectly on:

1. The extent and thickness of the denture borders
2. Denture base contour
3. Denture retention (stability)
4. Facial expression.

As the resorption of the ridges occurs the muscular forces become more important for denture retention.

Muscles of Facial Expression (Fig. 2.8)

The muscles of facial expression are responsible for various facial expressions like smiling, laughing and frowning. The facial expression is accomplished by the movable interactions of the muscles of facial expression. All the muscles of facial expression are not inserted into bone, so require tooth support for normal facial expression in edentulous patients. These muscles are inserted into skin and oral mucosa. If the muscles of facial expressions are not properly supported by artificial teeth, none of the facial expressions appears normal. The nasolabial sulcus, the philtrum, the commissures of the lips

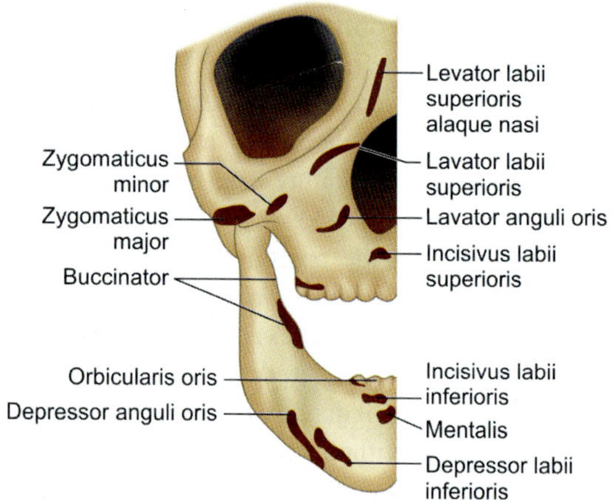

Fig. 2.8: Muscles of facial expression

and the mentolabial sulcus will not have their contours. Incorrect positioning of teeth incorrect vertical dimention or incorrect contouring of denture base can affect facial expressions adversely. Lack of support allows sagging of the soft tissues of face while over-supported inhibits the normal contraction of facial muscles and changes the greater stability in muscle tone.

The combined action of the muscles of facial expression has a profound effect on the contours, borders of the dentures. They should be considered in selecting impression materials and techniques. Selection of tray size and contour, border moulding and the flow of the impression material are all very important.

The residual ridges of adequate width and height will provide stability and retention to the denture base. The muscle of facial expression will not produce problem in proper border extensions except at modiolus. Only the elevator of the lower lip (mentalis) and the muscle of cheek (buccinator) have insertions on the jaws close to the denture border. All other facial muscles drape over the polished surface contours of the denture. When the residual ridges undergo resorption, the muscle origins become more intimately related to the borders. The insertion of the muscles of facial expression at the modiolus and particularly the position and action of the orbicularis oris influences the impression making.

Effect of the Muscles of Facial Expression on Denture Borders

Modiolus: One centimeter lateral to the corner of the mouth unilateral convergence of many muscles of facial expression form the bundle of tissues, called modiolus (Latin meaning "Knave" or "hub of a wheel"). Unless the denture borders are narrowed in the premolar region, functional movements of the modiolus may cause dislodgement of the lower denture. The upper denture is not affected by its movements due to greater stability (Fig. 2.9).

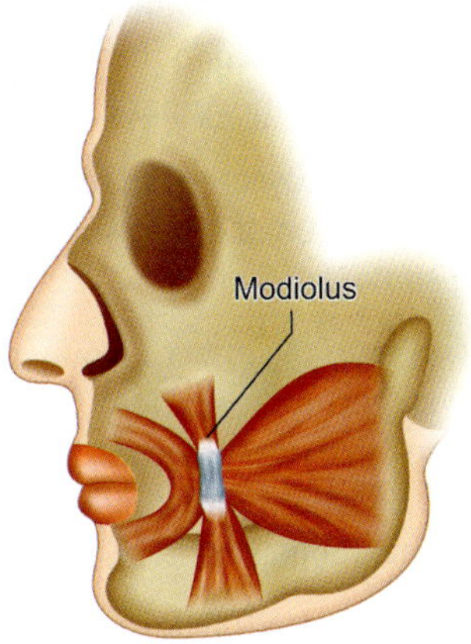

Fig. 2.9: Modiolus

Orbicularis oris: It is the principal muscle of the lips and inserted into the modioli with other muscles of cheeks—the buccinator, qudratus labii superioris and inferioris, zygomaticus, triangularis and incisive muscle.

The orbicularis muscle on contraction closes the lips against the teeth. The upper denture due to the greater stability is not affected as it does with the lower denture. The upper anterior teeth may, therefore, be placed more forward for esthetic need of the patient. The lower denture with poor ridge cannot withstand pressure and easily displaced posteriorly. This can be prevented by terminating the heal of the denture up to the ascending ramus acting as posterior stop.

Buccinator: It pulls the corner of the mouth during sucking, blowing, swallowing and maintaining food on the occlusal table. Contraction of buccinator muscle pulls the maxillary and mandibular buccal frenae backward. The polished buccal surface of the maxillary denture should be concave downwards and outwards so that the buccinator muscle on contraction forces the denture upwards. In mandibular molar region the polished buccal surface of the denture should be concave facing outwards and upwards so that the buccinator muscle on contraction forces the cheek inwards and press the denture downwards.

Levator anguli oris (Caninus): It elevates the corner of the mouth. It is attached to the maxillary buccal frenum and affects its movement.

Risorius: It pulls the corner of the mouth laterally. It may affect the position of the canine and premolar teeth during smile.

Mentalis: It elevates the lower lip outwards, rendering the lower vestibule shallow. The functional movements of the mentalis are essential for determination of length and contour of the labial flange of the mandibular denture.

Depressor labii inferioris: It depresses and elevates the lower lip. It may shorten the mandibular anterior vestibule.

Depressor anguli oris (triangularis): It draws the corners of the mouth downward. The muscle during sucking exerts pressure on the teeth and denture borders.

Quadratus labii superioris: The muscle is composed of three muscles—the levator labii superioris alaeque nasi, levator labii superioris, and zygomaticus minor, raises the upper lip.

The action of all three muscles is to raise the upper lip, shorten the nasolabial fold, and widens the nostril. It is responsible for size and contour of the maxillary labial flange.

Zygomaticus major: It draws the corner of the mouth upward and laterally during laughing or smiling. No direct action. The positioning of canine and premolars affects the function of the muscle.

Incisive muscles: There are four muscles, one in each quadrant. They contract to make the vestibular depth shallow. This may shorten the anterior flange extension and denture retention particularly in the lower jaw.

Muscles of Mastication

The primary muscles of mastication are the masseter, temporalis, internal pterygoid, and external pterygoid. These first three muscles close and make lateral movement of the mandible. The fourth acts as a guiding muscle.

Effect of Muscles of Mastication on Denture Borders

Masseter muscle: It affects the distobuccal border of mandibular denture pushing it against the buccinator muscle. It may affect the distal part of the maxillary buccal flange.

Temporalis muscle: It may affect the posterior border of mandibular denture by lifting it at retromolar pad.

It may affect buccal border of the maxillary denture by forcing buccinator muscle during lateral movement of the jaw.

Medial pterygoid: It may affect the denture border in the hamular notch area.

Lateral pterygoid: It has no action on denture borders.

Muscles of Mandibular Depression

Three groups of suprahyoid muscles are responsible for assisting in mastication. They are the mylohyoid, geniohyoid and digastric muscles. The muscles of suprahyoid group can elevate the hyoid bone and depress the mandible. The pull of suprahyoid muscles will cause opening (depression) of mandible provided infrahyoid muscles stabilized the hyoid bone. The geniohyoid and mylohyoid start the opening movements and the anterior belly digastric completes it.

Effect of Muscles of Mandibular Depression

Only two suprahyoid muscles—the mylohyoid and geniohyoid—have effect on denture borders. The infrahyoid group of muscles has no influence on denture borders. The mylohyoid muscles form the floor of the mouth. It elevates the hyoid bone, the tongue, and the floor of the mouth during swallowing. As the mylohyoid is a thin sheet muscle, it can easily be displaced during impression-making.

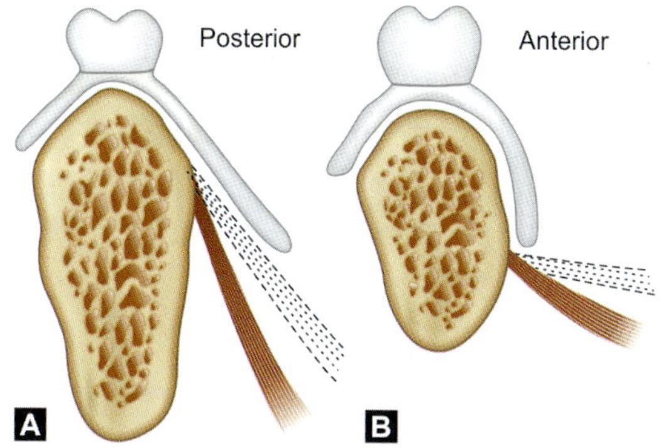

Figs 2.10A and B: Mylohyoid in anterior and posterior lingual region

The denture flange in anterior lingual region along the mylohyoid ridge can be extended vertically as the anterior fibers of mylohyoid extend horizontally (Figs 2.10A and B). In the posterior region if the denture flange is extended under the mylohyoid ridge, its movement will cause ulceration of the soft tissues on the bony prominence. The denture flange may be extended below the mylohyoid ridge as long as it slopes toward the tongue. It will help in stabilizing the mandibular denture by the tongue. The mylohyoid ridge in cases of extreme resorption of ridge can be surgically removed and repositioned at a lower level. By proper border moulding of the structures of this area, an S-shaped curve will be formed when viewing the lingual border of the impression from the tissue side.

The geniohyoid muscle usually presents no problem but in extreme resorption it may interfere with denture border. It may be then surgically removed and repositioned at a lower level.

Muscles of Soft Palate

The muscles of soft palate are the levator veli palatini, tensor veli palatini, musculus uvulae, palatoglossus, and palatopharyngeus. Out of these the levator and tensor veli palatini muscles elevate the soft palate and aid in determining the limit and contour of the posterior palatal seal.

Effect on Denture Border

The posterior border of the maxillary denture must end on a nonmobile part of soft palate. The action of palatal muscles is not disturbed unless the denture border is carried too far posterior.

Pharyngeal Muscles

The muscles of the pharynx are superior, middle and inferior constrictors, stylopharyngeus, salpingopharyngeus, and palatopharyngeus. The superior constrictor is the most important pharyngeal muscle in complete denture fabrication. Contraction of this muscle limits the posterior extent of the retromylohyoid space. This muscle exerts pressure against the distal extension of the mandibular denture.

Effect on Denture Border

Overextension in this area will cause the ulceration of tissues which produce a symptom of sore throat.

Muscles of Tongue

The tongue has two, groups of muscles, intrinsic and extrinsic.

The *intrinsic* muscles have both origins and insertions within the tongue they change the shape and size of the tongue.

The *extrinsic* muscles are responsible for the position of the tongue because they have attachments outside the tongue. They are genioglossus, hyoglossus, styloglossus and palatoglossus.

Genioglossus Muscle

It originates from the genial tubercles and passes to body of tongue.

Action: Protracts and depresses the tongue. Elevate the floor of the mouth with mylohyoid and, therefore, affects the length of the lingual flange.

Hyoglossus Muscle

It originates from the body and greater wing of the hyoid bone and inserted at the side of the tongue.

Action: It depresses the tongue.

Styloglossus Muscle

It originates from the anterior part of styloid process, enters the base of the tongue passes to its tip.

Action: It pulls the tongue upward and backward.

Palatoglossus Muscle

It originates from the anterior surface of the soft palate and inserted to the side of the tongue.

Action: It raises the tongue and forms part of the boundary of retromylohyoid fossa.

Effect of Tongue Muscles on Denture Flanges

The most difficult region in which to obtain a border seal is the anterior lingual border. The mylohyoid muscle acts anteriorly as well as posteriorly to raise the floor of the mouth, and the genioglossus muscle functions in the region underlying the lingual frenum (Fig. 2.11A). The superior fibers of the genioglossus muscle attach to the superior genial tubercles and function in depressing the body of the tongue. It is the action of the superior genioglossus muscle that pulls the tip of the tongue posterosuperiorly, depresses the center of the tongue to form a concavity during bolus formation, and pushes the anterior floor of the mouth to its superior position. To establish and maintain border seal throughout the functional range of movement of the anterior floor of the mouth the anterior lingual flange should be extended posteriorly to contact sublingual folds when floor of the mouth is at rest (Fig. 2.11B).

Tongue size and movement is also important in every step of denture fabrication. Tongue movements are necessary for mastication, deglutition, and speech. The denture flanges must be contoured to allow the tongue to have the wide range of movement.

The position and the size of tongue play an important role in the stability and retention of lower denture. An enlarged tongue in edentulous patient causes difficulty in making impression and jaw relation record. A retracted or small tongue creates problem in retention due to lack of peripheral seal.

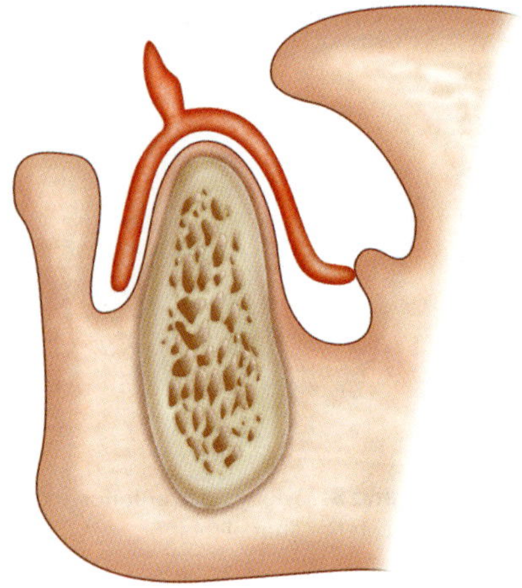

Fig. 2.11A: Peripheral seal at the anterior lingual border established by extending to most superior level of floor of mouth

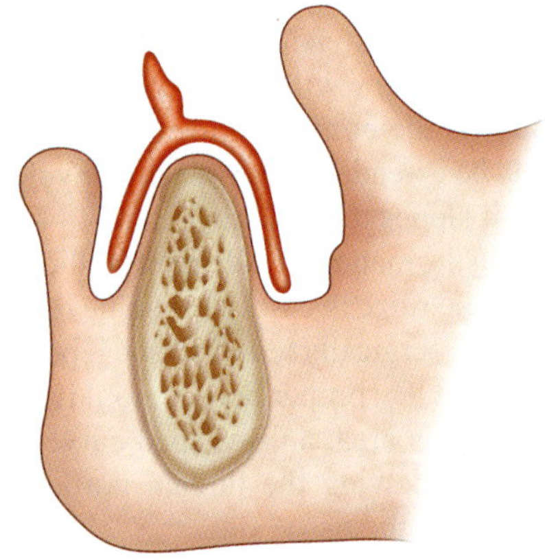

Fig. 2.11B: Peripheral seal at the anterior lingual border is established by the horizontal extension of the anterior lingual flange sublingually at rest position of floor of mouth

SALIVARY GLANDS AND SALIVA

There are three major salivary glands—parotid, submaxillary and submandibular glands and hundreds of minor glands in lips, cheeks and palate. The secretion of saliva by these glands is controlled mainly by the parasympathetic nervous system.

Saliva is a mixer of two types of secretions: (a) serous secretion, (b) mucous secretion. The serous is thin watery secretion containing enzyme ptyalin for digestion of starch. The thick mucous secretion acts as lubricant. The parotid and submandibular glands are fully serous whereas the sublingual glands and minor salivary glands are mainly mucous.

Functions of Saliva in Edentulous Mouth

1. Removal of debris
2. Antibacterial, antifungal, antiviral
3. Initiation of digestion
4. Perception of taste
5. Lubrication of the mucosa prevents abrasion by denture
6. Assistance in denture retention.

The quantity and quality of saliva are two important variables in denture retention. The retention is decreased in decreased salivation called xerostomia or in excessive salivation known as sialorrhea.

Clinical Significance

For successful full denture treatment, the rate of flow of saliva and its viscosity are important. Normal rate of flow is about 1 ml/ min. A saliva of medium viscosity with normal rate of flow helps in retention of complete dentures. Increased salivation or decreased salivation prevents the normal function of saliva to help in denture use.

1. *Excessive salivation of palatal glands*: The minor salivary glands in the posterior 2/3rd of the palate are particularly important in retention and impression making in maxillary complete denture. Excessive secretion of palatal glands in this region may distort the maxillary impression. To prevent this, the palate may be massaged to empty the glands, or wiped with gauge or astringent mouthwash can be prescribed.
2. Excessive salivation of submandibular and sublingual salivary glands may cause difficulty in impression making. Use of drugs reducing salivary secretion like pilocarpine can be used with some degree of success.
3. Xerostomia.

The cause should be investigated from the medical history and if possible therapy should be advised. In severe case artificial saliva (glycerin-based mouthwash) may be necessary. In case of an unfavorable case, the problem should be discussed with the patient before treatment. It may be advisable to limit the use of denture during meals or the diet containing more fluid may be advised.

Applied Anatomy in Jaw Relation Records

The masticatory system as a whole is a functional unit. The different components of the masticatory system are composed of the teeth and jaws, the temporomandibular joints, ligaments and muscles of mandibular movements, the tongue, cheeks and lips and neuromuscular system and vascular system. For fabrication of complete dentures, a close adaptation of the dentures with the structures of the masticatory system is essential. This is achieved by determination of the vertical dimension of occlusion that is harmonized with the temporomandibular joints and masticatory muscles and surrounding soft tissues. So, knowledge of (1) anatomy of temporomandibular joints, (2) muscles associated with mandibular movements, and (3) various movements of mandible are essential for the dentist for recording jaw relations.

Anatomy of the Temporomandibular Joint (Fig. 2.12)

The temporomandibular joint is a bilateral ginglymoarthrodial or sliding hinge joint (ginglymo = hinge, arthrodial = sliding joint). It is formed by the

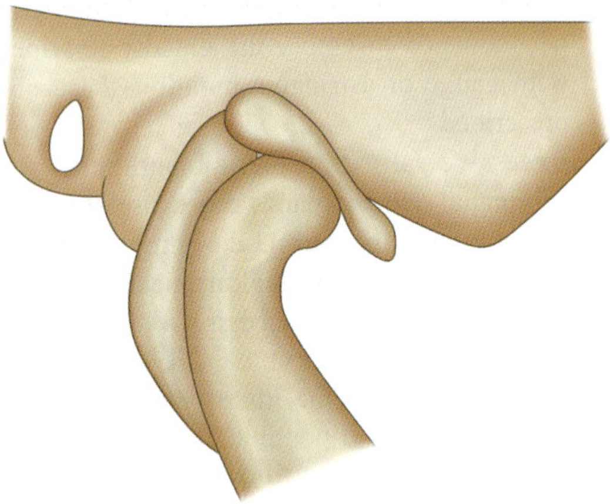

Fig. 2.12: Temporomandibular joint

articulation of the condylar process of the mandible with the mandibular fossa of the temporal bone. It is an integral part of the masticatory system. The movements of the joints are controlled by the muscles which have adaptability to changes in tooth occlusion with the help of neuromuscular mechanisms. The temporomandibular joint is a compound synovial joint but differs from other synovial joints in that the articular surfaces are covered by dense fibrous connective tissue in place of hyaline cartilage. It has a fibrous articulating disk interposed between the bony articular surfaces dividing the joint into two compartments, upper and lower. Each compartment acts as separate joint during function. Two types of movements occur in two joints. In the upper compartment it is primarily translatory while in lower compartment, it is primarily rotation. The joint consists of the condyle, articular disk, capsular ligament and the articulating surface of the skull.

The *condyle* is 2 cm mesiodistally and 0.5 cm anteroposteriorly. The distance between the centers of two condyles is variable with an average 10 cm. The *articulating disk* is saddle-shaped in its upper surface, concave anteroposteriorly and convex mediolaterally. The lower surface is concave in both directions. The muscle activity merely stabilizes the disk during mastication.

The *capsular ligament* is the fibrous, funnel-shaped ligament surrounding the glenoid fossa, articular disk and the condyle. It is triangular in shape the base at the cranial side and the apex at the neck of the mandible. It is attached anteriorly to the lateral pterygoid muscle and posteriorly it is attached to the articular fossa, the disk and the condyle. These ligaments restrict the amount of rotation of the mandible and protect the structures of the joint by limiting border movements. It defines the envelope within which all movements occur (Fig. 2.13).

The *articulating surface* consists of a concave fossa posterior known as the glenoid fossa and a convex anterior articular eminence. The condyle rests on the posterior slope of the articular eminence and moves forward along the articular eminence which bears the most of the load. The glenoid fossa is not a functional part of the joint. The fossa comes in contact with only posterior part of articular disk.

Clinical significance: Due to the complexity of the joint normal function of the joint is complex and there is difficulty in diagnosis and treatment planning of abnormal function of the joint.

For fabrication of complete dentures a close adaptation of the dentures with the structures of masticatory system is essential. This is achieved by determination of a vertical dimension of occlusion that harmonizes with the temporomandibular joint and masticatory muscles and the surrounding soft tissues.

Extracapsular ligaments: The mandible is attached to the base of the skull by two pairs of extracapsular ligaments: the sphenomandibular and the stylomandibular ligaments. Ligaments cannot stretch to support the movement of the joint (Fig. 2.13).

Muscles Associated with Mandibular Movements

The muscles that move the mandible are:

1. *Muscles of mastication*:
   a. Lateral pterygoids
   b. Medial pterygoids
   c. Temporalis
   d. Masseter

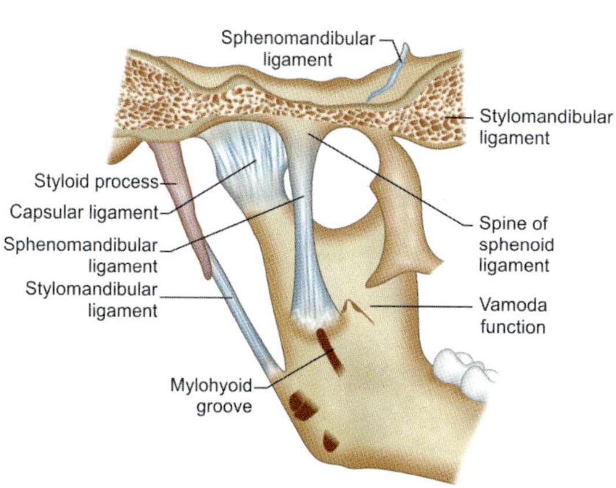

Fig. 2.13: Capsular and extracapsular ligaments of temporomandibular joint

2. *Suprahyoid muscles*
3. *Infrahyoid muscles*

All these muscles work together as one group.

Muscles of Mandibular Movement (Flow chart 2.2)

A. *Temporalis*: Retracts and elevates the mandible. It also helps in rotating and closure of the mandible.

B. *Masseter*: Retracts and protracts the mandible. It is the main power of mandibular closure.

C. *External pterygoid*: Superior head is attached to the articular disk and moves the disk forward. The right and left one either in unison or independently move the mandible forward. The inferior head also depresses and helps to rotate the mandible.

D. *Internal pterygoid*: Elevates and rotates the mandible and protracts and closes the mandible.

E. *Suprahyoid muscles*: Include the digastric, mylohyoid, geniohyoid, stylohyoid muscles. The last three mylohyoid, geniohyoid and stylohyoid help stabilize the hyoid bone. When the bone is stabilized, all suprahyoid depresses the mandible.

F. *Infrahyoid muscles*: Help to immobilize the hyoid bone, enabling the suprahyoid muscles to depress the mandible.

Clinical Significance

The muscles of mastication are capable of developing a force of 44 lb (20 kg) between opposing natural teeth within short range of normal vertical dimension. The closing force is less than 13 to 16 lb (6 to 8 kg) with complete dentures. If the vertical dimension is reduced much below normal there will be loss of power of mastication. This results in drooping of the corner of lips, puckering and wrinkling of lips and flattening of the philtrum

Flow chart 2.2: Muscles of mandibular movement

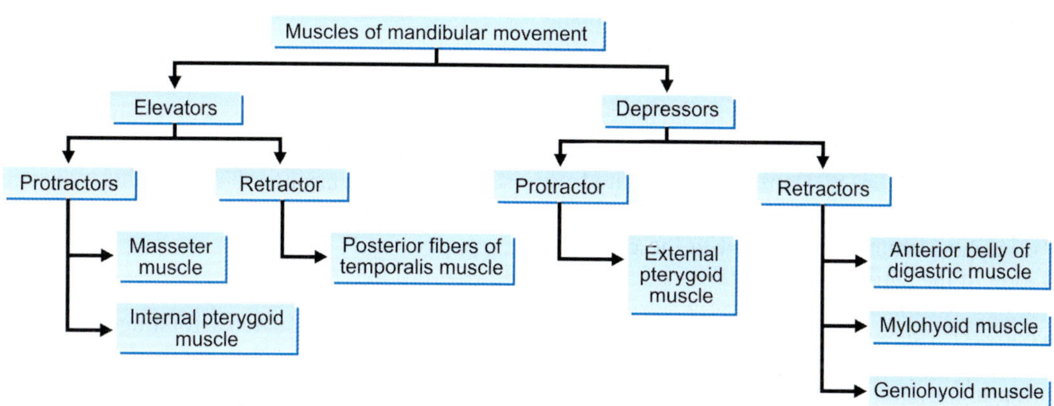

giving an old appearance. It can be only removed by restoring the normal vertical dimension of occlusion. All the muscles of mastication except lateral pterygoid have their origin and insertion in bone.

If dentures are made with increased vertical dimension heavy premature occlusal contact of teeth will occur to cause discomfort and damage to the underlying tissues. It is claimed that resorption of the ridges results from the forces of occlusion with excessive vertical dimension. This will ultimately results in loss of fit to the resorbed ridges.

When the posterior teeth are lost and mastication is performed with the anterior teeth or when complete denture is fabricated after a long complete edentulous period, abnormal chewing habits with the mandible in protrusion are acquired. It results in loss of delicate balance between protruding and retruding groups of muscle. The protruding group with excessive use becomes more dominant. In this case, difficulty in the recording of centric relation is anticipated and complete relaxation of the muscles of mastication with gentle hinge closure is used.

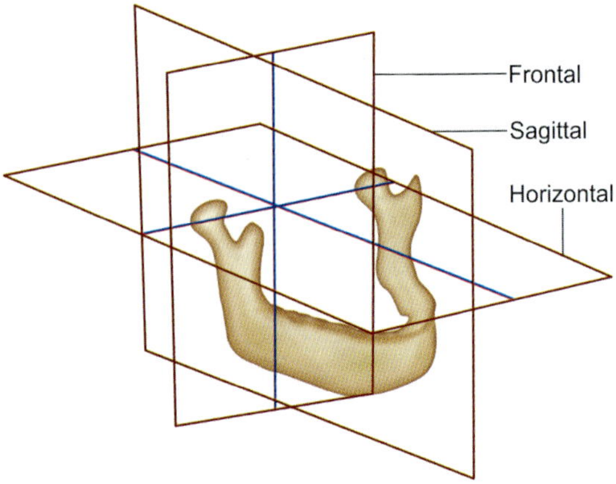

Fig. 2.14: Reference planes

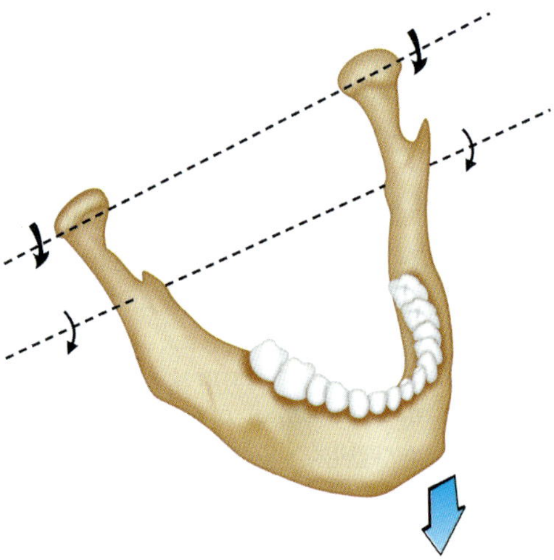

Fig. 2.15: Rotation around the horizontal or hinge axis

Mandibular Movement

All basic mandibular movement is either rotation (ginglymus or hinge action) or translation (diarthrodial action). So, the temporomandibular joint is classified as a ginglymoarthrodial joint. These movements take place with reference to three planes of the skull—the sagittal plane running vertically in the anteroposterior direction, the frontal plane running vertically from left to right, and horizontal plane (Fig. 2.14).

The mandible rotates in each of the three axes. The point of intersection of three axes is called *the center of rotation.* Dental cast mounted on articulator with a face bow record places the center of condylar elements correspond to the center of rotation of the patient.

Rotation

A rotation is one in which all points within a body move around a common axis produced by the interaction of three axes of rotation. It occurs around the rotational centers within the condyles and takes place in the lower chamber of the temporomandibular joint. It occurs up to 12 mm in separation of anterior teeth beyond this translation accompany rotation.

Horizontal Axis (Fig. 2.15)

The mandible is capable of rotating around this horizontal or hinge axis to produce opening and closing movements. This rotation can occur in any degree of protrusion and in centric relation.

Centric relation has been defined as the rearmost, uppermost and midmost position of the condyle in the glenoid fossa. Now the word rearmost is precisely omitted. So, centric relation is the untranslated hinge position of the mandible in the cranium.

Vertical Axis (Fig. 2.16)

The mandible moves around the vertical axis of one condyle, produces rotation of the mandible in the horizontal plane, resulting in a lateral excursion toward the side of the rotating condyle. The condyle around which the rotation occurs is known as rotating or working condyle. The opposite condyle is the orbiting or nonworking condyle.

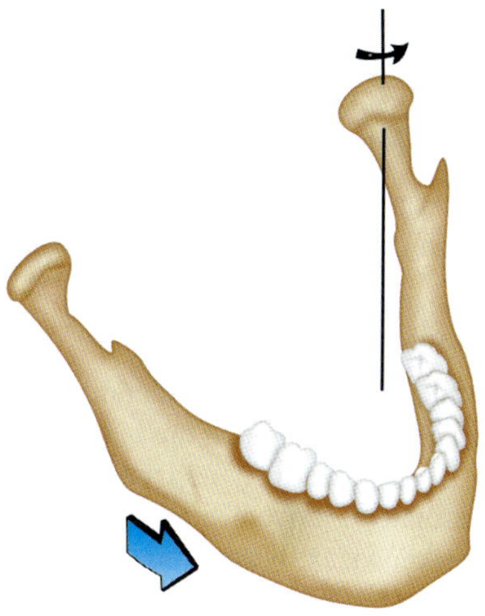

Fig. 2.16: Rotation around the vertical axis

Sagittal Axis (Fig. 2.17)

During lateral excursions of the mandible, the orbiting condyle travels downward and forward producing a rotation around a second horizontal axis that is called sagittal axis.

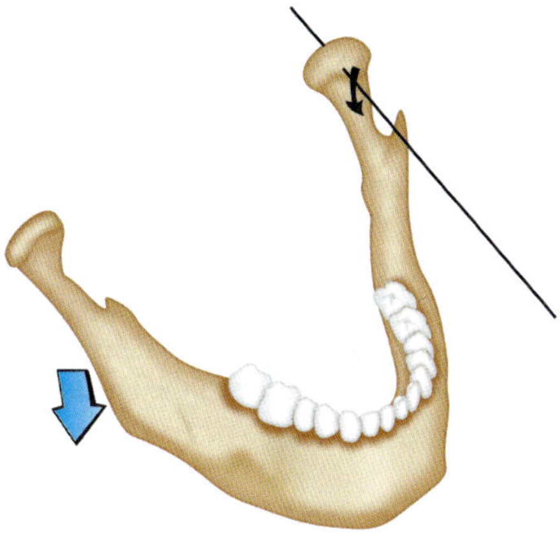

Fig. 2.17: Rotation around the anteroposterior sagittal axis

Translation

A translation is one in which all points within a body are moving at the same velocity and in the same direction. It occurs in relationship of condyle and its articular disk with the articular fossa. It takes place in the upper compartment of the temporomandibular joint and may occur simultaneously in all three cranial planes.

The *combination of rotation and translation* occurs during lateral movement of the mandible in the horizontal plane.

Types of Translation

There are various types of translation as follows:
- Protrusion
- Retrusion
- Lateral movement.

Protrusion

It is the forward gliding movement of the mandible from centric relation. During the straight protrusion, the condyles move forward and downward along the slopes of the articular eminence forming an angle with Frankfort plane. The angles can be registered with a fair degree of accuracy by means of protrusive checkbite and can be transferred to an articulator.

Retrusion

It is the backward movement of the mandible from centric relation. It occurs when the mandible is forced with the help of the fibers of the temporalis, digastric and masseter muscles. It is only about

0.5 mm and a strained position which patient cannot reproduce.

Lateral Movement

It is the forward translation of the working condyle and rotation of the nonworking condyle.

Bennett Movement (Fig. 2.18)

It is the lateral swing of the mandible when the working side (side in which the mandible moves) condyle moves anteriorly and laterally outward. This anterolateral movement of the working side condyle is known as **Bennett movement** which is a compartment of lateral movement.

Bennett movement is defined in glossary of prosthodontic terms as "Bennett movement is the bodily lateral movement or lateral shift of the mandible resulting from the movements of the condyles along the lateral inclines of the mandibular fossa during lateral jaw movements". Bennett movement was discovered by Dr Norman Godfrey Bennett in 1908. The nonworking condyle at the same time moves downward, forward and medially.

The angle formed by the nonworking condyle with the sagittal plane during Bennett movement is known as Bennett angle with the mean value of 128 degrees.

Bennett movement takes place in working condyle whereas the Bennett angle is formed by the nonworking condyle with the sagittal plane. Bennett angle may be present in the absence of Bennett movement.

Types of Bennett Movement (Fig. 2.19)

There are three types of Bennett shift or Bennett movement depending upon the timing and the amount of movement:

1. Progressive side shift
2. Precurrent side shift
3. Immediate side shift

Progressive side shift: The side shift of the orbiting condyle occurs throughout the range of the movement.

Precurrent side shift: The lateral shift occurs in the first 2 or 3 mm of forward movement of the orbiting condyle.

Immediate side shift: The shift occurs before any forward movement of the orbiting condyle.

Clinical Significance of Bennett Movement

Adjustable articulators possess settings for Bennett's movement. The Bennett shift is on an average about 1.5 mm towards the lateral position

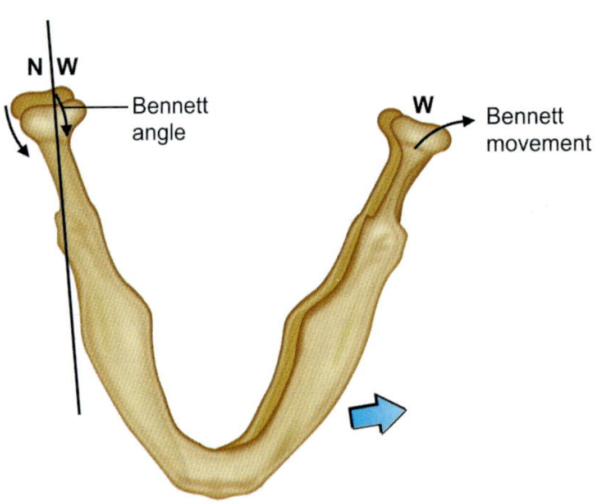

Fig. 2.18: Bennett movement and Bennett angle

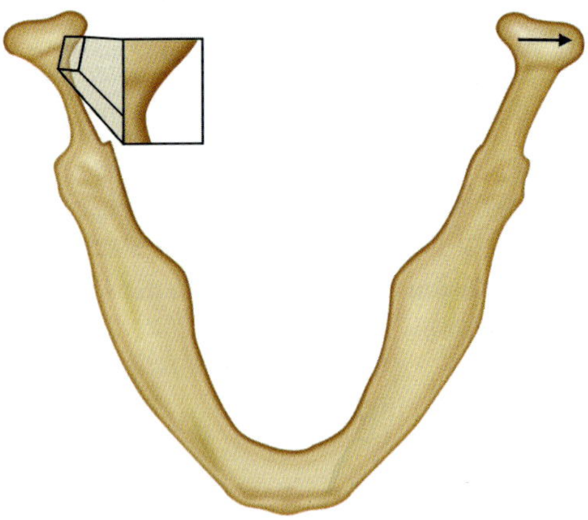

Fig. 2.19: Types of Bennett movement (horizontal plane)

where the buccal cusp of the working side are on the same position. Bennett movement from the centric occlusion is important if teeth contact is in gliding occlusion as they move from and to centric occlusion. Bennett's movement determines cusp height and morphology.

Border Movement

The extreme physiological movements of mandible are known as border movement. *Border movement* is defined as "mandibular movement at the limits dictated by anatomic structures as viewed in a given plane" (GPT). The three-dimensional space created by the combination of border movement is known as *space envelope*. It can be recorded with a pantographic apparatus. It is an extraoral tracing device attached to stabilized base plates. Envelopes of motion in the sagittal, frontal and horizontal planes in the pantographic tracing are shown separately in Figures 2.20 to 2.22.

Movements along Sagittal Plane

It represents pure rotation around a horizontal axis between the center of each condyle or it may represent translatory movement downwards, upwards, forwards, backwards or combination of these.

Movements along Frontal Plane

These may be rotatory, around a sagittal axis through the center of each condyle or they may be translatory—lateral, medial, upwards and downwards, or combinations of these.

Movements along Horizontal Plane

This can be rotations around a vertical axis passing through the center of each condyle, or they may be translatory—lateral, medial, forward or backwards, or combinations of these.

Movements within the boundaries of movement space are known as intraborder movements. Chewing cycle takes place within the envelope of motion. The mandible moves along three

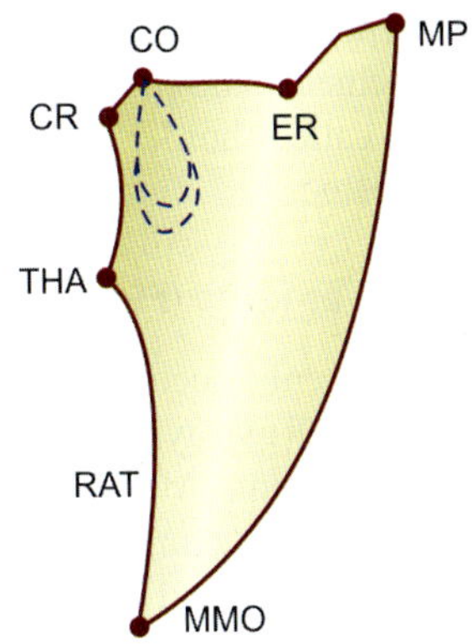

Fig. 2.20: Beak tracing: Border movements recorded in the sagittal plane
(Abbreviations: CO, centric occlusion; CR, centric relation; MMO, maximum mouth opening; MP, maximum protrusion; ER, edge to edge relation; RAT, retruded axis translation; THA, translation horizontal axis)

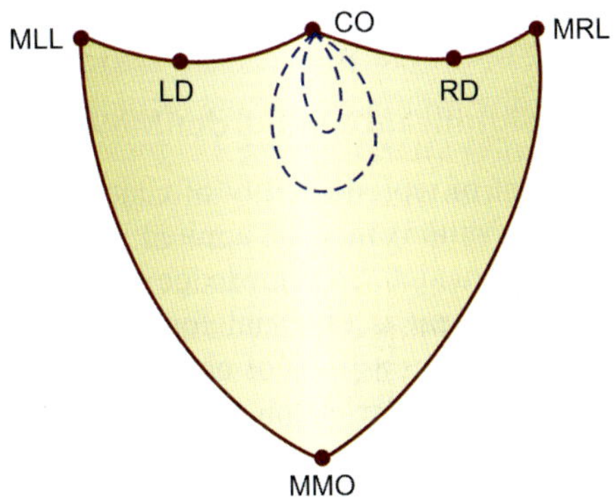

Fig. 2.21: Shield tracing: Border movements recorded in the coronal plane
(Abbreviations: MMA, maximum left lateral; MRL, maximum right lateral; LD, left deviation; RD, right deviation; CO, centric occlusion)

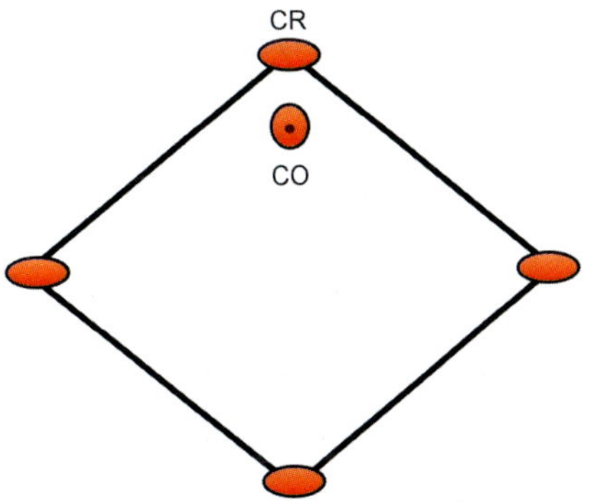

Fig. 2.22: Border movements in horizontal plane
(Abbreviations: CO, centric occlusion; CR, centric relation)

directions up to a point. The border limitation of the mandibular movements and moving the mandible to these points is called 'border movements of the mandible'.

Intraborder Movements (Fig. 2.23)

Intraborder movements occur within the *space envelope*. They are of two types—functional and parafunctional movements. Mandibular functional movements occur during mastication, speech, swallowing, respiration and facial expression. Mandibular parafunctional movements are clenching, grinning and bruxism. All functional mandibular movements do not require occlusal contacts. Many parafunctional movements occur with teeth contact. Most functional movements of the mandible occur within physiological limit and, therefore, rarely coincide with border movements.

Clinical Significance of Border Movement

The concept of reproducibility of centric relation (a border position) may be applied in complete denture construction. So, knowledge of mandibular border movement is essential for the dentist to understand various aspects of occlusion, artificial teeth arrangements, selection of recording devices and articulators. An ideal articulator is one which simulates the jaw movements within the contact range of teeth so that the occlusion built on the instrument will function properly in patient's mouth. However, no such instrument exists. Therefore, refinement of occlusion intraorally is essential.

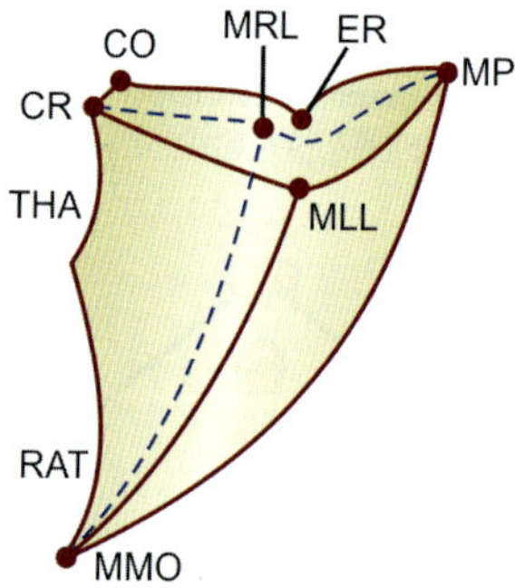

Fig. 2.23: Space envelope: Combination of border movements in all three planes

(Abbreviations: CO, centric occlusion; CR, centric relation; MMO, maximum mouth opening; MP, maximum protrusion; ER, edge to edge relation; RAT, retruded axis translation; THA, translation horizontal axis; MLL, maximum left lateral; MRL, maximum right lateral)

Factors of Regulation of Mandibular Movements

The factors of regulation of mandibular movements can be divided in two groups:

I. Neuromuscular regulation of movement
II. Determinants of mandibular movement.

Neuromuscular Mechanisms and Reflexes

The mandibular muscles do not function by themselves but are controlled by the "masticatory center" or neural network in the brain forming the complex neuromuscular mechanisms. The principal mechanisms are the proprioception and the jaw opening and closing reflex. The neuromuscular mechanism through proprioceptive nerve endings in the periodontal membrane, muscles, and joints monitors the position of the mandible and its paths of movement. It will program the most physiologic paths at certain circumstances. Dentists have indirect control over this by modification of teeth in harmony with temporomandibular (TM) joints.

Proprioception: Sensory receptors are located in the periodontal ligament, in the muscles of mastication and in the temporomandibular joints. They convey the information about the movements and position of the mandible. These receptors are known as proprioceptors. During chewing the signal from proprioceptors passes to trigeminal sensory nuclei and it cross over the motor centers and initiate or changes muscle activity.

Jaw opening and jaw closing reflexes: After obtaining the impulses from the proprioceptors one of the two reflexes will be activated depending upon the position of the mandible. In jaw closing if proprioceptors determine that greater force should be required, the jaw closing will be continued with greater force.

The loss of natural dentition with loss of the receptors in the periodontal membrane causes the patient loses the very sensitive mechanism feedback to the neuromuscular system. In a complete denture wearer such feedback is derived from mucous membrane receptors which do not provide the same level of sensitivity. This causes the reduced masticatory forces exerted by denture wearers. The new denture wearer must learn and develop adaptation to offset the displacing forces. The limited lateral movements are usually, therefore, allowed to the new complete denture wearers.

The lateral rudimentary movements with natural teeth are limited due to tooth morphology and large overbite of the anterior teeth. The complete denture wearer due to less masticatory forces may develop chewing with rudimentary lateral movement.

Determinants of Mandibular Movement

The anatomic structures that dictate or limit the movements of the mandible are known as determinants of mandibular movement.

The contacts of the opposing teeth is the **anterior determinant** and the temporomandibular joints anatomies (slope of the articular eminences, condyles and medial walls) are the **posterior determinants** of mandibular movement.

The mandibular movements are established by the temporomandibular joints posteriorly and tooth contacts anteriorly. These two combine to affect mandibular movement. These two end controlling factors determine the position of artificial tooth for developing an occlusion that helps in complete denture stability. The dentist has no control over the posterior determinants—TM joints but have direct control over the anterior tooth determinants.

Effect of Opposing Tooth Contacts

Natural teeth are the primary force in mandibular movements. The role of artificial teeth in complete dentures is considered as secondary force in mandibular movements as they are attached to a movable denture base on a displaceable tissues. If the teeth in maximum occlusal contact cause malposition of condyles and discomfort, neuromuscular mechanism will try to correct it. The effect is more on the denture, supporting structures than on the TM joint. To prevent this effect positioning of the teeth in relation to the rotational center of the condyles a face bow transfer to an articulator is required. This helps to position the teeth in relation to condylar center and eccentric movements can be performed without deflective contacts.

Effect of Temporomandibular Joint Anatomy

All functional movements begin with an opening movement of the jaw. Tooth position and developing occlusion should not interfere with the condylar controlled cyclic action of chewing. This requirement and the production of a stable closure of the mandible in centric relation are major factors required in complete denture construction. This will promote the health of supporting tissues, has reasonable performance and comfort for the patient.

Methods of Recording and Reproducing Mandibular Movements

It should be easy to understand methods of the recording and reproducing mandibular movements only after acquiring the knowledge anatomy. It should be clear that all possible mandibular motions and their effects cannot be reproduced by one instrument or technique.

Maxillomandibular Records

Static Records

a. Interocclusal records
b. Facial records

Dynamic Records

a. Functionally generated path
b. Pantograph tracing

CONCLUSION

All types of tissues are involved in the biologic environment of the complete denture. The oral mucosa provides the intimate contact with the denture. The thickness of the soft tissues and their tolerance to abuse is important in denture patient. Bone provides the ultimate support, muscles and saliva play in denture retention, function and esthetics due to their effect on the polished and fitting surfaces. Temporomandibular joint plays a significant role in mandibular movements and its positions particularly the condylar position are utilized in determination of jaw relation.

BIBLIOGRAPHY

1. Boucher LJ. Anatomy at temporomandibular joint as it pertains to centric relation. J Prosthet Dent. 1962;12:3.
2. Hanau RL. Occlusal changes in centric relation. JADA. 1929;16:903.
3. Mack A. Complete Denture. British Dental Journal. 1964;116:10.
4. Martone AL. An approach to prothodontics through speech appliance. J Prosthet Dent. 1962;12:3.
5. Martone AL. Anatomy of the mouth and related structure. J Prosthet Dent. 1962;12:1.
6. Martone AL. Clinical application of concepts of functional anatomy and speech science of complete denture prothodontics. J Prosthet Dent. 1962;12:5.
7. Robinson MJ. The influence of head position on TM joint dysfunction. J Prosthet Dent. 1966;16:1.
8. Sheppard IM. Anteroposterior and posteroanterior movements. J Prosthet Dent. 1962;12:1.
9. Shannon EJ, Leff A. Mandibular and articular movements. J Prosthet Dent. 1962;12:1.
10. Silverman SI. Denture prosthesis and functional anatomy of maxillofacial structures. J Prosthet Dent. 1956;6:305-31.

Chapter 3

Examination, Diagnosis, Treatment Planning and Prognosis

INTRODUCTION

The success or failure of complete denture treatment is usually determined at the diagnosis stage. To obtain predictable result, the dentist must apply his skill. Before applying his skill the dentist must diagnose each case of complete denture individually.

According to Devan, "The dentist should meet the mind of the patient before he meets the mouth of the patient."

DEFINITION OF DIAGNOSIS

Diagnosis is the examination of the physical state, evaluation of the mental or psychological make up and understanding the needs of each patient to ensure a predictable result.

Diagnosis in complete denture is a continuing process and is not accomplished in a short time. In many patients, the most pertinent/important finding escape the operator until the planned treatment near completion.

The diagnostic record for complete denture treatment can best be complied by using a systematic diagnostic form (Table 3.1). From this information a treatment plan and prognosis can be developed. The dentist must consider each patient as an individual. It is possible to categorize patients and anticipate certain problems, but always remember that not all patients will fit a predetermined group.

According to difficulty faced, patients can be categorized in the following types:

Group 1: Relatively easy, compromises can be made during the treatment (70%).

Group 2: Somewhat difficult, they make about 20% of all patients.

Group 3: Difficult, about 10% of the patients who have anatomical and psychological problems.

TREATMENT PLANNING

Developing a course of action that encompasses the ramification and sequelae of treatment to serve the patient's needs.

Treatment planning is a consideration of all of the diagnostic findings, systemic and local which influence the surgical preparation of the mouth, impression making, maxillomandibular relation records, occlusion to be developed, form and material in the teeth, denture base material and instruction in the use and care of dentures.

In evaluating a patient, a decision should be reached whether or not successful therapy can be instituted for that patient. This decision should be based upon the result of the examination. It should be based upon a physical examination; the patient's attitude may negate the construction of successful complete denture. On the contrary despite extremely unfavorable prognosis successful complete denture may result when patient truly desires to wear dentures. The patient's attitude is more difficult to overcome than the physical hazard of atrophic ridges.

The success of complete denture treatment depends on so many physical and mental variables. It is advisable to use a complete checklist to ensure that all the influencing conditions have been examined.

DIAGNOSTIC FORM

I. Patient Data

Name ____________________

Telephone no: (Home) —————— (Business) ——————

Age_______ Sex________ Occupation and social position__________ Tooth shade________ Mucosa shade________

Cosmetic index: Class I (High), Class II (Medium), Class III (Low).

Personality: Philosophic, Exacting, Hysterical, Indifferent.

II. Medical History

General health

Major ailments (if any):

Whether under any medication:

III. Dental History

1. Chief complaint____________________
2. Period of edentulousness____________________

Maxilla____________________Mandible____________________

3. Reason for extraction______________
   Caries____________________
   Periodontal diseases______________
   Others____________________
4. Previous denture history—number
   Satisfactory/Unsatisfactory____________________

If unsatisfactory, state the reasons____________________

Existing Dentures Experience

Retention

Stability

Extension

Esthetics

Phonetics

Occlusion

IV. Extraoral Clinical Examination

1. Face form: Ovoid______________ Square______________ Tapering______________
2. Profile_______Straight (see Fig. 3.2) ______________ Convex____________Concave _______
   (Class I) (Class II)
   (Class III)
3. Complexion: Fair______________ Medium______________ Dark______________
4. Lips Active______________ Flaccid ______________ Normal ______________
   Long ______________ Medium______________ Short______________
   Thick ______________ Thin ______________ Normal ______________
5. Muscle tone: Class I (Normal)________Class II (Slightly impaired)________ Class III (Greatly impaired).
6. TM joint: Normal________Cripitus________Clicking________ Deviation________

7. Neuromuscular coordination:
   Class I: (Excellent)
   Class II: (Fair)
   Class III: (Poor)

V. Intraoral Clinical Examination

1. Arch size:
   Class I: Large
   Class II: Medium
   Class III: Small
2. Arch form
   Class I: Square
   Class II: Ovoid
   Class III: Tapering
3. Shape of the ridge
   Class I: U-shaped square
   Class II: V-shaped
   Class III: Flat
   Class IV: Knife edge
4. Interarch space
   Class I: Ideal interarch space to accommodate the artificial teeth
   Class II: Excessive interarch distance
   Class III: Insufficient interarch distance
5. Ridge parallelism:
   Class I
   Class II
   Class III
6. Ridge relationship (Angle classification):
   Class I: Normal
   Class II: Retrognathic
   Class III: Prognathic.
7. Bony undercuts:
   Maxilla—Class I (None); Class II (Slight); Class III (More): Require removal
   Mandible—Class I (None); Class II (Slight); Class III (More): Require removal.
8. Tori:
   Class I (Absent)
   Class II (Mild): Surgery optional
   Class III (Large): Require surgical removal
9. Palatal throat form:
   Class I: Gentle (Large and normal in form with a relative immovable band of resilient tissue 5 to 12 mm distal to a line drawn across the distal end of the tuberosities).
   Class II: Medium (sized normal in form with immovable tissue 3 to 5 mm distal to a line drawn across the distal end of the tuberosities).
   Class III: Abrupt (drop of soft tissue 3 to 5 mm anterior to a line drawn across the palate at the distal end of the tuberosities).
10. Lateral throat form:
    Class I: Large
    Class II: Medium
    Class III: Small.
11. Mucosa condition:
    Class I: Healthy: Uniform thick and firm
    Class II: Irritated and thin
    Class III: Pathological thick and flabby

12. Border and frenum attachments:
    Class I: High
    Class II: Medium
    Class III: Low.
13. Saliva:
    Class I: Normal quality and quantity
    Class II: Excessive saliva with much mucin
    Class III: Scanty with mucin
14. Tongue size:
    Class I: Normal
    Class II: Large
    Class III: Small.
15. Tongue position:
    Class I: Normal
    Class II: Retracted
    Class III: Retracted
16. Gag reflex.

VI. Radiographic Examination

VII. Pre-extraction Records

VIII. Treatment Plan and Prognosis

Tissue conditioning—
Preprosthetic surgery—
Tooth selection shade mould and material

Tooth selection	*Shade*	*Mould*	*Material*
Maxillary anterior			
Mandibular anterior			
Maxillary posterior			
Mandibular posterior			

IX. Prognosis

Mandibular denture
Factors
____
____
____
____

Criteria for retention
Good Prognosis
____
____
____
____

Bad Prognosis
____
____
____
____

Factors
____
____
____
____

Criteria for stability
Good Prognosis
____
____
____
____

Bad Prognosis
____
____
____
____

Maxillary denture
Factors
____
____
____
____

Criteria for retention and stability
Good Prognosis
____
____
____
____

Bad Prognosis
____
____
____
____

From this checklist an accurate treatment plan and prognosis is formulated by collecting and interpreting diagnostic data. The problems should be identified early and explained clearly to the patient prior to the treatment. Problems that are explained after they occur, may delay treatment, will be considered by the patient as excuses for poor dental skill. It will have an adverse effect on doctor-patient relation.

A logical approach to diagnosis begins with a patient interview, which may also include a dental and medical history, followed by radiographic and oral examinations.

So, a proper emphasis should be given in collecting, interpreting, and transferring the diagnostic information into a treatment plan.

EXPLANATION OF DIAGNOSTIC FORM

The information required to interpret the diagnostic data properly is given above. The discussion is followed to fully correlate the diagnostic findings and clinical practice.

Patient Data

Name: It is necessary for the purpose of identification and record.

Age: The age of the patient gives an indication of his ability to wear and use dentures efficiently. Young patients are generally in good health, and this is reflected in the oral tissues. In young patient, resorption of ridges is rare and all the anatomical and physiological factors are more favorable than in older patients. The young people possess more powers of accommodation or adaptability, and learn to use artificial dentures with little apparent effort. An arbitrary change point is considered to be age 40. Patients younger than 40 are usually adaptable to change, their tissues heal rapidly and offer good resistance. Patients over 40 have tissues that do not heal as quickly and have a mental attitude not to adapt to new situation. Many patients over the age of 60 years find it difficult to adapt to new situations. Tissue repair is often slow, and in many cases there was extensive destruction of denture-supporting tissues. Age is also important in the selection and arrangement of artificial teeth.

Sex: In general, women are more difficult to please with appearance of their denture than are men. They are more aware of their face and lips than are men. Any change in this part of body is readily apparent to them. Women during menopause can be difficult to treat due to psychological problems, dry mouth, burning sensation in the mouth and general vague pain.

Men tend to be more occupied with their work and less concerned with their dentures. They do accept comfort and function.

Occupational and social position: Knowing the patient's occupation and social position helps the dentist in determining what the patient expects from his dentures. In general:

- Higher the social position, more demanding the patient is about esthetics.
- A patient who speaks before group of people would be concerned about speech patterns more than one who paints for living.
- Tooth position for a musician who plays a wind instrument would be more critical than for person who does not use the mouth in making a living.
- Person who works in cafeteria is in high-risk for frequent eating.

  At this time dentist should also identify discrepancy between expectations and reality before the start of treatment otherwise success will elude both dentist and patient.

Tooth shade: The preliminary shade selection should be made in the first visit without the patient participation as most patients have a wrong concept about the size and color of teeth. These require some patient education. The final selection of tooth shade and mould is usually done at third visit and patient's participation should be needed at that time.

Mucosal shade: The color of the denture base material should match with the color of the mucosa. For proper selection of shade manufacturers, supplied color tabs may be used at chair side.

Cosmetic index: It is the esthetic expectations of the patient. The patients are classified as high, medium and low cosmetic indices.

Class I: High cosmetic index: Patients with high cosmetic indices are often exacting, appreciative and cooperative.

Class II: Moderate cosmetic index: The patients are of moderate expectations.

Class III: Low cosmetic index: The patients with low cosmetic indices are often indifferent and uncooperative.

Patient personality: Meeting the mind of the patient is essential before institution of treatment. To understand a patient the psychological assessment is required. House (1937) classified the patient as philosophical, exacting, indifferent and hysterical.

Philosophical Patients

- These patients are with best mental attitude.
- These patients are rational, sensible, calm and well adjusted in difficult situation.
- Their motivation is generalized as they desire denture for the maintenance of health and appearance and feel that having teeth replaced is a normal, acceptable procedure. Prognosis is excellent.

Exacting/Critical Patients

- These patients are methodical, precise, accurate, and immaculate in dress and appearance at times make severe demands.
- They are dissatisfied, distrust and want guarantee or remake at no additional charge.
- A firm control of these patients is essential.

Indifferent Patients

- These patients have questionable or unfavorable prognosis. These patients have little concern for their teeth or health.
- They have little appreciation for the efforts of their dentist.
- Often seek treatment because of insistence of their family.
- They will give up early if problems are encountered in new teeth.
- Their attitude can be discouraging to the dentists who treat them.
- Education programmed in dental condition is recommended treatment plan.

Hysterical/Skeptical Patients

- They are those patients who have bad results with previous treatment and, therefore, are doubtful that anybody can help them.
- They often have a recent series of personal tragedies such as loss of spouse, business problems.
- Sometimes they demand unrealistic expectation, i.e. patients demand esthetic and function equal or greater than natural teeth. They have poor prognosis.

Medical History

General health: Generally, a patient who possesses a good general health will be able to accept and adapt to a complete denture better than those in poor health. So, the dentist must know about the systemic diseases that may affect complete denture therapy, e.g. AIDS, anemia, arthritis, Bell's palsy, carcinomas, tuberculosis, diabetes, lupus erythematosus, nicotinic stomatitis, Parkinson's diseases, Pemphigus vulgaris, Paget's diseases, Plummer-Vinson syndrome, scleroderma. The medical history questions are to alert the dentist to possible medical problems in dental chair. A positive answer indicates the necessity of further investigation.

The dentist should know what medicines the patient is taking. Some medicines have direct effect on the oral cavity. Tranquilizers and antidepressants may cause dry mouth. Hormone therapies often cause extreme sore mouth for edentulous patients. In many situations, it will be necessary to consult patient's physician before preceding with the treatment. Sometimes, a change in treatment plan will be beneficial.

Debilitating Diseases

Patients having debilitating diseases should be under medical control. Diabetes, tuberculosis and blood dyscrasias require extra instructions in oral hygiene, eating habits and rest of tissues. The patient's physician must be consulted before denture construction. The frequent recall visit is required to keep the adaptation of the denture base correct.

Diseases of Joint

Osteoarthritis of the temporomandibular joint presents a problem in complete denture construction as mandibular movements are painful. This causes jaw relation and impression procedures difficult.

Cardiovascular Diseases

In presence of cardiovascular diseases, the patient's physician should be consulted as denture appointments may be contraindicated or shortened, and along with premedication.

Neurological Diseases

Parkinson's diseases and Bell's palsy involve nerve and patients may be treated but the problems of denture retention and jaw relation records should be encountered with special attention.

Malignancies

The diagnosis of oral lesions should be done by biopsy, and treatment with surgery, and radiotherapy should be followed by denture construction only after proper healing. The clinical examination of the tissues after postinsertion of denture is essential.

Menopause

The hormonal changes cause bone changes, generalized osteoporosis. The mental changes may cause burning mouth, gagging and vague pain in the patients. Medical or psychiatric treatment may be required before dentures are constructed.

Diet: The patient should be questioned about his diet. Dentist must remember that a patient who has been edentulous may have unconsciously changed his diet due to his inability to masticate properly and if the nutritional intake of patient is found to be lacking, an adequate diet should be prescribed.

Dental History

Chief Complaint

It is the patient's reasons for seeking dental treatment or new dentures. The exact words of patient should be noted. This indicates the knowledge and patient's concern for a particular problem. The patients who seeks dentures as a result of family pressure is rarely a successful unless he is educated about denture during the treatment and supplied with written instruction for use and care of denture.

Dates of Extraction of the Teeth

This helps to ascertain the rate of resorption and gives an idea of stability of the denture-bearing tissues. The longer the patient been edentulous, the more bone resorption usually is noted. More resorption in one area than in other is difficult to treat with a complete denture. The patients who have been edentulous for a long time and did not wear artificial dentures are difficult to treat.

Reasons for Extraction of the Teeth

The reasons for loss of natural teeth help to ascertain the rate of resorption of ridges. The rate is more expected in tooth loss due to periodontal disease. Extraction due to caries usually produces less resorbed ridges.

Previous Denture History

The denture history is very important in evaluation of the prognosis of complete denture treatment. The patient should be asked whether the dentures were satisfactory or never satisfactory, previously satisfactory but now unsatisfactory, previous denture was satisfactory new denture unsatisfactory.

The number of dentures that the patient has had and the length of time each has been worn help in evaluating the anticipated prognosis. A patient with a successful denture treatment will probably be having good prognosis again. The type of teeth—anatomic or nonanatomic, porcelain or resin—should be determined according to the previous successful denture. The reasons for satisfaction or dissatisfaction with the previous dentures (i.e. with the masticatory efficiency, retention, stability, esthetics, phonetics, comfort and occlusion) may affect the type of replacement to the patient.

The loss of retention may be due to faulty occlusion or overextension or underextension of borders. The discomfort and difficulty in chewing may be due to fault in occlusion. The altered speech may be due to error in vertical dimension, poor retention, or error in placement of teeth.

Existing or Present Dentures

The reasons for dissatisfaction with the present dentures may also affect the type of replacement to the patient. The followings should be checked:

1. Occlusion
2. Retention
3. Stability
4. Esthetics
5. Phonetics
6. Extension

Extraoral Clinical Examination

Face form: Leon Williams (1914) and House and Loop (1939) were first to consider the importance of the outline form of the anterior teeth. They classified the outline form, or shapes, of the face and selected anterior teeth in harmony with the facial form. The face form is classified by connecting points on lateral aspect of face, i.e. the forehead, zygomatic arch, and angle of the mandible. There are four basic shapes of a person— (1) square, (2) square tapering, (3) tapering, and (4) ovoid (Fig. 3.1). The shape of the maxillary central incisor should be similar to that of face when placed upside down. This method is known as geometric theory. Artificial tooth manufacturers use this theory as the basis for tooth mould classification. Although the theory is not proven (Wright found 60,7% not correlate), the harmony between face and tooth forms enhances esthetics.

Facial profile (Fig. 3.2): The incisogingival and mesiodistal curvatures of incisor teeth are similar to the profile curvature of face. So, facial profile is helpful for selection of anterior tooth.

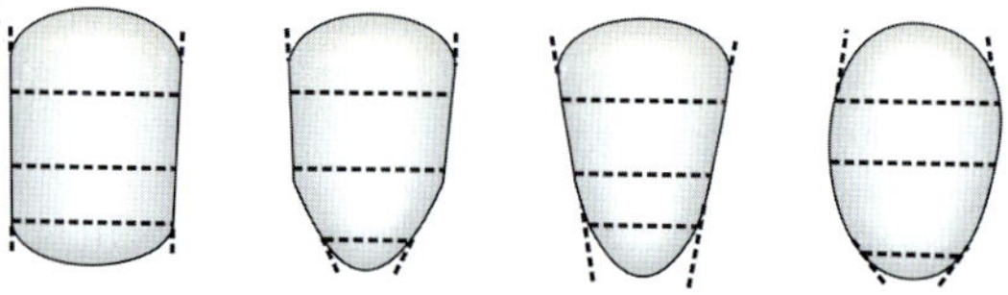

Fig. 3.1: Face form: Square, square tapering, tapering and ovoid

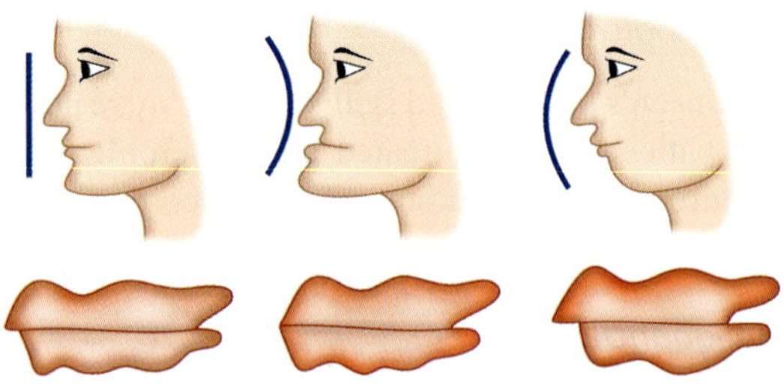

Fig. 3.2: Facial form (profile) and ridge relation (profile)
Classification according to angle:

Class I	Class II	Class III
Normal	Prognathic	Retrognathic

Complexion: It is important guide in the shade selection. The shade should have harmony with complexion. The relationship of color of hair or eye is questionable in shade selection.

Lips: Short lips show more tooth structure. The opposite is true for long lips. Thin lips are difficult to treat because the slight oversupport may greatly affect facial expression.

Muscle tone: Tone of muscles of facial expression is classified according to House:

*Class I:*The patient possesses normal tone, tension and placement of muscles. No degenerative changes have yet occurred. Only patients wearing immediate dentures have a class I muscle tone.

Class II: The patient possesses approximately normal function but slightly impaired muscle tone due to wearing of adequate dentures with correct vertical dimension of occlusion is of this type.

Class III: The patient possesses impaired muscle tone and function due to poor health and grossly inefficient dentures. This produces loss of vertical dimension of occlusion, decreased biting force and wrinkles. Excessive flaccidity reduces the ability to control the dentures. It also increases the possibility of denture base overextension. The proper tray fabrication, border moulding and impression is required for the correct extension of denture base.

Temporomandibular joint: The temporomandibular joint should be examined digitally by placing the fingers on the joints when the patient opens and closes the mouth. Any pain, clicking and crepitus or abnormal movements should be noted. Discomfort or pain has been associated with excessive increase or decrease of vertical dimension and arthritis.

Neuromuscular coordination: The mandibular movements should be coordinated. Uncontrolled movements cause difficulty in determining correct centric relation and protrusive records and forbid the use of a balanced occlusion with anatomic tooth.

Intraoral Clinical Examination

Arch Size

Class I (Large): Best for retention and stability.
Class II (Medium): Good for retention and stability.
Class III (Small): Poor for retention and stability.

Denture stability will be hampered if there is a great discrepancy between the upper and lower arch. The choice of cuspless posterior teeth will lessen the problem.

Arch Form (Figs 3.3 to 3.5)

Generally arch form is classified (House) as:

Class I (Square): The square arch is best form to prevent rotational movements and provides stability to the dentures.

Class II (Tapering): The tapering arch prevents rotational movements to a lesser degree.

Class III (Oval): The oval arch is round in shape and gives little or no resistance to rotational movements.

If the arch form is not same in the maxilla and mandible, there will be problem with tooth arrangement and stability.

Shape of the Ridge

The contour of the residual ridge determines the amount of vertical and horizontal the denture basis

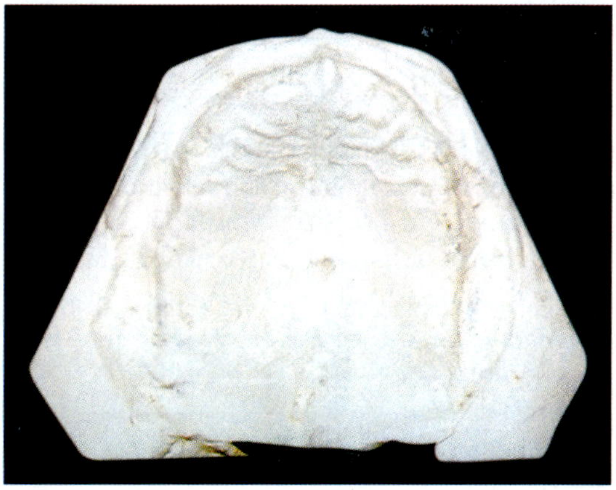

Fig. 3.3: Square-shaped maxillary arch

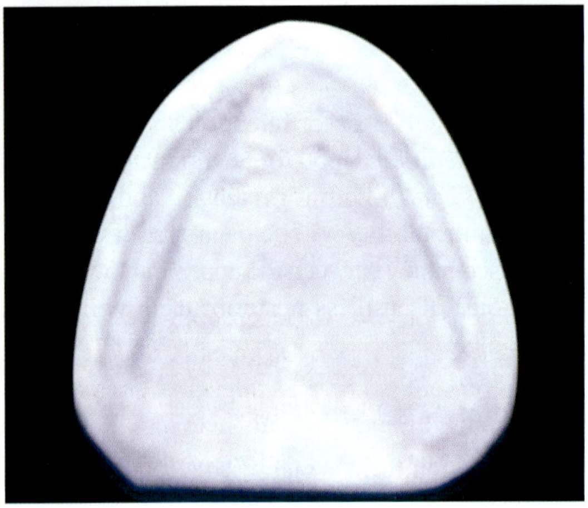

Fig. 3.4: Tapering-shaped maxillary arch

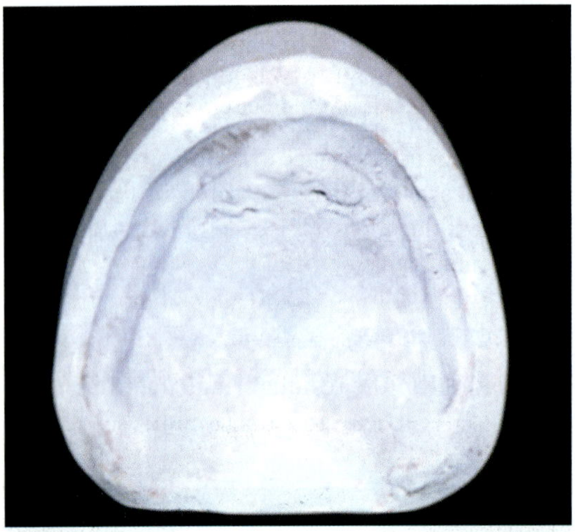

Fig. 3.5: Ovoid-shaped maxillary arch

Class I (Square): The square and is U-shaped ridges are best for denture stability and retention.

Class II (V-shaped): The V-shaped ridges are less favorable as slight pressure on the denture base causes displacement of the denture from the underlying soft tissues.

Class III (Flat): The flat ridges offer the poorest resistance to horizontal forces.

Class IV (Knife edge): The knife-edged ridges also can offer little resistance to vertical forces. The pressure on the ridges traumatizes the mucosa covering the top of the ridge and sufficient relief should be provided on it.

Interarch Space

The interarch distance between the ridges approximately parallel. In case of normal interspace the arrangement of teeth is easy and stability of the denture is good.

Excessive interarch space is usually accompanied by severe resorption and produces leverages on the denture base and decreases stability.

Insufficient interarch space creates difficulty to accommodate the artificial teeth.

Ridge Parallelism

Class I: When both the ridges are parallel, no sliding movement of the denture occurs during function.

Class II: When the mandibular ridge is divergent from the occlusal plane anteriorly one denture will slide forward.

Class III: When the maxillary ridge is divergent from the occlusal plane anteriorly or both the ridges are divergent anteriorly both the dentures will slide forward.

Ridge Relationship (Figs 3.6A to C)

Class I (Normal): The maxillary ridge crest is directly above the mandibular ridge. In this case, anterior teeth are set with an object and overbite of 1 to 2 mm. In this case, usually the posterior teeth can be set in normal position with 1 mm overjet. This is most favorable ridge relation for complete dentures and balanced occlusion is possible.

Class II (Retrognathic): The mandibular ridge is narrower and shorter than the maxillary ridge that makes the setting of posterior teeth difficult. These patients often have wide range of mandibular movement that makes the balance occlusion necessary. They frequently show habitual closure position anterior to centric relation.

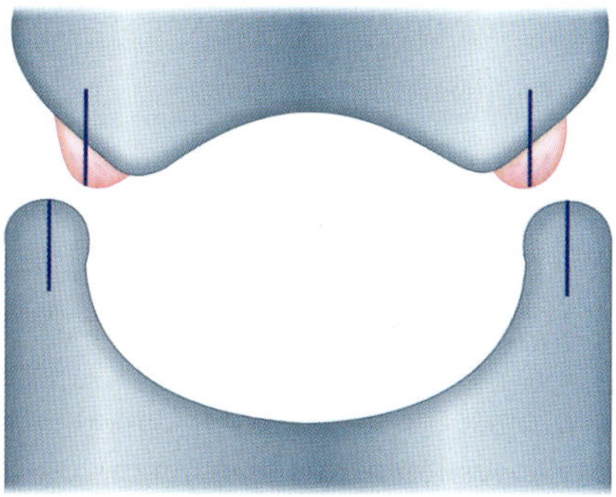

Fig. 3.6A: Normal (class I) ridge relation—posterior view

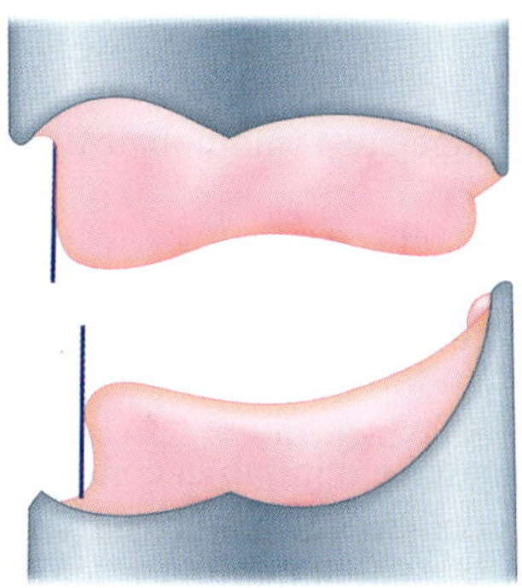

Fig. 3.6B: Normal (class I) ridge relation—buccal view

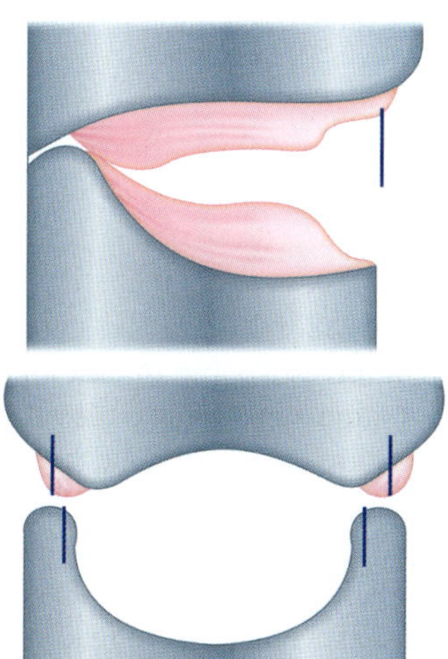

Fig. 3.6C: Prognathic (class II) ridge relation—buccal and posterior view

Class III (Prognathic): The mandible is larger and wider than maxillae. These patients show no excursive movement but only open and close hinge jaw movement. This makes balance occlusion unnecessary. These patients show a posterior, and sometimes, an anterior cross-bite.

Bony Undercuts

Bony undercuts are found on both the maxillary and mandibular ridges. On maxilla undercuts are usually present in anterior ridge and lateral to the tuberosities. Undercuts do not help in retention but cause loss of border seal. Selective relief of denture is the treatment. Surgical removal is rarely needed.

Tori (Fig. 3.7)

Small mandibular or maxillary tori usually present no problem in denture fabrication. If undercuts are present in tori, they should be removed surgically. If very thin mucosa overlies, the tori relief in denture should be provided.

Palatal Throat Form (Fig. 3.8)

According to House, classification of the soft palate is based on the degree of palatal flexure which is important to the formation of the posterior palatal

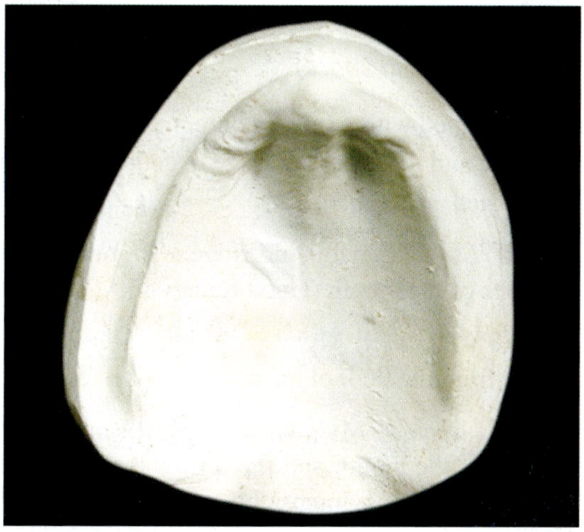

Fig. 3.7: Torus palatini

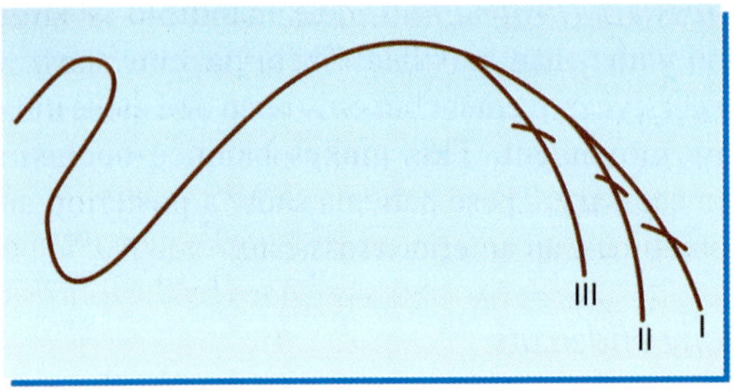

Fig. 3.8: Palatal throat form classes I, II and III

seal in the maxillary denture. The junction of hard and soft palates is marked with an indelible pencil when the patient blows through nose while holding it closed. The line of palatal flexure/vibrating line is then marked when the patient say "Ah".

Class I: Gradual flexure of soft palate 5 to 12 mm behind the junction of hard and soft palates. It is very favorable as it is wide.

Class II: Turns down approximately at an angle of 45° of tissue 3 to 5 mm behind the junction of the hard and soft palates.

Class III: Turns down abruptly at an angle of 70° just behind the hard and soft palates. It is most critical situation to locate the seal area and movement of soft palate may result in a loss of retention.

Lateral Throat Form (Retromylohyoid Space)

It is examined with a small mouth mirror placed in the space and the patient is asked to gently protrude the tongue.

Class I (Large): Mylohyoid ridge is10 mm above the floor of the mouth (Good retention).

Class II (Medium): Mylohyoid ridge is less than 10 mm from the floor of the mouth (Fair retention).

Class III (Small): Mylohyoid ridge at same level to floor of the mouth and the mirror is displaced. Retention is almost impossible for lower denture.

Mucosa Condition

Class I: Healthy

Class II: Irritated

Class III: Pathologic, e.g. papillomatous

Border and Frenum Attachments

Class I (Low): The border or frenum attachments close to the vestibule (less than 6 mm).

Class II (Intermediate): The border or frenum attachments close to the ridge crest (between 6–12 mm).

Class III (High): The border or frenum attachments high up the ridge crest (more than 12 mm).

Saliva

Class I: Amount and consistency of saliva is normal.

Class II: Excessive thin saliva containing water or thick saliva contains much mucus. Excessive saliva may cause gagging and interface with impression making.

Class III: (Xerostomia) Saliva is scanty and mucinous may reduce retention of denture.

Tongue Size (House)

Class I: normal in size

Class II: Large in size

Class III: Excessive large

The tongue gives trouble in case of large and small sizes. A large-sized tongue may displace the mandibular denture. A small tongue fails to produce border seal for the lower denture. The enlarged tongue makes the impression and jaw relation records difficult, however, once the denture is worn by the patient for several days, tongue adapts to the denture.

Tongue Position

Wright (1949) classified tongue position as follows:

Class I: The tongue completely fills the floor of the mouth. The lateral borders of the tongue rest on or against the residual ridges. The tip of the tongue rests just lingual to anterior mandibular ridges. This is the normal position of tongue and is the most favorable for denture border seal. Wright states that 65% of all the patients have a normal tongue position.

Class II: The tongue is flattened and broad with its apex in normal position.

Class III: Retracted tongue—The apex is curled upward or downward and depressed in the floor of the mouth. The retracted tongue fails to provide a seal and also unseat the mandibular denture. A retruded tongue position (in 35% of all patients) causes the tissues of the sublingual gland to move posteriorly and inferiorly to break the seal of the lingual flange and retention is sacrificed.

In extreme resorption of anterior ridge where the lip falls back, a tongue with a forward position may act as a balancing force preventing the backward displacement of the denture.

To help control the tongue the patient may be advised tongue exercises two or three times daily as follows:

Exercise 1. The tongue is swing sideways and placed outside the lower lip about half an inch. This is repeated.

Exercise 2. The tongue is thrust out and pulled back quickly.

Exercise 3. The tongue is thrust out rapidly.

The preprosthetic "bubble-gum" therapy for a period of week is advised by some clinicians. The patient chews gums for weeks and increases its size gradually. It is thought that the patient will adapt to restricted tongue space before the dentures are delivered.

Some patients will never be able to master to control the denture with tongue. So, the importance of tongue control should be pointed out to the patient prior to construction of the denture to make the patient know about his failure to master the normal tongue position and not the fault of the dentist in case of a denture problem.

The dentist must be careful in designing the denture so that they prevent the movement of tongue as little as possible which is gained by the following rules:

1. Teeth must never be set inside the ridge to cramp the tongue causing movement of the dentures and trauma to the patient. The tongue space should be measured from the old successful dentures and copied in the new one.
2. The tongue should rest on the lingual flanges which slope slightly inwards and downwards.
3. The palate of the maxillary denture should be as thin as possible as permitted by the strength of the denture base material.
4. The posterior edge of the maxillary denture should not be thick and square-edged to cause retching. Instead, a thin posterior edge post-dammed properly will sink into the compressible tissues of the soft palate and prevent retching.
5. The occlusal plane of the mandibular denture should be kept at the level of the tongue so that the lateral borders of the tongue rest on the occlusal surfaces of the teeth when the mouth is opened. This will prevent rising of the lower denture while receiving food.

Gag Reflex

Gagging is due to psychological and somatogenic causes. The gag reflex is assessed by gently touching the palate with a mouth mirror. The patient may gag during impression making. To prevent that, sedatives may be employed, but the medicines should be avoided. The patient should be kept in an upright position and his attention is distracted. The use of first setting impression material and quick manipulation is essential.

Radiographic Examination

The panoramic radiographs are valuable to examine the osseous structures that support the denture. The nature of the supporting bony structure has been classified by Wical and Swope as follows:

Class I: Approximately 2/3rds of mandibular alveolar bone remains.

Class II: Approximately 2/3rds to 2/9th mandibular alveolar bone remains.

Class III: Approximately 1/3rds or less mandibular alveolar bone remains.

This classification is based on the measurement of the distance from the inferior border of mandible to the lower edge of the mental foramen devided by three.

Approximately 25% of edentulous mouths show the presence of some types of retained pathology like roots, unerrupted teeth, cysts, etc. A pantographic X-ray is valuable in estimating the bone quantity but it has little value in evaluating bone quality. An image of retained root or unerrupted tooth in a pantographic X-ray should be viewed in a periapical X-ray. If the retained root or tooth is present for many years symptomless, and shows no pathology, removal may not be necessary. Of course, a regular yearly check-up is necessary (Fig. 3.9).

Pre-extaction Records

All types of pre-extraction record is helpful. Study casts and close up photographs are most useful but radiographs and patients recollection can also be used.

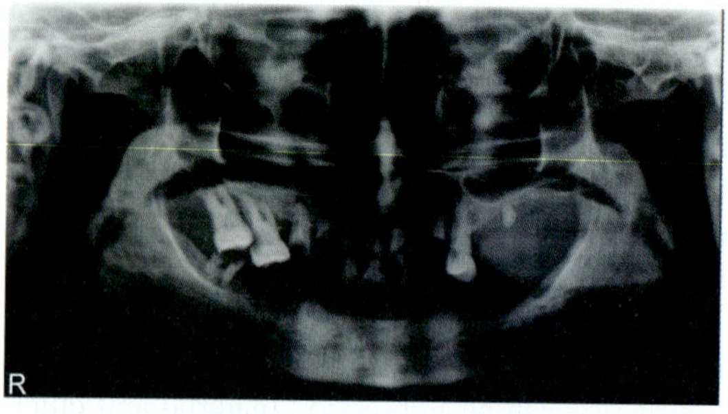

Fig. 3.9: Pantographic radiograph

Treatment Plan and Prognosis

After all the relevant information has been gathered in the form of a chart, prognosis a treatment plan should be formulated. Treatment plan is the sequence of procedures planned for the treatment of a patient after diagnosis. A treatment plan includes necessary preprosthetic surgery and tissue conditioning. It should include the procedures to be followed, materials to be used, and time schedule required for treatment. It should be presented to the patient along with the prognosis, and the fee to the patient for approval. After obtaining the patient's consent, treatment should be started. Treatment without such plan makes it impossible to obtain the informed consent of the patient. Without informed consent, problems like loss of patient, loss of fees and even litigation may occur. The mere listing and accumulation of diagnostic data are insignificant unless the information obtained is correlated, evaluated and integrated in the plan of treatment. Successful treatment of the complete denture problem depends upon the sound planning, dentist's skill and ability along with the patient's mental attitude.

The construction of a set of denture is divided into several visits. There is very little variation in basic planning in the construction of dentures. Where a particular difficulty may be anticipated, the normal routine may be changed. A basic plan is as follows:

Adjunct Care

In the first visit, a list of proposed adjunct therapy as finger massage, tissue conditioning, prescribed medicines to combat infection as candidiasis, denture stomatitis is prepared. The occlusal adjustment and relining of the denture may cause recovery. The antifungal drugs as nystatin and amphotericin B result in tissue recovery to normal in 14 days. The denture should be immersed in 1%

sodium hypochloride solution at night during this period.

Tissue Conditioning

In the first visit, types of tissue treatment material to be used and frequency of tissue treatment should be determined. If examination of the mouth reveals that the state of oral tissue is unsatisfactory for supporting dentures, some preliminary mouth preparation may be necessary. The wearing of ill-fitting dentures for sometimes causes some deformation of the soft tissues. If the dentures are withheld from the patient for 48 to 72 hours, this tissues trauma recovers. As most patients would be unwilling to accept such a course, temporary lining materials known as "tissue conditioners" have been devised to allow the tissue recovery to occur while the denture continue to be worn. After an initial set, these materials remain plastic up to 3 to 4 days, therefore, soft tissue which has been distorted may recover. Where excess pressure is being applied the tissue conditioner will be displaced and the fitting surface of the denture base will show through the area of excessive pressure thus revealed can be reduced (Figs 3.10 and 3.11).

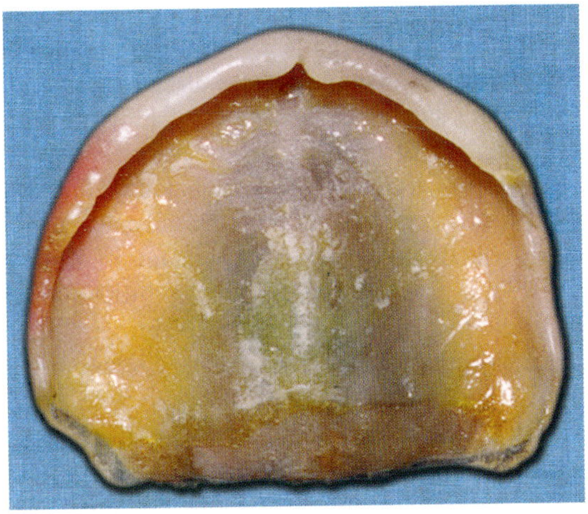

Fig. 3.10: Complete upper denture refined with tissue conditioner

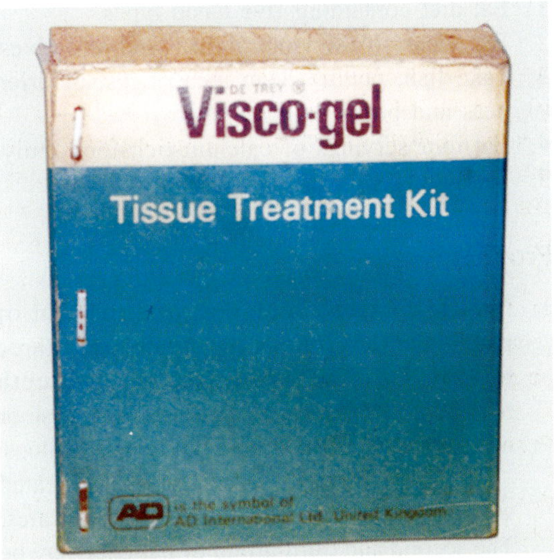

Fig. 3.11: Tissue treatment or conditioner kit

Surgical Mouth Preparation

The prosthodontic should be aware of the situation before the extraction of teeth and perform the preparation accordingly following the list of staging of the surgical procedures.

- *Surgical preparation during extraction of teeth:*
  - Removal of sharp bony spicules and tips of interdental septum using the ronguer forceps.
  - Application of sharp pressure between thumb and index finger after all extraction of teeth to even contouring the ridge.
- *Surgical preparation of edentulous mouth:*
  - Removal of retained roots or unerrupted teeth, dental cysts
  - Reduction of sharp bony mass, e.g. mylohyoid ridges, sharp ridges, enlarged tuberosities, torus.
  - Removal of soft hyperplastic tissues caused by denture hyperplasia or flabby anterior ridges.
  - Removal of high frenum attachments.
  - Deepening of shallow sulcus to increase denture-bearing area.
  - Orthognathic surgery to improve ridge relation.
  - Important denture procedures.
  - Surgery of congenital defects.

Nutritional Counseling

Nutritional counseling is a very important step in treatment planning of a complete denture patient. The quality of diet for such patient can be improved with nutritional counseling. An unbalanced diet that lacks fruits, vegetables or proteins and calories can turn perfectly made denture into an unsatisfactory one. So, a properly guided balanced diet should be included in prosthodontic treatment. The main objective of nutritional council is to correct nutritional imbalances that interfere with body and oral health. The dentist need not diagnose specific nutritional deficiency but can help the patient providing with nutritional guidelines. This can be done using five basic food guide pyramid as follows:

1. Eat diet containing five basic types.
2. Eat at least five servings of fruits and vegetables.
3. Take fish, poultry, lean meat, eggs, or dried peas and beans daily.
4. Eat four servings of calcium-rich food daily.
5. Take eight glasses of water.

Prosthodontic Care

1. **Nature of treatment:** Patients in need of prosthodontic care can be divided into three general groups: Those with natural teeth remaining, those wearing dentures who wish or need replacements, and those who are edentulous.

   The first group of patients may be treated with removable partial denture, or overdentures. The second and third group of patients may be treated with conventional soft tissue supported complete denture or implant supported complete denture.
2. **Articulator used:**
   a. Manufacturer and instrument number
   b. Control settings: Horizontal condylar guidance (right and left); incisal guide angle; and incisal guide lateral angle (right and left)
3. **Tooth selection:** The shade, mould and material of anterior and posterior teeth should be selected.
4. **Denture base material:** Available materials like heat-cure or microwave cure or soft base.
5. **Denture base shade:** Pink, special pink, veined matching the patient's gingiva.
6. Anatomic palate including rugae or conventional palate.
7. **Characterization:** Choice of stain, drawing proposed plan.
8. List of items to improve the new dentures.
9. List of items not to be changed in new dentures.

Patient Appointments

In the first visit, a set of preliminary impressions may be obtained. In addition, surgical procedures are discussed and planned and preoperative therapy may be given.

This therapy needs the use of any medicine or rest to the mouth to produce ridges which are well healed and the gingival are in good tonus.

During the second office visit the final impression is taken and the cast poured using dental stone. Bite rims are made prior to the third visit.

The third visit is concerned with obtaining vertical dimension centric relation and orientation relations which is transferred to an articulator. In addition, eccentric relations are obtained and the condylar guidance is established. The selection of anterior teeth is possible in this stage.

The fourth visit is to trying of dentures to verify records and to satisfy the patient's esthetic need.

The fifth visit is the insertion of the dentures.

The sixth visit is the first postoperative visit after 24 hours for sore spot adjustment, remounting of casts and final occlusal adjustment.

Then any subsequent visit required for oral examinations and treatments. When the periodic recall for oral examination and the necessary postinsertion appointments are completed the patients are instructed to call for an appointment if there is any problem.

Every denture patient should be placed on a regular recall program at a 12-month interval. The necessary occlusal corrections, relining and new denture should be made as required as changes in the mouth occur continuously.

PROGNOSIS

The determination of the prognosis of every complete denture case is important to both operator and patient. The examination both visual and digital will bring out all the favorable and unfavorable circumstances under which the problem is to solve. An analysis of the situation will show the operator the extent of favorable and unfavorable conditions and assess his ability to reduce the unfavorable conditions using certain techniques. On this assessment of the possibilities and limitations the prognosis of the case is graded as being simple, average, and extreme difficult. In a difficult case, a fee twice as higher may be quoted by the operator. The cost of production in this case may increase due to mouth preparations, relining, rebasing, or even remaking the dentures. The unfavorable oral condition of the patient must be informed before the start of treatment and with the cooperation of the patient the operator can utilize his skill to produce successful dentures. There are a number of salient features in the mouth to be taken into consideration before determination of prognosis.

Ridge Relationship (Anteroposterior)

a. Class I (Angle's classification) jaw relation.
b. Class II (Angle's classification) jaw relation.
c. Class III (Angel's classification) jaw relation.

In case of class II and III, the dentist has to encounter great difficulties during placement and arrangement of tooth for balanced occlusion. On the contrary, in class I jaw relation, the problem of arrangement of teeth is comparatively simple procedure.

Ridge Relationship (Lateral)

a. Mandibular ridge is much wider than maxillary ridge.
b. Maxillary ridge is much wider than mandibular ridge.
c. Maxillary and mandibular ridges are almost of same width.

In the first two cases, difficulties will be encountered in setting up the teeth. In the first case, it may be necessary to arrange the teeth in cross-bite relation. In the second case, the occlusion may be limited to the second premolars and molars only.

Interarch Distance

An ideal interarch distance at vertical dimension of occlusion is 16 to 18 mm.

a. *Normal*: When there is a normal distance between the ridges, the conditions are favorable for arrangement of anterior and posterior teeth.
b. *Excessive*: When there is an excessive distance between the ridges, it is very difficult to get stability of the dentures during mastication because of the large distance between the occlusal surfaces of the upper and lower teeth to their respective ridges.
c. *Inadequate*: When there is very limited space between the ridges, setting of teeth may have to be mutilated to arrange them in proper position.

Nature of Denture-bearing Tissue

The denture-bearing mucosa and submucosa overlying the bone are not of uniform thickness. They may be classified into three groups:

a. Thick and compressible mucosa because of their extreme resiliency returns to their original position when compressed. They may loosen the dentures after the pressure is released. An extensive papillary hyperplasia due to traumatic ill-fitting denture should require surgery. A moderate papillary hyperplasia can be treated with tissue conditioner until healing has taken place. A new denture should be constructed then.
b. Thin uncompressible mucosa never allows the dentures to brought into intimate contact with soft tissues lessening retention. Therefore, the prognosis is poor.
c. Average thick mucosa allows the dentures to brought into intimate contact with the soft tissues and good retention and prognosis is obtained.

Maxillary Ridge Prognosis (Table 3.1)

The prognosis for the maxillary complete can be divided into factors that can affect retention and stability. The factors are as follows:

a. Size of ridge
b. Shape of palatal vault
c. Bilateral tuberosity undercuts
d. Size of tuberosity
e. Maxillary torus

a. *Size of ridge*: The degree of success with complete denture can be made for a patient depending upon the anatomy of the edentulous jaws. The prognosis depends upon the factors of retention and stability. Adhesion and cohesion are directly proportional to the area covered. Therefore, a larger jaw offers more favorable prognosis. But larger jaws have got the difficulties in manipulation of trays and impression materials. So, a medium-sized mouth is easiest to work with.

b. *Shape of ridge and palatal vault*: The shapes of palatal vaults may be of three types:
   - Excessively deep and triangular, V-shaped palatal vault. This is usually associated with very heavy ridges and a thick, yielding mucosa. This type will cause difficulty in retention for the maxillary denture. The excessive thick mucosa after being compressed will tend to return to its original position and causes loosening of denture. Moreover, the forces of adhesion and cohesion are not acting at right angles to the surfaces to be separated. Lastly the heavy ridges act to support the denture rather than to retain it. These types of ridges require good peripheral seal and balanced occlusion for good prognosis. The posterior palatal seal area presents an abrupt drop of soft palate, thus providing less space for adequate palatal seal. Any movement of the denture in function may break the seal, as there is no horizontal bearing area.
   - Palatal vault of average depth and square in shape is favorable to retention of denture, therefore, the prognosis is favorable.
   - Flat palatal vault with small ridges and shallow sulcus due to resorption is not favorable because ill-developed ridges do not resist lateral or anteroposterior movements. But when all other conditions are normal, it is decidedly favorable.

c. *Bilateral tuberosity undercuts*: Bilateral bony undercuts occurring on the labial and buccal surfaces of maxillary tuberosity present problems in the insertion of correctly extended denture flanges. These may be blocked out of one or both on the master cast before processing the denture if not much. These are unfavorable because this reduces the peripheral seal. In very much pronounced undercuts surgical removal on one or both sides may be necessary.

Table 3.1 Prognosis for maxillary complete denture

Factors	Good prognosis	Worst prognosis
Form of ridge and palatal vault	Broad, U-shaped or flat	Deep V-shaped
Tuberosity undercut	Non-undercut	Undercut
Depth of gingival sulcus	Normal resilient mucosa, deep sulcus	Taut, shallow sulcus, thin, in elastic sub-mucosa
Size of ridge	Medium	Large and small
Arch form	Square or ovoid	Tapering
Palatal throat form	Gradual flexure or moderate flexure out	Abrupt flexure
Maxillary torus	Absent	Present with undercut

d. *Size of tuberosity*: The enlarged maxillary tuberosities encroaching on the interridge distance cause problem in denture construction. The maxillary tuberosities often extend inferiorly to occlude with the third molar or retromolar pad of the mandible. The maxillary sinuses occasionally extend deep into the tuberosity and complicate a surgical removal of the tuberosities. In such case, both the dentures need not be extended to the areas of contact.
e. *Maxillary torus*: A good denture can be made in the presence of a maxillary torus if it is not extended up to the vibrating line. If the torus is accompanied by undercut, it creates problem, then surgical reduction is necessary (see Fig. 3.7).

Mandibular Ridge Prognosis (Table 3.2)

The prognosis for mandibular denture depends on stability and retention. The retention and stability of a denture varies from patient to patient and depends upon the anatomic and physiologic factors as follows:

a. Type of mandibular ridge
b. Nature of sublingual fold space
c. Tongue position
d. Buccal shelf
e. Buccal pad of fat
f. Muscle tone.

a. *Type of mandibular ridge*: The mandibular ridges may be divided in three types:
   - High and heavy mandibular ridge: This type of ridge is very favorable because it affords an excellent bearing area for the mandibular denture.
   - Flat ridge: The extremely flat ridge due to complete resorption of the alveolar process is usually favorable, provided the denture is properly extended.
   - High but thin and sharp mandibular ridge: The "knife-edged" ridge offers the poorest prognosis because the mucosa, placed between the sharp bony ridge and the rigid denture base, is constantly traumatized. Sometimes, this type of ridge is covered with fibrous tissues that are easily displaced. Failures are very common with this type of ridges.
b. *Nature of sublingual fold space*: This is the potential space between the lower anterior ridge and sublingual gland where the denture border lies in. This space may be either well developed or poorly developed. A well-developed and resilient sublingual fold spaces are favorable as a seal of denture base extension can be achieved. In case of a poorly developed sublingual space fold, the prognosis is poor.
c. *Tongue position*: It is the position of the tongue at rest and in function.

Table 3.2 Prognosis for mandibular complete denture

Factors	Good prognosis	Worst prognosis
Type of ridge	High	Knife edge
Nature of sublingual fold space	Well defined	Ill-defined
Tongue position	Normal	Retracted
Buccal shelf	Flat and wide	Concave and narrow
Tissue tone	Resilient	Tense and taut
Tissue support	Elastic tissue	Thin or movable
Buccal fat pad	Rests on masseteric notch	Does not rest on notch
Interarch space	Adequate	Inadequate

A normal tongue position according to Wright's classification is one where the tip of the tongue rests forward in a position just lingual to the mandibular anterior teeth. The prognosis is good due to maintained peripheral seal in the sublingual fold space.

In case of a retracted tongue position the border seal in the sublingual fold area is lacking causing worst prognosis.

d. *Buccal shelf*: The buccal shelf area is the key area for mandibular denture stability due to its large flat surface. A broad flat buccal shelf area provides better prognosis than a sharp sloping, narrow, or concave buccal shelf.
e. *Position of buccal pad of fat*: The buccal pad of fat is composed of areolar connective tissues found in posterior cheek. In the mandibular denture this tissue rests over the denture border in the masseteric notch area to stabilize it as well as achieve a seal for good retention.
f. *Tissue tone*: The tissue tone is the relative resiliency or tautness of the muscles of cheek and lips. If the denture border is slightly over-extended, and the tissues are taut, the denture stability will be affected. But if the tissue is resilience, it will provide cushioning effect for the denture.

CONCLUSION

The mere listing and accumulation of diagnostic information are pointless and of no significance unless data obtained is carefully correlated, critically evaluated and intelligently integrated in treatment plan.

A thorough knowledge of subject, an adequate degree of skill and experience, sound clinical judgment and a maximum effort constitute dentist's ultimate success in serving the edentulous patients.

BIBLIOGRAPHY

1. Barone JV. Diagnosis and prognosis in complete denture prosthesis. J Prosthet Dent. 1964;14:207-13.
2. Chester P. Examination diagnosis and treatment planning. J Prosthet Dent 1960;10:1004-10.
3. Ellinger CW, Rayson JH. Diagnosis and treatment planning. Lea and Febign Philadelphia. 1975;49-67.
4. Freidman S. Effective use of diagnostic data. J Prosthet Dent. 1959;9:729-37.
5. Henry S. Roentgenographic Examination of edentulous patient. J Prosthet Dent. 1961;18:304-7.
6. John A, Thomas T. Simplified complete dentures. DCNA. 2004;40:625-40.
7. Robert E. Patient evaluation and treatment planning for complete denture therapy. DCNA. 1996;40:1-17.
8. Sharry JJ. Complete denture prosthodentics. Mcgrow Hill Book company, 3rd edn, 1962.
9. Sheldon W. Essentials of complete denture prosthodontics. AIIBS Publishers, 2nd edn. 1996;39-55.
10. Wial KE, Swope CC. Studies of residual ridge resorption; Part I use of panoramic radiographs for evaluation and classification of mandibular resorption, J Prosthet Dent. 1974;7-12.
11. Zarb-Bolender. Prosthodontic treatment for edentulous patients. 12th edn; Mosby; 2004.

Chapter 4

Retention, Stability and Support of Complete Dentures

INTRODUCTION

The optimal complete denture treatment requires good qualities of retention, stability and support. They are interrelated. Some physical, mechanical and biological factors of retention, stability and support are the determinants that enhance the properties of retention, stability and support in the complete denture through their influence on the relationship between the denture base and the edentulous ridges. There are controversies regarding the roles played by these factors, and there relative importance in clinical applications in various impression techniques. So, a thorough study and discussion is needed for proper understanding of the problems related to them and selection of procedures and techniques for the fabrication of successful complete dentures.

RETENTION

The main objectives of complete denture fabrication are to restore a patient's appearance, mastication and speech. If a denture is easily dislodged during speech or eating, it will create an embarrassing situation that may cause psychological trauma. A retentive denture dramatically contributes to patient acceptance of the finished prosthesis.

DEFINITION

The Glossary of Prosthodontic Terms (GPT-7), defined retention as the resistance in the movement of a denture away from its tissue foundation, especially in a vertical direction. It is the quality inherent in the prosthesis acting to resist the forces of dislodgement along the path of placement, e.g. the forces of gravity, the adhesiveness of foods, or the forces associated with opening of the jaws (GPT-7). It provides psychologic comfort and prevent mental trauma to the patient.

The relation of a complete denture is determined by the fit of the tissue-bearing surface so alteration of the dimensions of this surface affects the retention. When the denture is worn, saliva fills the space between the denture and the tissue.

FACTORS AFFECTING COMPLETE DENTURE RETENTION

The factors that affect retention can be classified as:

A. **Physical factors:** The primary retention of complete denture is obtained from various physical factors. They act just after the insertion of the denture in the mouth.
B. **Biological factors:** The secondary retention is obtained by acquired muscular control gradually acquired by the patient after wearing the denture a period of time.
C. **Mechanical factors:** Those are aids in retention when applicable.

Physical Factors

The physical forces of adhesion, cohesion, gravity and atmospheric pressure play an important role in denture retention.

1. *Adhesion*: It is defined as the molecular attraction between unlike molecules to bind them together and form a larger mass. A drop of water introduced on the surface of a solid glass plate will resist movement away from the glass. This occurs between the denture base and saliva, and mucosa and saliva. The physical laws of adhesion are as follows:
   - Adhesion is indirectly proportional to the areas in contact, i.e. the more the area covered, the greater the adhesion. Hence, the maxillary dentures covering the larger surface area than mandibular denture will have greater retention than a mandibular denture. The patients having small jaws or very flat alveolar ridges have less retention comparing to the patients with large jaws or prominent ridges. Hence, the impression must be in maximum intimate contact with the tissues and extend fully to the limits of the health and function of the oral tissues.
   - Adhesion is increased in proportion as the contact is closer.
   - Adhesion is increased as the contact is prolonged.
   - Adhesion is inversely proportional to the film thickness of saliva.

   Adhesion is also occurring between denture bases and the mucosa. In xerostomia the denture base adhesion with mucosa will be more but it will cause ulceration of oral tissues due to lack of lubricating action of saliva. A saliva substitute containing carboxymethylcellulose (CMC) or oral pilocarpine 5–10 mg three times daily may be effective in xerostomia.
2. *Cohesion*: It is the physical force of attraction between molecules of the same material.

   A molecule of same material has an attraction on the neighboring molecules. It occurs in the intact film of saliva in between the mucosa and the denture base. The average amount of saliva excreted by the salivary glands is 1.5 liters per day. The half of this amount is secreted during meals when the salivary glands are stimulated maximum. The quantity and quality of saliva play a very vital role in complete denture retention. The quantity of the saliva and its quality (viscosity) are very closely interrelated. The viscosity of saliva is important in cohesion. Normal quality and adequate quantity of saliva is cohesive. When the quantity of saliva is excessive and quality is watery, cohesion is decreased. When the quantity of saliva is decreased and its viscosity is increased, cohesion is decreased due to increase in the film thickness of saliva. The force of cohesion is less than the force of adhesion. The saliva acts as "glue" that pastes the denture to the mucosa. A concave meniscus should be formed between the two surfaces, mucosa and denture. The gap between the polished surfaces of denture and lips or cheeks, if narrow and long, increases the resistance of denture to displacement. The flanges of the denture must be thick enough to contact the cheek and lip mucosa to provide valve-like seal effect of the soft tissues. The denture flanges and borders should not be reduced while polishing and finishing (Fig. 4.1).

   The viscosity of saliva is of importance in the phenomenon of cohesion. The flow of saliva depends on its viscosity. Thus, increase

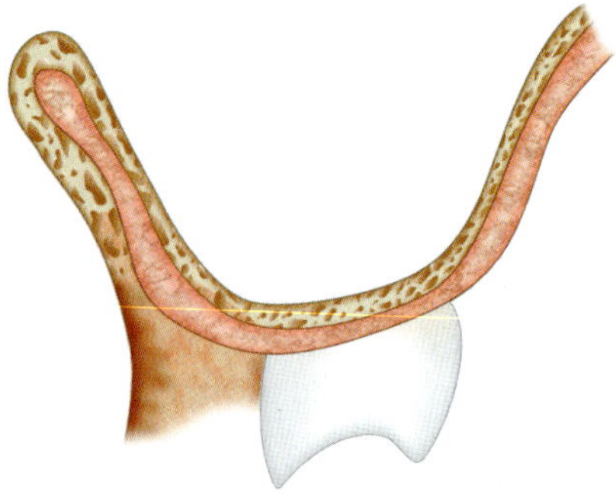

Fig. 4.1: Thin saliva film (spotted area) between denture meniscus develop at the border of denture and soft tissue draping of cheeks also

in viscosity of saliva should increase the retention. But in practice such never happens and as excessive viscous saliva accumulated beneath the denture traps air and retention is lost.

3. *Surface tension*: Interfacial surface tension acts by virtue of a thin film of saliva between two intimately contacted fitting surfaces of denture and oral tissues. It is the resistance to separation in the film of liquid between two well-adapted surfaces of rigid material. Thinner the fluid film, the greater will be the surface tension. That is why an accurate fit is necessary. The retention of a mucostatic base is based on interfacial surface tension. It is effective in the maxillary denture. In mandibular denture, the amount of saliva in the border of the denture eliminates the effect of interfacial surface tension. It results in less retention.
4. *Gravity*: The force of gravity aids in retention of lower dentures. Conversely, it acts as a displacing force in upper dentures, but it is not of sufficient magnitude to be considered as an important factor. In mandibular denture incorporating lead shots in the lingual polished surface of the denture base may increase the weight of the denture. In maxillary denture, especially large and complicated obturators, gravity acts as dislodging force. These should be made as light as possible by thinning out the peripheral borders, or making the palatal part of the denture too thin. In either case, these cause loss of retention of maxillary dentures so, this is not advisable. Thin peripheral borders of maxillary denture will permit the entrance of air between the denture and the palate causing equalization of air pressure under and outside of the denture. The vital role of atmospheric pressure in denture retention will be lost completely.

   An excessively thin palatal portion of maxillary denture also undergoes frequent fracture. The golden rule is the best to follow here in that the maxillary and mandibular dentures should be made neither very thick nor very thin. The denture when dislodged can be reseated by closing the mouth. If the opposing teeth are even due to balanced occlusion, the denture can be reseated easily by closing the mouth.

   The force of gravity is an unimportant factor in denture retention. If a maxillary denture has a tendency to drop it is not due to its greater weight. Similarly, mandibular denture is not retentive not because it is lighter in weight than the average. It is due to poor stability of the dentures and a more complex phenomenon that will be discussed next.
5. *Atmospheric pressure*: It is the physical factor of hydrostatic pressure. It is due to the weight of the atmosphere on the earth's surface. At sea level this force amounts to 14.7 psi. The physical property of atmospheric pressure is taken as an aid in complete denture retention. The retention of denture by atmospheric pressure is directly proportional to the area coverage by the denture base. For atmospheric pressure to be effective, the denture must have a prefect peripheral seal. The pressure between the denture and basal tissue drops below atmospheric pressure. The difference between these two pressures gives a positive force holding the denture in place. The use of selective pressure impression technique with proper functional border moulding, proper shaping of labial surface, and postdamming of posterior palatal area, is essential for the atmospheric pressure to be effective in denture retention.

Atmospheric pressure is an adjunct in denture retention. So relief chambers to increase atmospheric pressure effect should be avoided as they soon become ineffective due to tissue growth into them.

The thickness or depth of sulcus varies from mouth to mouth but it should be 1 mm in an average.

A lower denture may be postdammed at the distal part of the denture on the keratinized tissue of the 'pear-shaped pad' and not on compressible retromolar pad.

The border molding and postdam will contribute to the retention of denture by atmospheric pressure.

Biological Factors

1. *Neuromuscular control*: Neuromuscular control is the functional forces exerted by the muscles in denture retention. The acquired muscular control develope at the reflex level to retain denture rather displace it as a foreign body. It becomes effective after the denture has been worn for a period of time. In younger patients, the required conditioned reflexes will be developed more rapidly than in older patients. This is one reason why younger people are usually more tolerant of new dentures than are older patients. For muscular control to exercise the maximum effect on retention, the dentures themselves must be shaped to assist this action. If the buccal flanges of the maxillary denture slopes up and out from the occlusal surfaces of the teeth and if the buccal flanges of the mandibular denture slope down and out from the occlusal plane, the contraction of the buccinators muscles will tend to seat both the dentures on their basal seats.

   The lingual surfaces of the lingual flanges should slope towards the center of the mouth so that tongue can fit against them and perfect the border seal on lingual surface.
2. *Intimate tissue contact*: Intimate tissue contact is a biologic factor that refers to the close adaptation of the denture base to the underlying soft tissues. The technique of impression will determine the degree of intimate tissue contact obtained with the tissues at rest and during function.

   An impression material with adequate flow should be used to avoid uneven pressure during impression that may cause a localized rebounding effect of the compressed tissues under the denture base and denture 'sorespots' are produced.

   This does not advice mucostatic impression but a slight generalized pressure on the soft tissues is desirable. The use of medium viscous light bodied impression material with sufficient flow in a nonperforated tray eliminates the need of full arch relief spacers in the tray. This ensures close adaptation of the denture-base and may compensate to a degree for the dimensional changes in the finished dentures. Lammie recommended slight pressure on periphery through border molding ensuring positive contact of the denture border at delivery.
3. *Peripheral seal*: The border seal affected by intimate contact of both the upper and lower denture borders with the surrounding soft tissues. The seal around the posterior palatal seal area enhances its effectiveness. The soft tissue area at or beyond the junction of the hard and soft palates on which pressure, within physiologic limits, can be applied by a denture to aid in its retention. The retention of a complete upper denture is largely dependent upon the establishment of an effective seal against the ingress of air around its border. In the sulci the seal is developed by the elastic displacement of the soft tissues by the rounded border of the base but it must be continued across the palate at the posterior border. So, this may be achieved in the impression procedures or be created impirically by cutting the posterior palatal bead on the final cast. This postdam displaces the palatal mucosa when the denture is seated in the mouth, restricting the flow of saliva and air beneath this border.

   The postdam extends across the pterygomaxillary notches and along the vibrating line. It should be about 4 mm wide in its widest part. Due to normal variations in the thickness of the soft tissues in different parts, it is customary to be made moderately narrow in its central part, wider and deeper as it extends laterally on each side, and narrow again as it proceeds towards the pterygomaxillary notch, to fade out behind the tuberosity. Generally, a wide postdam has the advantage that if it subsequently becomes necessary to shorten slightly the length of the denture, the postdam should not be destroyed during the initial "learning period" while the patient is acquiring skill in manipulating the dentures.

4. *Shape of the ridge*: The success in denture retention is achieved when the edentulous ridges are firm and regular and covered with firmly attached dense mucoperiosteum. Patients possessing high V-shaped palatal vault present the retention problem. The processing error may be so severe that postpalatal seal cannot compensate for the resultant lack of intimate tissue contact. In such situation, either a metal base or a cold cure relining will be necessary.

   In case of a large buccal space in the maxillary denture it must be made to fill space to produce adequate border seal in the buccal space or retrozygomatic space. The area should be border moulded so that this is recorded with the normal functional movement of the coronoid process.

   The mandibular denture generally presents retention problem because of the difficulty in establishing the lingual border seal due to movable floor of the mouth which rises and falls during speech and eating.

Mechanical Factors

1. *Undercut areas*: The undercuts are frequently found at labial side of maxillary ridge and buccal to one or both *tuberosities*. Generally, undercut ridges do not aid in retention of dentures. In case of unilaterally undercut, it is possible to rotate the denture into position. The presence of undercut helps in retention if they possess some compressibility to allow the denture to be inserted. The undercuts exist labial of the maxillary alveolar ridge and buccal to one or both tuberosities, prevent vertical displacement of denture. In case of bilateral undercuts, one of the bilateral undercuts may be utilized by blocking the other with plaster or cement on final cast before processing.
2. *Denture adhesives*: The adhesive in powder form contains natural gums as tragacanth or acacia or Karaya with cellulose. The powder is sprinkled on the moist fitting surface of the denture and fitted in the mouth where it sticks to the tissues for several hours. The gum is gradually washed away due to flow of saliva and its effect is lost. So, it is effective in upper denture but not effective in lower denture where salivary flow is more. Creams and gel forms of adhesives are also available.

   Adhesives turn to pastes viscous when mixed with saliva. The viscosity of the paste between the denture and the tissue is much higher than that of the film of saliva. Retention is related to viscosity so retention is increased with a poorly fitting denture. In a well-fitting denture, the use of an adhesive increases the film thickness, and retention is not improved.

Advantages

1. It is useful during jaw relation records with temporary base, and its verification afterwards.
2. It can be used to wear old denture when the current denture is being repaired.
3. It can be used for short period in immediate denture which becomes loose due to alveolar resorption.
4. It can be advantageous to use adhesive by public speakers, e.g. singers, teachers, actors, etc.

Disadvantages

1. It is not much effective in lower denture.
2. It works as a temporary measure.
3. It produces an unpleasant feeling.

Uses

1. Theoretically denture adhesives should not be needed with a well fitted denture, except in case where conventional method of developing retention cannot be achieved. Dentures made over inferior qualities of basal tissues like

tapering arch form, high frena when worn with denture adhesive, increase retention to the range of denture made over adequate denture-bearing tissues. Denture dislodgement during chewing and talking are reduced using denture adhesives according to Tarbet WJ, Silverman G and Schmidt NF (1981), Kapur K (1967). Their use can be advised temporarily in initial learning period. Various studies have showed that denture adhesives are of immense help during various stages of fabrication of complete denture treatment procedures also. In United Kingdom and in United States of America, tons of denture adhesives are sold to large number of patients who find their old dentures lacking retention following normal slowly progressive alveolar resorption, or to use with immediate dentures.

2. *Springs*: Coiled stainless steel springs fitted with swivels in the premolar region of both the dentures are used where retention is extremely poor, particularly in hemimaxillectomy or congenital defects in maxilla. The dentures are attached with each other and have to be inserted in the mouth by holding in intercuspal position.
3. *Suction disks*: These aid in retention by creating partial vacuum. Rubber suction disks are held by a metal stud inserted into the fitting surface of the palate of the maxillary denture (Fig. 4.2). It often causes ulceration and ultimate perforation of the palate due to bone resoption (Fig. 4.3).
4. *Suction chambers*: A relief chamber is created on the fitting surface of the palate, produce partial vacuum and may help in denture retention. It should be of no use when tissue grows down into it to obliterate it.
5. *Surface acting treatment*: The fitting surfaces of the dentures are treated with hydroxy containing polymers in dental laboratory to increase the wettability and adhesion of saliva to the denture base to improve retention. These materials wear out within a short time during routine denture cleansing by the patient rendering them ineffective.

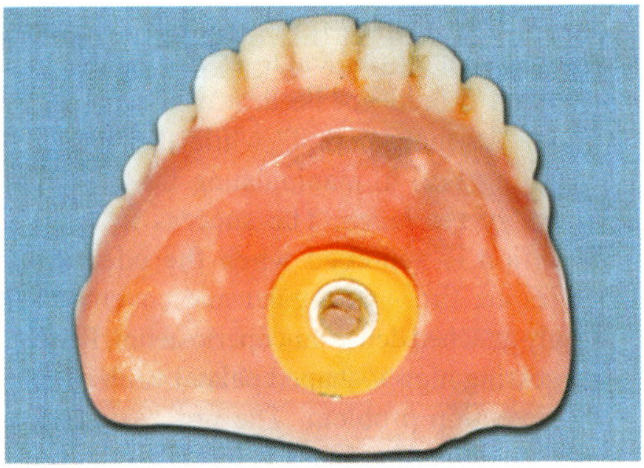

Fig. 4.2: Rubber suction disks are held by metal stud attached to maxillary denture fitting surface

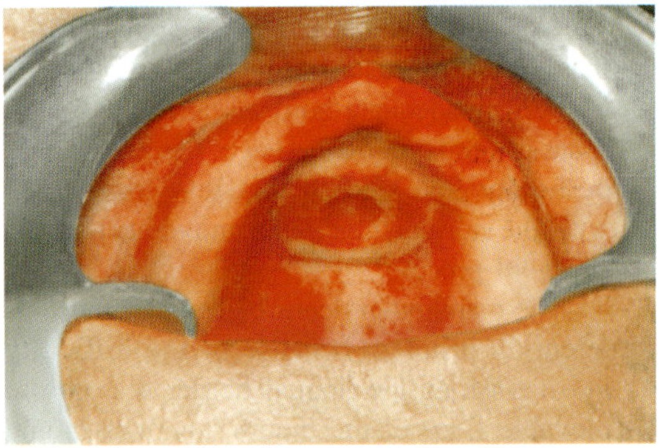

Fig. 4.3: Ulceration of palate due to use of rubber suction disk

6. *Magnets*: Small magnets of similar polarity may be placed opposing each other beneath the posterior teeth of opposing dentures. The repulsive forces of the like magnetic poles keep the dentures in place. These forces, however, will be negligible when the teeth are separated by a few millimeters.

STABILITY

Stability is defined as the quality of prosthesis to be firm, steady, or constant to resist displacement by functional, horizontal and rotational stresses (GPT-7).

Any movement of the complete denture in a horizontal direction either anteroposterior or laterally is its instability. Denture instability robbed the patient of physiologic comfort. In practice poor stability due to unfavorable residual ridge affects support and retention and results in destructive forces on the edentulous ridges during function.

Factors affecting Stability

1. Residual ridge height and contour.
2. Adaptation of denture base to the underlying tissues.
3. Residual ridge relationship.
4. Contour of polished surfaces.
5. Relationship of the opposing occlusal surfaces.
6. Tooth position and occlusal plane.

Residual Ridge Height and Contour

The stability of the complete denture depends upon the anatomic variations of the patient determined by residual ridge height and contour. A large, square, broad ridge offers a greater resistance to lateral forces than a small, narrow, tapered ridge (Fig. 4.4). Small rounded irregularities often contribute to better stability than a ridge smoothened by alveoplasty.

Square and tapered arches resist rotational forces more than an ovoid arch.

A steep palatal vault may provide greater stability than a flat vault due to greater surface area of contact at right angle to the direction of force.

Adaptation of Denture Base

The close adaptation of the denture base to the underlying healthy mucosa is most important for stability. Adequate extension of the denture base for maximum coverage within ridge physiological limits and positive and intimate contact of the denture base with facial and lingual ridge slopes is essential for denture stability. The nature of the soft tissue in the palatal inclines is ideal to resist horizontal or rotating forces due to their thickness whereas thin mucosa of mandibular lingual inclines is less ideal to resist force due to thinness. The flabbiness of tissues over the ridge also lessen stability.

The development of stability is limited by the anatomic variations that determine the residual ridge height. The lingual slope of the mandible is almost 90 degrees to the occlusal plane. This successfully resists horizontal forces. Large, square and broad ridges provide a greater resistance to horizontal force than small, round, narrow and tapered ridges. Small smooth irregularities of residual ridge favor stability. The surgical removal will decrease stability.

Residual Ridge Relationship

The horizontal ridge relation is usually rated by Angle's classification.

In class I ridge relation the stability is better for complete dentures as the maxillary ridge crest is directly above the mandibular ridge.

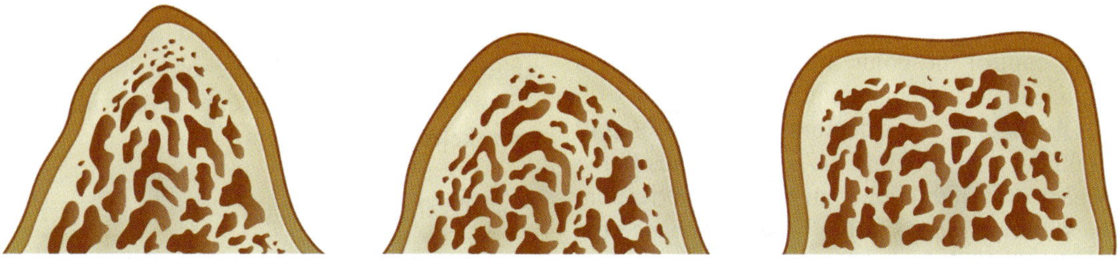

Fig. 4.4: Square ridges offer greater resistance to lateral forces than smaller round or tapered ridges

In class II the mandibular ridge is narrower and shorter than the maxillary ridge and also often has a large excursive movement. That causes loss of stability and makes balanced occlusion important.

In class III the mandible is longer and wider resulting in anterior and posterior cross-bite that causes denture instability. The posterior cross-bite can be treated with nonanatomic (zero degree) teeth to enhance stability.

Contour of Polished Surfaces

The contour of the external polished surface provides the principal factor for complete denture stability. The shape of the denture bases should be triangular in cross-section. The maxillary buccal flange should incline laterally upward. The mandibular buccal flange should incline laterally and downward and its lingual flange should incline medially and downward. The buccal and labial flanges of the maxillary and mandibular dentures should be concave so that the cheeks and lips will exert sitting force to enhance stability. The main muscles of cheeks and lips are buccinators and orbicularis oris respectively. During speech, mastication and deglutition these muscles contract to transmit vertical forces tending to seat the dentures.

The modiolus is the node near the corner of the mouth formed by eight muscles like orbicularis oris, buccinators, caninus, triangularis, zygomaticus and quadratus muscles. It functionally separates the labial vestibules from buccal vestibules. The denture base must be so shaped to allow the modiolus to function properly.

According to Fish, the superior fibers of buccinator seat the maxillary denture while the middle fibers control the bolus and the inferior fibers stabilize the mandibular denture.

The shaping of the denture bases according to the functionally molding the muscles leads to the concept of "neutral zone" in denture fabrication. The teeth are placed in this zone to enhance the stability of the dentures. The general cross-section of the polished surface of a denture through the residual ridge area should be triangular. This permits forces to direct against these surfaces for best stability.

Relationship of the Opposing Occlusal Surfaces

The presence of balanced occlusion reduces lateral destabilizing forces and helps in stability of dentures. The simultaneous contacting of the maxillary and mandibular teeth on right and left and in the posterior and anterior occlusal areas in centric and eccentric positions are developed to lower or limit the tipping or rotating of the denture bases in relation to the supporting structures.

Irrespective of the type of posterior teeth form or occlusal concept used, the dentures must be free of occlusal interferences within the functional range of movement of the patient. The function of speech, swallowing, and mastication are considered as the normal range of function. The premature contacts during various functional and parafunctional movements developed lateral forces and affect the stability. Bilateral occlusal contact in centric relation is essential to limit the dislodging forces. Many patients have mandibular horizontal range of movement limited to centric relation. This is true for skeletal class III (prognathic) patients. Excursive balance is not necessary for them. Only balance in centric is sufficient. A balance occlusion is limited by the buccolingual and mesiodistal dimensions of anatomical cuspal inclines of teeth. Patient with a functional range of movement beyond the limits of balance will not be benefited with balance occlusion arrangement. So, a bilateral fully balanced occlusion is not indicated for a skeletal class II (retrognathic) patient with a functional range of lateral and protrusive excursions of 4 to 6 mm or greater. Bilateral balance is only important for a skeletal class I patient.

Tooth Position and Occlusal Plane

The superoinferior position of the occlusal plane is a factor for stability. A mandibular occlusal plane that is too high can result in reduced stability. It is due to two reasons. First, lateral lifting forces directed against the teeth are magnified as the plane is higher. Second, the mandibular denture needs to be controlled by the muscles of tongue, lips and cheeks. A high occlusal plane prevents the tongue from placing food on the occlusal table from the buccal vestibule. Bisecting the interridge distance improves the mandibular denture function and stability.

SUPPORT

Complete denture support is the resistance to the vertical movement of the denture base towards the ridge. It counteracts those forces directed toward the ridge. Support is the foundation, on which a dental prosthesis rests, or to hold up and serve as a foundation. This helps in maintaining the occlusal relationships established during tooth setting on the articulator. A complete denture could perform function ideally as long as the proper support is present to resist tissue ward movement during functional loading.

Support is defined as, "The resistance to vertical forces of mastication, occlusal forces and other forces applied in a direction towards the denture-bearing area."

Methods to Obtain Support

Effective support is realized in a denture as:

1. The denture is extended to cover a maximum surface area without impinging on movable or friable tissues,
2. Selectively loading the tissues most capable of resisting resorption during function,
3. Tissues most capable of resisting vertical displacement are allowed to make firm contact with the denture base during function.
4. Compensation is made for the varying tissue resiliency to provide for uniform denture base movement under function and maintain a harmonious occlusal relationship.

Factors affecting Support

Factors within Tissue

1. Fit of dentures to the underlying tissues so that occlusal surfaces can correctly oppose one another at the time of initial closure and under functional loading.
2. Nature of supporting tissues.
   Soft tissues: The soft tissues should be firmly bound to underlying cortical bone and should contain a resilient layer of resilient submucosa. It should be covered by keratinized mucosa. The bone beneath it should be resistant to pressure induced remodeling. These properties minimize base movement, lessen soft tissue trauma and reduce long-term pressure induced bone resorption.
   Hard tissues: The rate and amount of bone resorption and remodeling occur more in the anterior part of mandible and maxilla. Minimizing the pressures in those regions and directing the forces toward the areas of relative resistant to resorption may help to maintain healthy residual ridges.
   The pressure: 'Tension concept' holds that pressure simulates resorption whereas tension maintains the integrity and causes deposition of bone. A complete denture in function cannot transmit tension to bone and can produce only pressure underneath to cause resorption.
3. *Health of tissues*: The maximum support obtained from any denture-supporting area largely depends upon the health of the supporting tissues. The tissues should be as healthy as possible while supporting prosthesis. They may have been abused by wearing ill-fitting dentures for many years. Tissue treatment is required prior to construction of new prosthesis in these cases. This is usually done by providing rest to the abused tissues by keeping the dentures out of mouth for a week. Many patients will not follow this advice and moreover hyperplastic tissue may not resolved

within this period. This requires correction of ill-fitting denture by adjustments of denture base as well as the occlusion followed by use of tissue treatment material. The denture base may have to add up with cold cure resin or to reduce by trimming. The occlusal adjustments for inadequate vertical dimension as well as correction of centric relation are mandatory before the tissue treatment material is used to treat the abused tissue. As soon as the tissue health is restored, an accurate impression of the whole denture support area should be recorded and a bubble-free cast is produced. This cast should be handled with care during all laboratory and clinical steps to prevent damage that prevent the denture construction on it.

4. *Anatomical structures of supporting tissues*: The success of complete denture depends largely on the relation of dentures to the supporting and limiting structures. The denture- bearing tissues can be divided into primary and secondary support as well as tissues that require relief to minimize pressure. The primary stress-bearing areas in mandible include the pear-shaped pad and the buccal shelf area. The retromolar pad is not a stress-bearing area. The distal extension of the lower denture is the junction of pear-shaped pad and retromolar pad. The ridge crest area and genial tubercles may be treated as secondary stress-bearing areas (Fig. 4.5A).

   The primary stress-bearing areas in maxilla include horizontal anterolateral hard palate. The ridge crest acts at best as secondary stress-bearing area. The midpalatine line and incisive foramen are relief areas (Fig. 4.5B).

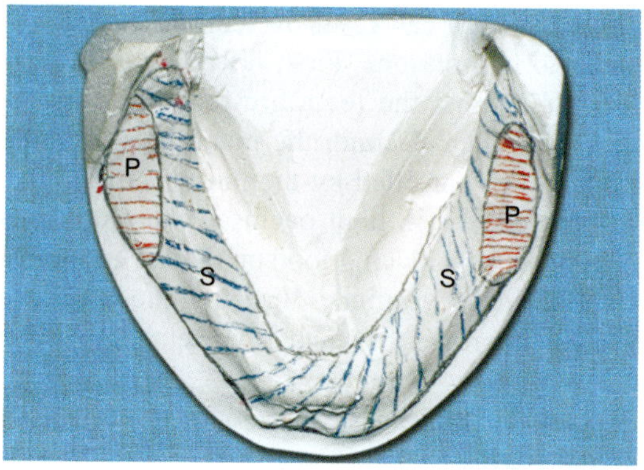

Fig. 4.5A: Primary stress-bearing area (P) and secondary stress-bearing area (S) of mandibular ridge

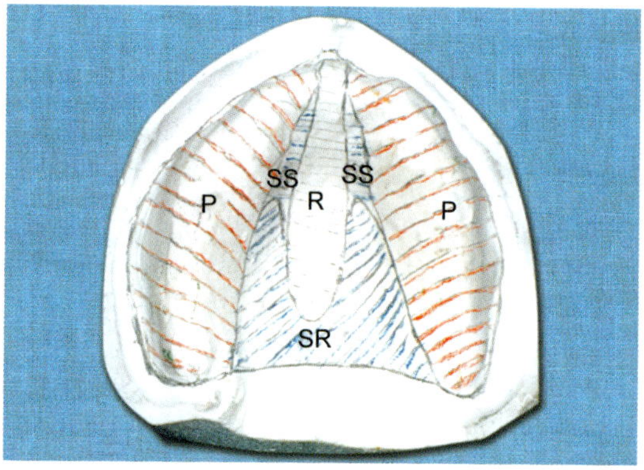

Fig. 4.5B: Primary stress-bearing area (P), secondary stress-bearing areas (SS), relief areas (R) in maxillary ridge and secondary retentive area (SR) of maxillary ridge

Factors in Denture and its Base

1. *Area of coverage*: The denture is extended to cover a maximum surface area without impinge on movable or friable tissues. These help to distribute forces over a wide area. The basic "snow shoe principal" of maximum extension decreases the stress per unit area under the denture base, decreasing tissue displacement, and reduces denture base movement.
2. *Area of occlusal table*: The force of mastication on supporting tissues is more if the occlusal surfaces are broad than if they are narrow.
3. *Fitting surface of denture base*: It should be as smooth as possible or the rough fitting surface of the denture will have sand paper-like rubbing effect on the mucosa causing ulceration.
4. *Impression technique*: A true mucostatic or pressure-less impression is virtually impossible. The fluid impression material is rigid and causes some pressure. A denture base records the functional form of tissue by displacing

the resilient tissues. At rest that denture base may rebound from the underlying tissues. So, no technique can provide an equal distribution of pressures both at rest and under function. A composite technique incorporating of both pressureless and selective pressure procedures can provide a desirable impression for a long-lasting prosthesis. This is done by (1) Impression materials exhibited least pressure, i.e. zinc oxide eugenol paste, (2) Equalization of pressure at crest of the ridge and palatal area by incorporating escape holes or wax spacers.

CONCLUSION

The optimal complete denture treatment needs good retention, stability and support. These are interdependent. There are some physical, mechanical and biological factors that promote the properties of retention, stability, and support in the finished dentures. The understanding, recognizing and incorporating these factors are necessary for complete denture fabrication.

BIBLIOGRAPHY

1. Barbenel JC. Physical retention of complete dentures. J Prosthet Dent. 1971;26:592.
2. Brill N. Factors in mechanism of full denture retention. Dent Pract. 1967;18:9.
3. Jacobson TE, Kroll AJ. Contemporary review of the factors involved in complete denture retention, stability and support. J Prosthet Dent. 1983;49:1-5.
4. Kabeenell JI. "More retention in complete dentures." JADA. 1970;80:116.
5. Lindstorm Re. Physical Aspects of Denture Retention and Stability. J Prosthet Dent. 1979;42:371.
6. Pleasure MA. "Impression procedures for stability of complex dentures." Dent, Clin N Am. 1968;653.

Chapter 5

Principles and Techniques of Impression Making

INTRODUCTION

Complete denture is an appliance which replaces all missing natural teeth and associated structures of the oral cavity. Impression making is the first and foremost step in complete denture fabrication. Impression material is essentially required for making the impression. In the year 1700, Wax was used to make impressions from which plaster models of the gums and teeth were formed. Replacement dentition was curved in ivory or animal bones on these models. After the introduction of impression materials, impression has been made in the early eighteenth century.

IMPRESSION

An impression is a negative likeness or copy in reverse of the surface of an object: an imprint of the teeth and adjacent structures for use in dentistry. It is made to produce a positive form or cast of the recorded tissues.

COMPLETE DENTURE IMPRESSION

A complete denture impression is a negative registration of the entire denture-bearing, stabilizing, and border seal areas present in the edentulous mouth (GPD).

Types of Impressions

There are two types of impression:
1. Preliminary impression
2. Master impression

Preliminary impression: It is defined as, "an impression made for the purpose of diagnosis, treatment planning, or the fabrication of a tray" (GPT). The preliminary impressions of the edentulous mouth are made for producing a diagnostic cast on which special trays will be fabricated. The preliminary impression should: (1) record the all denture-supporting area; (2) record the peripheral oral tissues around the denture-bearing area.

Master impression: It is the negative likeness made for the purpose of fabricating a prosthesis. The dentures are fabricated over the master casts.

Necessity of Two Stages Impression

Due to limitations imposed by the use of standard stock impression trays it is preferable to record the complete denture impressions in two stages—the primary impression in first visit and the master or final impressions at a subsequent visit. In primary impression, displacement of border tissues is acceptable to obtain certain landmarks. But denture made from such impression will be displaced during function or produce sore in the border tissues. The primary impressions are made for producing diagnostic casts and the second or the final impressions are made with more precise border extension in special trays fabricated on these casts.

Advantages of making impression in two stages:
1. Accurate determination of the peripheral border extensions.

2. Gaining the control of pressure applied in making final impression.
3. It helps in easier control the flow of an impression material.
4. It helps in dimensional accuracy of the impression material due to uniform thickness inside the tray.
5. To control the movable soft tissues around the impression with little distortion of these tissues.

"Making versus Taking" Impressions

The taking an impression is the recording negative imprint of tissues in a static and nondisplaceable form. But the tissues around the denture-bearing areas are resilient and dynamic in nature. So, we do not "take", but we "make" an impression. When the impression of a model is made, it can be "taking" of impression.

Objectives of a Complete Denture Impression

There are five primary objectives in an impression making. They are:
1. Retention
2. Stability
3. Support
4. Esthetic
5. Preservation of residual ridge.

Retention

Retention of denture is "the quality inherent in the prosthesis which resists the forces of dislodgement along the path of placement" (GPT-7). It is the resistance to the vertical displacing forces that are produced by gravity, adhesive foods, and the forces form the oral musculature. There are many dislodging forces which cause dislodgement of denture during speech or eating, causing psychologic discomfort and mental trauma. A retentive denture prevents the embarrassing situation of denture dislodgement. It also helps in patient's acceptance during delivery of the denture. Retention of a denture is indirectly proportional to the amount of healthy tissue that can be covered without impingement. Among all the objectives of complete denture, impression retention is considered as the least important. However, it gives psychological comfort to the denture wearer. Adhesion, cohesion, atmospheric pressure, mechanical locks, muscle control, and patient tolerance affects retention.

Stability

Stability is defined as, "the quality of prosthesis to be firm, steady, or constant, to resist displacement by functional horizontal or rotational stresses" (GPT-7).

It is the ability of the denture to withstand horizontal forces. For this, close adaptation to the undistorted mucosa is the most important. The lack of stability of denture seems to cause most of the gross soft tissue and bone changes that occur under denture. Stability of denture is, therefore, very important to the preservation of the ridge. Stability decreases with the loss of vertical height of the ridges or with the increase in flabby, movable tissues.

Instability robbed the patient of psychological comfort. In practice, poor stability affects support and retention and results in destructive forces on the edentulous ridges.

Support

It is defined as, "the resistance to the vertical forces of mastication, occlusal forces and other forces applied in a direction towards the denture-bearing area". Therefore, the greater the amount of area covered, the greater will be the support. The best support for the denture is compact bone covered with fibrous connective tissue. It is increased by selective placement of pressure on stress-bearing areas and relieving the nonstress-bearing areas of the basal seat that are in harmony with the resiliency of basal seat. This helps in maintaining the occlusal relationships established during tooth setting on the articulator. A complete denture could perform function ideally as long as the proper support is present to resist tissue ward movement during functional loading. This helps in retention, stability and preservation

Esthetics

Esthetics begins with the impression. A well-filled border, particularly in the maxillary impression, will fill out the cheeks and lips and give support to the lip muscles. In accordance with the amount of residual ridge loss of each patient, the border thickness should be varied. So that before accepting the final impression the vestibular sulcus should be filled, to restore the facial contour. Therefore, esthetic is another reason for a properly filled border.

Preservation of Residual Ridges

Though some physiological change is expected in edentulous mouths, the preservation of existing ridges is possible. It is done by maximum area coverage, reducing the force per unit area delivered to the supporting structures and by close adaptation to the tissues minimizing the movement of denture over the basal seat. The less the horizontal movement, less will be bone resorption under the dentures. M De Van (1952) stated that, “the preservation of that which remains is of utmost importance and not the meticulous replacement of that which has been lost”.

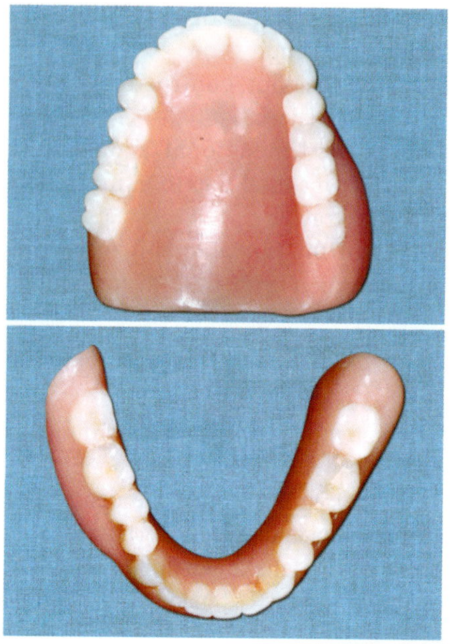

Fig. 5.1A: Complete dentures—occlusal and polished surfaces

ANATOMIC LANDMARKS

Before fabrication of the complete dentures the knowledge of oral anatomy of the supporting and limiting peripheral structures are essential because these are the anatomic landmarks of the denture-bearing area.

Complete dentures have three surfaces (Figs 5.1A and B)—(a) occlusal surface, (b) polished surface, and (c) basal or fitting surface or impression surface. The impression surface is produced from the impression of the denture-bearing area. The denture base must extend over the denture-bearing tissues as far as possible without interfering the health or function of the tissues.

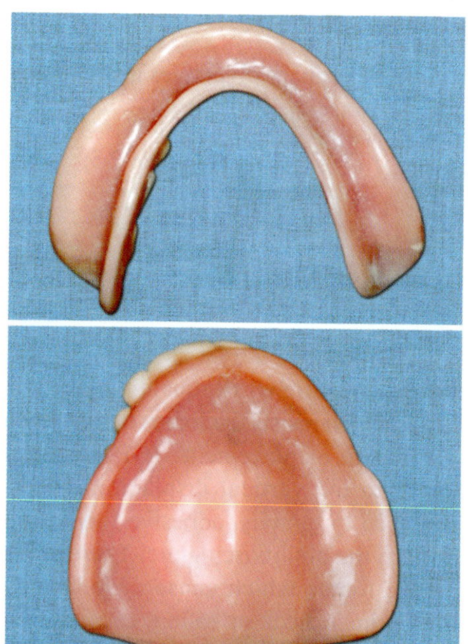

Fig. 5.1B: Complete dentures—basal surfaces are fitted to the basal seats

DENTURE-BEARING AREAS

The denture-bearing area covered by denture base consists of two areas:

a. **Stress-bearing or supporting area** which is a relatively static area and present minimal problems to record
b. **Peripheral or limiting area** although they are inseparable, they will be discussed separately for convenience.

Maxillary Denture-bearing Area (Fig. 5.2)

Average denture-bearing area of edentulous maxilla is 24 cm^2.

Maxillary Supporting Structures

1. Residual ridge
2. Hard palate
3. Rugae area
4. Incisive papilla
5. Median palatine raphe or suture
6. Zygomatic process/crest
7. Maxillary tuberosities
8. Torus palatinus.

Maxillary Peripheral or Limiting Structures

9. Labial frenum
10. Labial vestibule
11. Buccal frenum
12. Buccal vestibule
13. Pterygomaxillary (Hamular) notch
14. Postpalatal seal area
15. Fovea palatine.

Anatomy of Maxillary Supporting Structures

Residual Ridge

The crest of the residual ridge is considered as the primary support area for the maxillary denture as it is covered with a layer of masticatory mucosa and the underlying bone is compact cortical bone. The palate is usually regarded as the primary stress-bearing (support) area, as it is resistant to resorption.

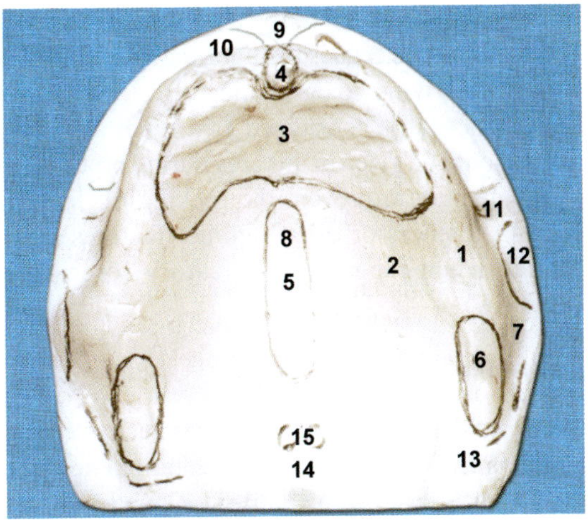

Fig. 5.2: Maxillary denture-bearing area

Hard Palate

The anterior 1/3rd of hard palate, the rugae area, the crest and slope of the residual ridges including the attached gingiva is composed of "masticatory mucosa". It is composed of highly keratinized stratified squamous epithelium and a thick and dense layer of connective tissue, the lamina propria supported by firm submucosa. In the middle 1/3rd of the hard palate, there is increase in adipose tissue except the midline. In the posterior 1/3rd of the hard palate, the adipose tissue is largely replaced by the glandular tissues. These tissues provide cushioning effect for the dentures.

Significance: The palate is usually considered as secondary support area, but it may become the primary denture support area if the residual ridges undergo resorption.

Median Palatal Raphe or Suture

It is the area extending from the incisive papilla to the distal end of the hard palate. It forms an irregular groove anteroposteriorly in or near middle

of the palate. The submucosa covering this area is very thin. The mucosa is tightly attached to the periosteum giving no cushioning effect.
Significance: It is considered as a relief area. So, relief should be given in this area during processing of the denture to prevent the rocking of denture causing soreness or even midline fractures from fatigue when repeated masticatory forces are applied.

Rugae Areas

These are raised areas of dense connective tissue radiating from the midline in the anterior one-third of the palate. The rugae appear as small grooves radiating from a central groove like branches of a tree.

Significance: It is the secondary stress-bearing area, as it resists anterior displacement of the maxillary denture.

Incisive Papilla

It is a pad of fibrous connective tissue overlying the opening of the nasopalatine canal for corresponding nerves and vessels. It is located between the two central incisors on palatal side in edentulous mouth. In edentulous mouth, it may lie on or labial to the crest of the ridge as a small round depression.

Significance: It is a relief area and undue pressure on it by the denture may cause burning sensation in the distributing area of the nerves emerging from the foramen.

Zygomatic Process/Crest

It is a process of maxilla inferior and lateral to the first molar. This crest like the buccal shelf area of mandible is a stress-bearing area in maxilla. Though the bone is good, yet the mucosa covering is very thin and failure to provide relief may cause ulceration in the area.

Maxillary Tuberosity

It is the bulbous extension of the residual ridge in the second and third molar region ends in hamular notch.
Significance: It supports the maxillary denture against horizontal and torquing forces. So the maxillary denture should cover the tuberosity. The tuberosity hangs down to occupy the space of the opposing teeth if retained after the mandibular molars are extracted and not replaced. The over hangs often contain excessive fibrous tissues which need surgical removal before denture fabrication.

Torus Palatinus

It is a hard bony mass that occurs in the midline of the palate in about 20% of patients.

Significance: It is covered by thin mucosa, so relief in the denture base is required to prevent the rocking of denture causing trauma to the supporting tissues or even midline fracture of maxillary denture.

Anatomy of Maxillary Limiting Structures

It is essential for the dentist to have knowledge of anatomy of the edentulous jaws and their limiting structures which act as positive guides to the limits of the impressions before making the impressions. The following limiting structures should be recorded accurately in impression of a maxillary complete denture.

Labial Frenum

The maxillary labial frenum may be single or multiple, narrow or broad, fold of mucous membrane extending from lips to crest of the residual ridge at the median line. It contains no muscle fibers, and therefore, can be surgically removed if attached very near the crest of the alveolar ridge.

Significance: As it inserts vertically, it has very little lateral movement, thus forms notch in the denture.

Sufficient relief, but not excessive, should be provided to allow normal functional movement of it.

Labial Vestibule

It is located between the labial and buccal frenae and contains no muscle fibers. It extends on both sides from the labial frenum to the buccal frenum.

Significance: The height and width of the impression is reflected by the activity of the orbicularis oris muscle. This muscle when contract presses the lips against the teeth does not affect the upper denture as much as it affects the lower because of the greater stability of the former. The upper anterior teeth together with sufficient width of labial flange will restore lips to their correct relationships.

Buccal Frenum

It may be single or multiple, contains no muscle fibers usually, but occasionally includes fibers of the caninus muscle, buccinator and orbicularis oris muscles.

Significance: It requires adequate anteroposterior relief during functional movement affected by the buccinator and orbicularis muscles.

Buccal Vestibule

It is the space between the ridge and the cheek distal to the buccal frenum to the hamular notch.

Significance: This space should be recorded properly in height and thickness, as it is essential for the downward, forward, and medial movement of the mandible. The height is determined by the attachment of the buccinator. The space is defined distally by the mandibular coronoid process and buccally by the contracting masseter muscle as they move.

Pterygomaxillary (Hamular) Notch

It is the depression distal to the alveolar ridge and mesial to the pterygoid hamulus indicating the lateral posterior border of the maxillary denture. The pterygomandibular raphe remains in close proximity as it arises from the hamular process.

Significance: The posterior palatal seal must be placed through the center of it. It is the area representing the posterior limit of the maxillary denture. If the denture is overextended here, on opening the mouth it will impinge on the tough pterygomandibular raphe either causing inflammation as sore throat or droping of the denture.

Postpalatal Seal Area

The posterior palatal seal area is defined in the "Glossary of Prosthodontic Terms" as "the soft tissues along the junction of the hard and soft palates on which pressure within the physiologic limits of the tissues can be applied by a denture to aid in the retention of the denture". It is not straight but follows the contour of the palatine bones.

In the mouth we observe vibrating line across the posterior part of the palate marking the division between the movable and immovable tissues of the soft palate. When patient say "ah" the maxillary denture terminates at this line so that it ends in soft movable tissues. The area consists of a thick submucosa containing glandular and loose areolar tissues which can be slightly displaced allowing the formation of the posterior palatal seal.

Significance: The labial and buccal borders of the maxillary denture fill functional depth and width of the sulci and prevent the ingress of air and saliva to the fitting surface of the denture and improve retention. The exposed posterior border of the denture cannot be enfolded by soft tissue and, therefore, must displace the mucosa of the palate to the complete the functional peripheral seal. The displaceability of the tissues just anterior to the vibrating line across the width of the palate is determined by digital palpation or by a ball barnisher. The groove for the postdam is cut into the master cast with a wax curving instrument just anterior to the vibrating line drawn previously. The depth and width of the groove is dependent on the displaceability of the tissues, will produce a "cuspid bow" shape. The groove moves through the hamular notch into the buccal sulci.

Fovea Palatini

The coalescence of the minor salivary gland ducts generally located slightly posterior to the junction of hard and soft palates near the midline. Their position is variable and, therefore, cannot be used to delineate the posterior border of the denture.

Mandibular Denture-bearing Area (Fig. 5.3A)

Mandibular dentures like maxillary should be extended as far as possible within the limits of health and function of the tissues and structures that support and surround them. But it is more complicated in a mandibular denture than the maxillary denture because in addition to labial and buccal surfaces, the lingual surface is to be considered. Moreover, the structures of the lingual side of the mandible are more complicated to control due to the greater range of movement and the speed of their actions. The support for the mandibular denture comes from the body of the mandible. Average denture-bearing area for edentulous mandibule is 14 cm^2.

Mandibular Supporting Structures

1. Residual ridge
2. Buccal shelf area
3. Mylohyoid ridge
4. Mental foramen

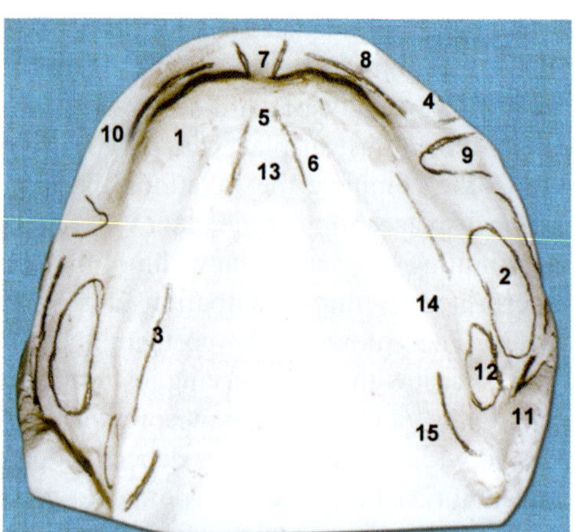

Fig. 5.3A: Mandibular denture-bearing area

5. Genial tubercles
6. Torus mandibularis.

Mandibular Limiting Structures

7. Labial frenum
8. Labial vestibules
9. Buccal frenum
10. Buccal vestibules
11. Masseter muscle
12. Retromolar pad
13. Lingual frenum
14. Alveolingual sulcus
15. Retromylohyoid space.

Mandibular Supporting Structures

Residual Ridge

The mandibular ridge crest is covered by a keratinized mucosa and firmly attached submucosa to the underlying periosteum providing good support to the denture. But the underlying bone is cancellous and not favorable as primary stress-bearing area for lower denture. It acts as secondary stress-bearing area.

Buccal Shelf Area

It extends anteriorly from mandibular buccal frenum, posteriorly to the anterior border of the masseter muscle. It is bounded medially by the crest of the residual ridge and laterally by the external oblique ridge.

Significance: It is composed of smooth, dense cortical bone which is at right angles to the vertical occlusal forces. So, it acts as primary stress-bearing area. The buccinator muscle is attached to the external oblique ridge and lies under the denture flange, but will not cause dislodgement of the denture as its fibers run parallel to the denture border.

Mylohyoid Ridge

It is a rough bony crest extending from the third molar to second bicuspid region. The mylohyoid muscle is attached to the mylohyoid ridge. In the anterior region the mylohyoid ridge with attached mylohyoid muscle lies close to the inferior border of the mandible. Posteriorly, it is superior in position and the lingual flange of the denture may extend below the mylohyoid ridge if it drops vertically or slopes at 45° toward the tongue. This will allow the mylohyoid muscle to function without dislodgement of the denture.

Significance: The lingual flange of mandibular denture should extend below the palpable portion of the mylohyoid ridge to avoid direct contact of border during chewing. This will provide adequate border seal and guide the tongue on top of the flange.

Mental Foramen

The foramen in a resorbed ridge will locate close to the crest in the premolar region. Through this passes the mental nerves and vessels which may be compressed to cause numbness of the lower lip.

Significance: The relief should be provided in the area to avoid compression on the nerve and vessels in highly resorbed ridges.

Genial Tubercles

The depth of the anterior lingual is influenced by the muscles attached to these. The resorption causes the genial tubercles to move upward which causes soreness in tissues in this area.

Significance: In a highly resorbed ridge, relief must be provided in denture base to avoid ulceration.

Torus Mandibularis

It is the bony prominence usually found bilaterally in the premolar region lingually in dented mandible. In edentulous mandible, where resorption has taken place it is on the crest of the ridge. As it is often covered by thin mucosa, it needs surgical removal because it is difficult to provide relief.

Anatomy of Mandibular Limiting Structures

The following limiting structures should be incorporated in the extension of mandibular complete denture impressions (Fig. 5.3B):

Mandibular Labial Frenum

It is a fold of mucous membrane between the alveolus and labial mucous membrane. It may be single or multiple and usually not as pronounce as the maxillary labial frenum. It may contain a band of fibrous connective tissue attached to the orbicularis muscle and may be very active during

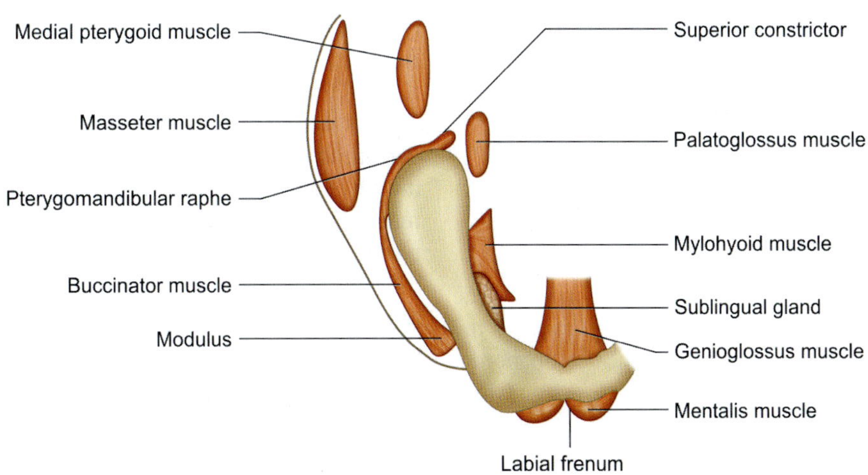

Fig. 5.3B: Structures limiting the borders of lower complete denture

speech and mastication. It forms labial notch when careful relief is given.

Mandibular Labial Vestibules

It is extended from the labial frenum to the buccal frenum in the premolar areas. It is limited in extension because the fibers of the orbicularis oris, incivus inferioris, and mentalis lie close to the crest of the ridge.

Buccal Frenum

It is a fold or folds of mucous membrane extending from the lip to buccal mucosa of the residual ridge in the premolar region. It overlies the levator anguli oris, the buccinators, and orbicularis oris muscles so must be functionally moulded. The notch formed should allow relief for the frenum, will prevent dislodgement during facial expression.

Buccal Vestibule

It runs downwards and outwards from corner of the retromolar pad to the buccal frenum following the attachment of the buccinator muscle which extends from the modiolus anteriorly to the pterygomandibular raphe posteriorly. The buccinator muscle forms a pouch in the cheek and the denture can be extended laterally to produce a large posterior buccal flange. The polished buccal surface faces outwards and upwards so that the contracting buccinator forces the cheek inwards to keep the denture in place. The buccinator affects both the lateral and the distal extension of the denture with the help of the pterygomandibular ligament.

Masseter Muscle

The periphery at the distobuccal corner of the buccal vestibule, the masseter muscle overlies the buccinator muscle and influences the denture border forming the masseteric notch.

Retromolar Pad

Distal to the crest of the edentulous ridge there is an elevated soft pad of mucosa, the retromolar pad. It is oval or round in outline lying on the retromolar fossa. The submucosa contains loose glandular and areolar tissue, pterygomandibular raphe, buccinator, superior constrictor, and temporal tendon fibers. The action of these muscles limits the extension of the denture at the distal part of the retromolar pad. So, the denture base should extend up to half or two-thirds of the retromolar pad. The posterior border of denture should be on the retromolar pad in order to have the denture end in soft movable tissues for additional retention and support. Failure to extend the denture up to the pad may increase resorption of alveolar ridge.

Pear-shaped Pad

In front of the retromolar pad and often attached with it is a firm fibrous pear-shaped pad. It arises from the collapse of the distal papilla into the socket on extraction of the last molar tooth. The distal papilla is often inflamed and leads to the formation of the fibrous pad. It is not always clearly visible, as the forward migration of the third molar reduces the inflammation and prevents the fibrous tissue formation that gives rise to this pad.

Lingual Border Anatomy

It is apparent that the lingual border of the mandibular impression is difficult to record and must be done in its functional form. To do this, the mandibular impression should be taken with the floor of the mouth raised to the functional position. This is done by protruding tongue gently to the vermilion border of the upper lip, with half closed mouth. Forceful protrusion of tongue against the maxillary ridge is avoided as it results in a short recording.

Mandibular Lingual Frenum

It is wide midline fold of mucous membrane as the anterior attachment of the tongue to the alveolar mucosa and the floor of the mouth. It lies over the genioglossus muscles. It is well above the genial tubercles, the attachment of genioglossus muscles in case of normal ridge but at the level of the genial tubercles in case of extreme resorption. It should be recorded in function as it is often close to the crest of the ridge during function though much lower at rest. The denture border cannot be extended beyond the highest level of tongue function. So, there is lack of seal in the anterolingual area which is compensated by the surrounding tissues affecting seal against the polished surfaces of the denture.

Lingual Vestibule/Alveolingual Sulcus

The space between the tongue and the alveolar ridge is called alveolingual sulcus. It extends from lingual frenum to the retromylohyoid curtain. It is divided into anterior and posterior parts:

a. *Anterior part*: The anterior part extends from the lingual frenum to the premylohyoid fossa. The structures in that area are the sublingual fold and the sublingual papilla (opening of Wharton's ducts) and sublingual glands rest on the mylohyoid muscle.
b. *Posterior part*: The posterior part extends from the premylohyoid fossa to the postmylohyoid fossa. The mylohyoid muscle determines the lingual flange of the denture. The lingual flange may extend 4 to 5 mm below the mylohyoid ridge if it drops vertically or slopes towards the tongue at 45 degree. It should not be extended below the mylohyoid ridge forming an undercut.

Retromylohyoid Space

It lies at the end of the alveolingual sulcus. It extends from end of the mylohyoid ridge to the retromylohyoid curtain. It is bounded lingually by anterior tonsillar pillar, distally by the retromylohyoid curtain and superior constrictor muscle, and on the buccal side by the mylohyoid muscle, the ramus, and the retromolar pad. The denture border should be extended posteriorly to contact the retromolar curtain when the tip of the tongue is touching the anterior maxillary residual ridge. By proper border molding of this area, a typical S-shaped curve will be formed when viewed from the tissue side.

THEORIES OF IMPRESSION MAKING

Final impressions for complete dentures are made in many kinds of materials and many widely different techniques. The technique to use for each patient should be selected on the basis of the diagnosis of the basal seat and border tissues. The controversy exists over:

1. The amount of pressure applied to the tissues while making the impression.
2. The degree of tissue detail to be captured.
3. The type of impression material selected.
4. The type of impression tray used.
5. Open or close mouth impression is made.
6. Peripheral borders either functionally moulded or arbitrary location.

IMPRESSION TECHNIQUES

There are various techniques of impression for complete denture construction depending on prosthodontist concept. They are classified in various ways as follows:

1. **According to degree of compression**
   - Minimum pressure/mucostatic technique
   - Mucocompressive technique
   - Selective pressure technique
2. **According to the position of the mouth**
   - Open mouth technique
   - Close mouth technique
3. **According to the types of impression tray**
   - Spaced tray technique
   - Close-fitting tray technique

ACCORDING TO DEGREE OF COMPRESSION

The denture-bearing areas are covered by soft tissues that vary in depth and quality in different areas.

There are three basic impression philosophies/theories related to compensation for these differences:

1. The minimal pressure technique
2. The definite pressure technique
3. The selected pressure technique.

Minimal Pressure/Mucostatic Impression Technique

An impression that is registered with a very minimum of pressure is known as a mucostatic impression. In this technique, an impression is obtained with low viscous material, little or no displacement of the soft tissues overlying the alveolar ridges and palate will occur. This technique is advocated for two reasons. First, the dentures are under pressure from occlusal load only for a relatively small amount of time, so dentures should fit the relaxed, unloaded tissue surface. Second, it is seen if the tissues are recorded in an undisturbed state with a free-flowing impression material, a thin film of saliva between the mucosa and the fitting surface of the denture increases retention and stability. The advocates of this technique believe that mucosa contains 80% water, acts as a liquid in a closed vessel so pressure on it is transmitted in all directions (Pascal's law) and thus cannot be compressed.

The impression is recorded of the mucosa in absolutely rest or static state so it is obtained with impression material softer than soft tissue in an oversized or spaced tray with no border moulding. No digital or occlusal pressure of any form is to be applied to the impression trays during impression procedure. Metal bases should be used as they are dimensionally stable than acrylic resin. Most of the clinicians consider that the mucostatic technique is superior to mucocompressive and makes impressions with minimum pressure.

Indications

1. Evenly thick alveolar mucosa.
2. Smooth surface alveolar bone.
3. U-shaped alveolar ridge.

Advantages

1. Minute details of resting tissue surfaces are recorded.
2. An even space of thin film of saliva exists between the mucosa and denture surface contributes to good retention.
3. Minimum pressure avoids distortion of the soft tissue.
4. Smaller flanges give comfortable functional wear.

Disadvantages

1. The mucostatic principle ignores the principle of dissipating occlusal forces over a large area to maintain the health of the basal seat.
2. It lacks necessary lip support, as the dentures are not extending into the labial and buccal vestibules.
3. The musculature is not being utilized fully for retention of the dentures.
4. The mucosal surface is not static over 24 hours; it is changing so the details of impression will lose during denture insertion.
5. The mucosa is not a closed vessel, as tissue fluids can escape under the border during chewing with the dentures.
6. The mucostatic principle does not consider peripheral seal in denture retention.
7. The mucosa of denture-bearing area itself is changing over 24 hours due to change in peripheral blood volume which creates a loss of retention of a denture in early morning.
8. A rigid denture base constructed on a cast obtained from such an impression will transfer the masticatory load to the centrally located unyielding areas of ridges. Rocking of the dentures may occur about this fulcrum.

Technique

1. Primary impressions are made with a low viscosity alginate or plaster to produce mucostatic impression which will include denture-bearing area.
2. A cast is poured out of these impressions.
3. A spacer of 3 mm thickness is adapted over the denture-bearing area. Four stops are prepared, two at canine region and two at molar region. The trays are prepared in shellac base plate or self-curing acrylic resin.
4. The trays are checked in the mouth for proper extension and adjusted if required.

5. A low viscous impression material is used to record the final impression with minimum pressure. No border moulding is done because adhesion is the only factor considered for retention.
6. After the material has set, the impression is removed and checked.

MUCOCOMPRESSIVE IMPRESSION TECHNIQUE

It is an impression made under load such that the mucosa is uniformly compressed and evenly condensed. The denture-bearing areas are not covered evenly with soft tissues but with variable depth and quality. So, if the denture under no occlusal load touches the soft tissues entirely, on occlusal loading, the denture will apply more force to the harder areas covered by thin tissues without submucosa. This may cause 'rocking' of upper denture in the midline. This effect, when marked, may result in midline fracture after slight resorption of ridges. The principal of the pressure technique is to record the soft tissues under a force similar to the occlusion and mastication, so that the softer areas are compressed by the impression. This is done to compensate the differences in the depth of soft tissue covering from one area to another. A denture made on a cast from such an impression touches the soft tissue at rest only. On occlusal loading, all the tissues are compressed. Impression compound due to its viscosity and varying degree of softness and flow is the material suitable for this technique. Craddock marked an "automatic relief" over hard palate to displace tissues using more viscous impression material.

Techniques

The mucocompressive technique can be applied both in open mouth and close mouth techniques.

Open Mouth Impression Technique

1. Primary impression is made with a low viscosity alginate to obtain mucostatic impression.
2. The cast is poured with good surface details.
3. Special trays are prepared with 3 mm thick spacer of wax over the primary casts.
4. The trays are loaded with an even thickness of new composition softened.
5. The surface of the composition is coated with Vaseline and impression of the cast is made so that it flows to the sulcus.
6. The compound is pressed around the tray edge and chilled in cold water.
7. The excess composition is cut out with a knife.
8. The surface of the composition is softened by dipping in hot water and seated in the mouth until hardens.
9. The set impressions are removed from the mouth and chilled in cold water in a bowl.
10. The impressions are dried; the surface is heated with pinpoint flame for uniform softening, dipped in hot water before insertion in the mouth to record the impression. This produces greater compression than equally soften compound used before.
11. The retention is tested by asking the patient to dislodge the impression by normal movement of the lips and cheeks.
12. The refining of the impression is done with a very thin layer of zinc oxide noneugenol paste (less viscous than eugenol paste).

Close Mouth Impression Technique (Functional Impression Technique)

This technique utilizes well-fitted occlusal rims prepared on primary cast prepared from a low viscosity alginate. The jaw relation is recorded first. The fitting surface of the rims are loaded with impression paste. The patient closes the mouth and performs functional movements allowing the tissues to be recorded in function. The completed impression is then transferred to denture base that duplicates the functionally loaded tissues. It is an impression of tissues purposefully made under a significant load so that the peripheries of the dentures are established during functional loading.

The material of choice is either mouth temperature flourable wax or soft liners.

Indications

1. Unevenly thick mucosa.
2. Flat alveolar ridge.
3. Even surface of alveolar bone.

Advantages

1. Peripheral seal is developed through compression of the soft tissues.
2. More stable denture during function due to intimate contact during function.
3. Load distribution is more even.
4. A more viscous impression material displaces the strong lip and tongue muscles during seating.
5. The denture made from a compressive impression has better retention as it is doubtful if that the compressed mucosa ever returns to its resting form.
6. With tissue in resting state an uneven space exists between the mucosa and the denture base, which prevents the development of an intact saliva film essential for good retention.

Disadvantages

1. The displaced soft tissues will rebound at rest causing dislodgement of dentures.
2. The dentures made from such impressions may compress the ridge beyond its physiologic limit, resulting in interfere with the blood supply to the tissues of basal seat and rapid resorption of the residual ridges.
3. Often the dentures made with closed mouth impression are overextended and need arbitrary trimming. It requires great skill to prevent damage to the residual ridges.

Selective Pressure Technique

Selective pressure technique is a combination of extension for maximum coverage with intimate contact with the movable tissues and light contact in nonmovable tissues. Selective pressure impression technique is based on the assumption that certain oral tissues can tolerate functional load better than others. The selection of "stress-bearing" or supporting and "relief area" and "limiting areas" is determined by clinical examination. Selective pressure impressions are made in custom trays which have less space in the primary denture stress-bearing areas, and greater space (more impression material) in the nonstress-bearing areas. Stress-bearing areas will be recorded with pressure (over the ridge) whereas the nonstress-bearing areas (middies and incisive papillae) will be recorded with minimum pressure. The selective pressure technique tries to create a denture base that selectively loads the oral tissues during function of the dentures with maximum stability and retention. It provides maximum coverage of tissues within the physiologic limits.

Technique

1. A preliminary impression is made in a stock edentulous tray to capture the whole denture-bearing areas.
2. A cast is poured in these impressions. The outline for the spacer is made 2 mm short of tissue reflection point.
3. A sheet of modeling wax is adapted and trimmed up to this line.
4. A custom acrylic resin tray is made which is border molded with stick compound.
5. A final wash impression is recorded with a free-flowing impression material like zinc oxide eugenol impression paste.

The principle of selective pressure technique is applied here, because zinc oxide paste in a spaced tray records the attached mucosa with minimum pressure, while compound pushes the more movable tissues and peripheral sulcus areas with additional pressure to the underlying bone. The final denture made out of this impression will selectively apply pressure to the peripheral tissues. The ridge crest areas (attached gingival) will receive less pressure.

Areas Requiring Some Pressure

Border Seal Area

Areas requiring some pressure are the alveolar mucosa at the border of the denture and the posterior palatal seal area which should be recorded with slight pressure to maintain a valve-like seal for retention. The pressure may be selectively applied along the border by eliminating the tray relief wax in that areas. It may also be done by using very soft modeling compound applied to the tray border.

Buccal Shelf

The buccal shelf is normally a secondary stress-bearing area for the mandibular denture, whereas the crest of mandibular ridge is the primary stress-bearing area. But in an excessively resorbed knife edges mandibular ridge covered with soft and easily displaced tissues, the roles of these two areas are reversed, and buccal shelf becomes the stress-bearing area. The border molding material can be then extended inward to produce tissue adaptation. The escape holes or slots are employed to provide relief over the ridges.

Retromylohyoid Fossa

The area that needs gentle pressure is the alveolar mucosa of the retromylohyoid fossa which should be in contact of the tray by adding a little soft tracing compound.

Areas Requiring Little Pressure

Areas requiring little pressure are the residual ridges and palate and the displaceable areas found often in the maxillary anterior ridge which cannot be corrected with surgery, should not be displaced during impression. A tray with relief space and escape holes with least compressible impression material should be used. The selective pressure technique tries to create a denture base that selectively loads the oral tissues during function of the dentures with maximum stability and retention. The ridge crest area will be less displaced when the denture is in function.

Indications

1. Normal healthy ridges
2. V-shaped alveolar ridge
3. Cancellous and sharp alveolar ridge
4. Resorbed ridges.

Advantages

1. Tolerance of the basal seat to pressure helps in obtaining maximum support for the denture within the limits of functional adaptation.
2. Maintenance of the peripheral seal is better.
3. It takes into consideration the differences in tissue compressibility and produces maximum palatal adaptation of denture base.

Disadvantages

1. It is impossible to record some of the areas with different pressure from the others.
2. A denture base made with functional recoding displaces the more resilient tissues. At rest the denture base may rebound away from the underlying tissues.

Comparisons of Three Techniques

The philosophies of three techniques of complete denture impression differ. They possess some advantages and disadvantages so to choose an ideal technique is difficult. It is seen from the above discussion that the mucocompressive impression technique results in bone loss. The minimum pressure technique produces dentures with inadequate retention. So, the need for a new technique was felt and gave rise to a combination of the two techniques—the selective pressure technique. But the selective pressure technique has limitations and disadvantages. A denture base made with functional recoding displaces the more resilient tissues. At rest, the denture base may rebound away from the underlying tissues. At present no single technique can provide an equitable distribution of pressures both at rest and during function. So, the choice is made by the dentist based on the condition of the (a) oral tissues, (b) concept of function of the tissues surrounding the denture, and (c) his ability to manipulation of the available impression materials.

Practical Significance

The minute inaccuracies which creep in our techniques of denture fabrication which produce a change in denture shape are greater than the difference between a mucostatic and muco-compressive impression. These inaccuracies occur due to contraction of wax, heat cure denture bases. Only where, there is marked difference between hard and soft tissues, a mucostatic and a mucocompressive impressions have any practical significance.

In patients with normal compressible mucosa any technique results same but in adverse conditions, mucofunctional (Close mouth) technique is preferable.

ACCORDING TO THE POSITION OF THE MOUTH

Open and Closed Mouth Impressions

Open Mouth Impression

In open mouth technique the operator will support the tray carrying the impression material in the mouth with some degree of mouth opening. The term 'open mouth' refers to a half-open position and no impression is made with the mouth widely open as this changes the sulcus shape. The facial musculature is stretched and reduces the sulcus width besides making it difficult for insertion of the impression tray. On half opening the mouth there is no change in sulcus shape. In cases where the elasticity of the mucosa is reduced as a result of atrophy, there is little difference in sulcus depth between the closed and half open positions. Open mouth impression is preferred to prevent a displacing force on the denture periphery when opening the mouth. In most of the cases, no significant change in sulcus form is effected by contraction of the facial muscles, in these an open mouth impression with the muscles in relaxed condition can be recorded with less difficulty.

Advantages

1. The operator can see the border moulding procedure.
2. The border moulding movements can be done more easily.
3. The denture is retained both in open and close mouth movements.

Disadvantages

1. The correct shape of the anterior region of sulcus is difficult to attain as the operator has to hold the tray by handle.
2. In a few cases where, there is functionally a large difference in sulcus position during contraction of the facial muscles it is difficult to record the functional position accurately.

Closed Mouth Impression

The impression is recorded with mouth closed in the closely adapted custom tray fitted with occlusion rim. Close mouth technique records the tissues in their functional form. In the first stage of the technique, the jaw relation is recorded. The rims are trimmed to the correct vertical dimension to support the upper and lower trays during impression procedures.

Advantages

1. In a few cases where there is functionally a large difference in sulcus position during contraction of the facial muscles, the closed mouth technique is preferred.
2. This method helps to border mold the periphery of the impression through the patient's own movements than by the operator and permits to record the exact functionally contracted sulcus through the entire length.
3. It is argued that close mouth impression causes the tissue compression under the dentures. This, however, is fallacious reasoning as impression material as a viscous fluid does not cause

the same amount of force to the underlying mucosa as the denture base does. In fact, the close mouth impression uses normal closing of the jaws to the centric occlusion.

Disadvantages

1. The soft tissues displaced by the impression tend to rebound to their undisplaced position when the forces are removed. This cause unseats the denture.
2. The denture held in a displaced position limits the normal blood flow.
3. The bone resorption due to lack of blood flow.
4. The resorption causes looseness of denture.
5. The complete dentures made with closed- mouth impressions are often overextended and require arbitrary trimming.

ACCORDING TO THE TYPE OF IMPRESSION TRAY

Spaced Trays and Close-fitting Trays

1. *Spaced trays*: These trays are used with elastomeric material or irreversible hydrocolloid impression material needed to accurately record undercut areas frequently buccal to edentulous tuberosities. The spacing provide sufficient thickness of the material to deform elastically so as to pass over the most bulbous part of tissues and then spring back into a correct negative replica. These types of trays must be used, even in absence of undercut, when the impression material (plaster or elastomers) requires sufficient thickness to resist breakage or tear during removal from the mouth. Two sheets of modeling wax may be placed over the outlined area of the primary cast, thus providing a space between cast and impression tray.
2. *Cloase-fitting trays (for use with zinc oxide paste)*: These trays are used to take impressions of nonundercut edentulous arches using a very thin layer (a 'wash') impression material. The impression made in trays is adapted directly over the primary casts. The undercut areas are blocked out before making close-fitting tray. The cast is coated with separating medium and a sheet of self-curing resin is adapted over the cast.

Advantages of Using Closely Adapted Tray

1. As the trays are less bulky they are more easily inserted into a small oral aperture, giving a clear intraoral view, and less discomfort to patient.
2. As there are less chances of displacement of cheek in sulcus areas, a more accurate impression of the sulcus is obtained.
3. They are very useful in cases where the mandibular rami are in close approximation to the maxillary tuberosities on both sides. The space is insufficient for a wide conventional tray.
4. In a case of strong musculature in lips and tongue which contracts reflexly during working in the mouth, placement of the tray is easier when the closely adapted tray is used.

Disadvantages of Closely Adapted Tray

The limitations of the zinc oxide impression paste are the only disadvantage of the method.

PRINCIPLES OF IMPRESSION MAKING

In making an impression the dimension and details of the fitting surface and periphery should simulate the space occupied by the denture. Slight pressure should be created against the sulcus mucosa to obtain border seal.

The surface of an impression may be divided into:

1. Supporting areas.
2. Peripheral or sulcus areas.

Recording of both needs different approach so should be discussed separately.

Recording of Supporting Structures

The impression of these areas may be recorded by either (a) Mucocompressive method or (b) Mucostatic method.

Recording of Peripheral Sulcus Areas

Stock trays are inaccurate in their adaptation to the sulcus. It may impinge in the sulcus and distort it giving overextension. There is also some outward distortion of the alveolar mucosa occurs by pressure of the tray on the cheeks and lips. A denture constructed on such impression does not fit at the periphery and retention is lacking.

There are two ways to record the functional sulcus shape with slight elastic compression of the mucosa.

a. A spaced (3 mm) tray 2 to 3 mm away from the depth of the sulcus is used with an impression material of moderate viscosity and slight compression for the sulcus recorded.
b. A more precise method of recording sulcus consists of a close spaced (0.5–1 mm) used with a thin layer of zinc oxide eugenol paste.

CLINICAL PROCEDURES OF IMPRESSION MAKING

Definition of impression technique—A method and manner used in making a negative likeness (GPT-4).

Impressions are made using various techniques and a variety of materials that can be used in constructing a complete denture. Prior to the impression procedure the patient's oral health should be optimum. A generally accepted technique will be described step-by-step. The complete denture impression procedure can be divided into the following steps:

Preliminary Impressions

1. Selection of impression tray
2. Selection of impression material
3. Positioning of the patient
4. Positioning of the operator
5. Procedure of preliminary impression.

Final Impressions

1. Tray adjustment
2. Selection of impression material
3. Border moulding of trays
4. Making of final impressions.

PRELIMINARY IMPRESSIONS

Definition

A negative likeness made for the purpose of diagnosis, treatment planning or the fabrication of a tray.

The first, the preliminary (or primary) impressions of the edentulous mouth are made in stock trays for diagnosis and for construction of custom tray.

To avoid confusion a standard conventional technique based on selective pressure theory is described, one using impression compound and one using irreversible hydrocolloid (alginate) as the preliminary impression material.

Instruments and Materials (Fig. 5.4)

1. Edentulous impression trays
2. Compound knife
3. Water bath (composition heater)
4. Impression compound
5. Bowl for hot water
6. Mirror and probe
7. Hanau alcohol torch
8. Bunsen burner

Selection of Stock Tray

The shape, size and form of the alveolar ridges and palate are examined for selection of tray from

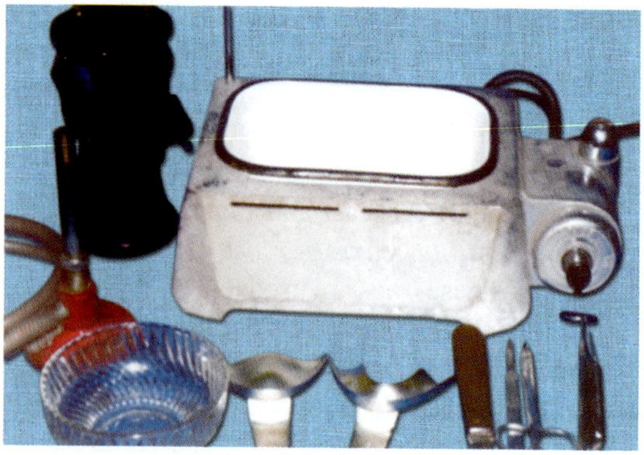

Fig. 5.4: Instruments and materials needed for primary impression

a range of stock metal trays. The upper and lower trays should cover the entire denture-bearing area and provide 6 mm space for impression material. They are chosen and tested in the mouth for their conformation to the anatomical form of the edentulous ridges. Care should be taken to avoid too large tray that will distort the border tissues and cause patient discomfort. If tray is too small, border tissues will collapse inward which results in underextended impressions causing problem in recording final impressions. Patient's existing denture can be used as a guide. The operator should examine the edentulous mouth and assess the length and width of the arch to be recorded (Figs 5.5A and B).

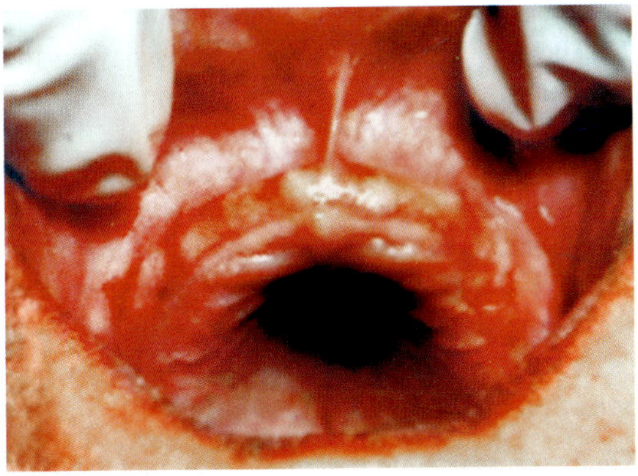

Fig. 5.5A: Examination of edentulous mouth to assess the length and width of the arch to be recorded (upper arch)

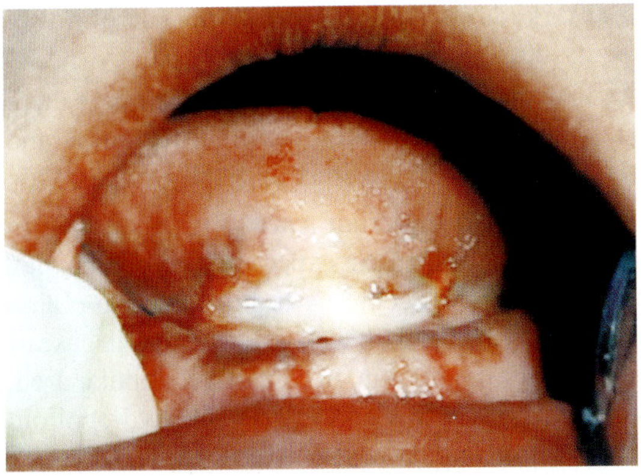

Fig. 5.5B: Examination of the edentulous mouth to assess the length and width of the arch to be recorded (lower arch)

Upper Tray

1. Selection of upper tray is done by comparing the measurement between the buccal surfaces of the maxillary tuberosities using callipers (Figs 5.6A and B).
2. The tray is inserted into the mouth and the posterior border is raised to contact the hamular notches.
3. The tray is then slowly raised anteriorly and visualizes the width of the tray required to record the functional width of the sulcus when patient half closes his mouth.

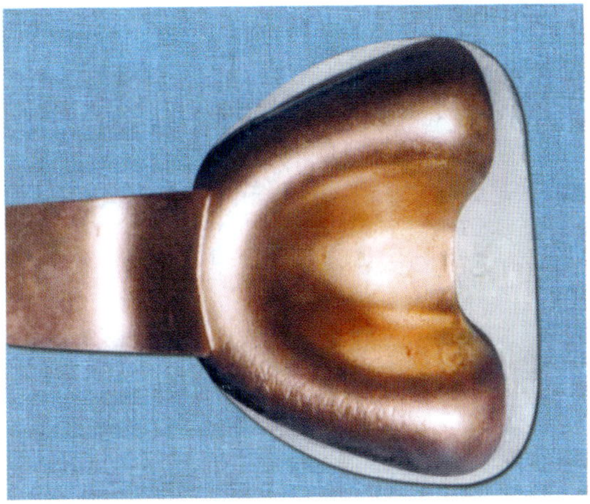

Fig. 5.6A: The desirable relationship between the upper tray and the hamular notches on a cast

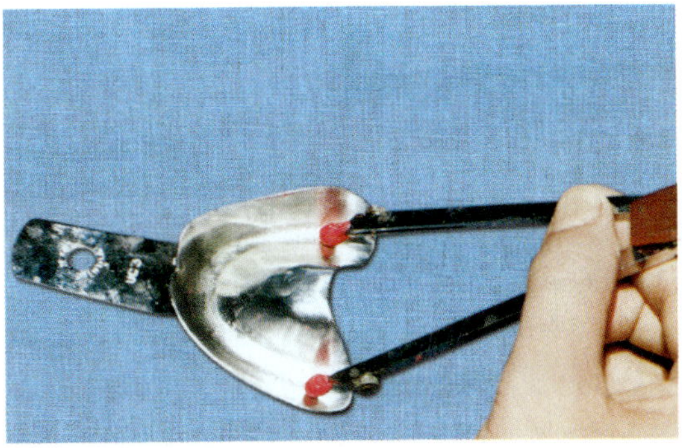

Fig. 5.6B: Selecting an upper tray by comparing the measurement with the distance between the buccal surfaces of the maxillary tuberosities

4. The tray should extend 5 mm beyond the external surface of the residual ridge. The flanges of the tray must be at least 2 to 3 mm short of the muscle attachment when the muscle attachments are in a state of rest.
5. If required, bending of the flanges slightly with pliers will provide adequate space. The tray should be checked for its proper contact with the hard palate without causing rocking.

Lower Tray

1. Selection of a lower tray is done by comparing the measurement between the lingual surfaces of the retromolar pads (Figs 5.7A and B).

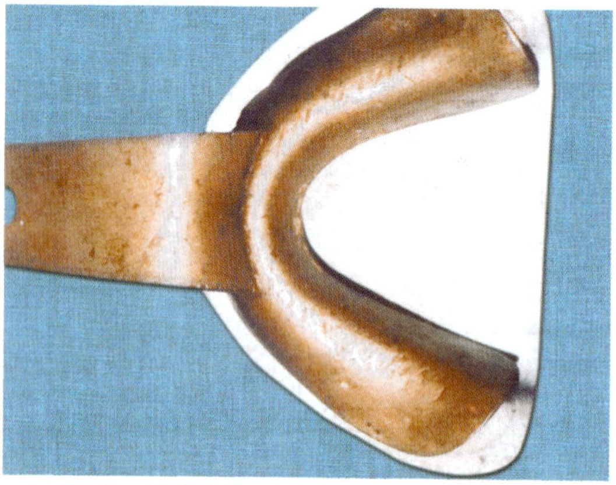

Fig. 5.7A: The desirable relationship between the lower tray and the retromolar pads on a cast

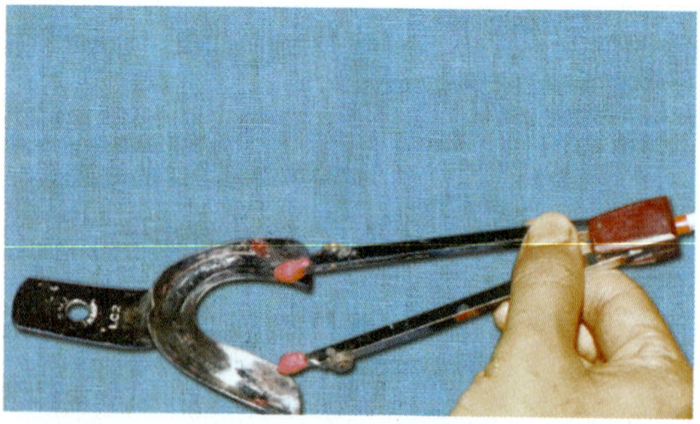

Fig. 5.7B: Selecting a lower tray by comparing the measurement with the distance between the lingual surfaces of the retromolar pads

2. The lower tray should be held with the handle pointing to the patient's left.
3. The left heal of the tray is inserted into the mouth with the right cheek retracted and the left heel is rotated and positioned with heals covering the retromolar pads.
4. The tray is lowered anteriorly to cheek the adaptation of the tray to the alveolar ridge. The space of 5 mm should exists between the tray and the ridge.
5. The flanges of the metal stock tray must be short of the muscle attachments lingually, labially and buccally by 2 to 3 mm when the muscle attachments are in a state of rest.
6. The flanges are checked visually for overextension into the labial and buccal sulci.
7. The lingual sulcus is checked by having the patient to raise the tip of the tongue to the palate. Only slight finger pressure in the premolar area will be needed to keep tray in position if the tray is not overextended. If the tray is overextended bending of the metal trays flanges with pliers may be required or another tray is choosen.

Selection of Impression Materials

The preliminary impression material may be:

1. Impression compound, a thermoplastic material, particularly indicated in the lower jaw with marked resorption where the surrounding tissues encroach the denture space.
2. Irreversible hydrocolloid (alginate) where there are large undercuts in the anterior region and around the tuberosities or flabby ridges.

These two materials vary in their ability to displace soft tissues. An experienced clinician may use any of them according to his choice to obtain acceptable results with well-selected tray in case of a maxillary impression. In case of mandibular arch, a poorly chosen tray and irreversible hydrocolloid impression may not give the acceptable result obtained with impression compound.

The impression compound is highly viscous, therefore, has sufficient body to flow beyond the tray without support into the sulcus against the pressure of lips or cheek, beneath the tongue or soft palate. It is correctable by cutting back or by addition. It has the advantage of allowing functional border moulding procedure definitively in the first impression, requiring only minimum corrections during the final impression procedure. The tissues of basal seat areas in the region of loosely attached mucosa exhibit extreme changes in shape and size according to mouth position (open or close) and muscle functions. So, an impression material must be selected that is correctable, as it permits the operator to record the moving tissues in a static impression so that the denture will have border extensions in harmony with function, maximum retention and stability, the potential for reducing bone loss (Table 5.1).

Patient's Position

The patient should be seated upright with the head in line with the body supported on the head rest in order to prevent the impression material flowing down the throat. When making the lower impression, the patient's mouth should be at the level of operator's shoulder. When taking the upper impression, the patient's mouth should be at the level of operator's elbow. The impression procedure should be explained to the patient to make the patient cooperative.

Operator's Position

For lower impression, the operator should be in front and on right side. For the upper impression, the operator should be behind and right of the patient.

Modeling Compound Preliminary Impression

The preliminary impression with modeling compound allows the complete border moulding procedure in one appointment along with it. The cast can be poured and custom tray is fabricated for the final impression.

Mandibular Impression

The mandibular impression should be made first so that patient becomes accustomed with the procedures and materials before the more difficult maxillary impression due to gagging reflex. The reflex salivation makes the mandibular impression difficult.

1. The lower impression tray should be inserted by rotating at right angle to its position into the mouth, with the cheek retracted by the operator's finger.
2. The tray is placed in the mouth with the heels covering the retromolar pads. The anterior part of the tray is lowered to see the proper adaptation of it to the alveolar ridge.
3. The compound is softened in a hot water bath at 55–60°C preferably thermostatically

Table 5.1 Choice of impression material and techniques

Type of ridge	Primary impression	Final impression	Technique
Healthy ridge, no undercut	Impression compound	Zinc oxide/eugenol, medium bodied elastomer	Conventional
Healthy ridge with undercut	Alginate	Alginate or elastomer	Conventional
Displaceable upper ridge	Alginate	Two-staged impression	Selective pressure impression
Knife-edge/fibrous ridge	Alginate	Zinc oxide/eugenol or light bodied rubber base	Selective pressure impression
Flat ridge	Impression compound	Tissue conditioning material	Functional impression

controlled, to maintain the recommended temperature. The compound is kneaded between the operator's fingers before use, being folded so that any creases produced will go inside the material.

4. The inner side of the tray is heated over flame.
5. The compound for the lower impression tray should be rolled to a rope of 1.5 cm diameter and long enough to reach around the heel of the tray (Figs 5.8A and B).
6. The compound is adapted to the tray by grooving with the finger to receive the crest of ridge. The compound should be longer in the lingual side than in the buccal side.
7. The surface of the compound is quickly flamed to ensure accurate surface detail of the tissue (Fig. 5.9).
8. The flamed surface is tempered by immersing the whole impression in hot water bath momentarily to prevent burning of patient's mouth (Fig. 5.10)
9. The tray is rotated into the patient's mouth, centered and the patient is instructed to raise and relax the tongue, and the tray is seated firmly downwards with first and second index fingers on premolar areas and patient is asked to protrude the tip of the tongue, move it from side to side, close the mouth and swallow, and suck in the cheeks. This

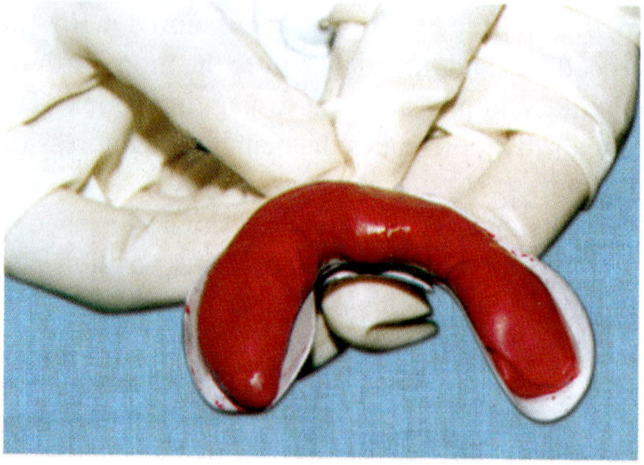

Fig. 5.8A: The compound is moulded into a rope for lower tray

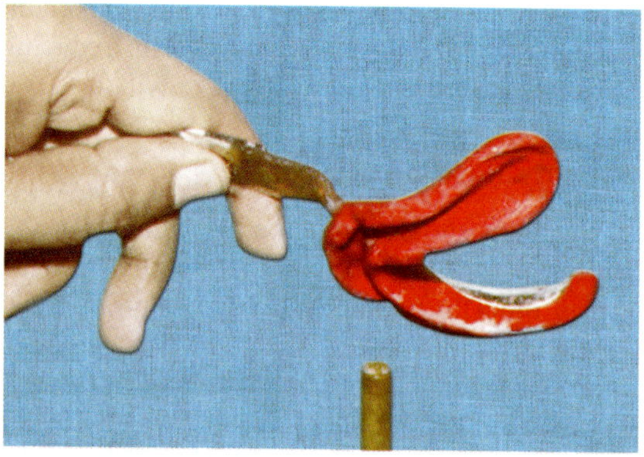

Fig. 5.9: The surface of the compound is further softened over a bunsen flame

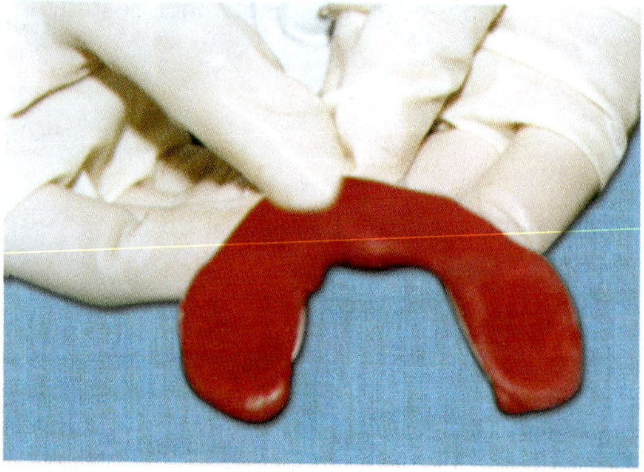

Fig. 5.8B: The compound has been adapted to the ridge form

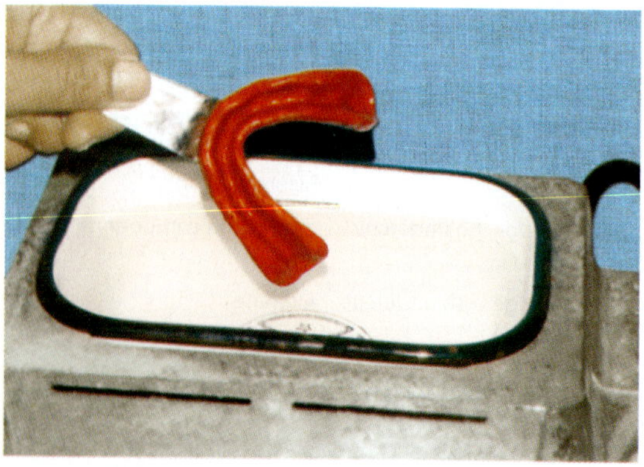

Fig. 5.10: Tempering the surface of compound by dipping in water at 60°C to prevent injury to the patient's oral soft tissue

movement activates the palatoglossus muscle, draws forward the palatoglossus arch forming the distolingual denture border. This exercise also moulds the anterior lingual border by activating the mylohyoid and the genioglossus muscles. When the flange is developed in this manner, the border of the lingual flange has a typical S-curvature.

10. The tray is held stationary while the compound cools with the thumb of right hand below the patient's chin and the first and second fingers on top of it in the premolar areas.
11. The impression is removed by upward and backward force after breaking the border seal. The impressions are checked for necessary landmarks. If the impressions are satisfactory, they are dipped in 1 in 20 aqueous solution of chlorhexidine for disinfection.

Checking of Mandibular Impression for Necessary Landmarks (Fig. 5.11)

1. Residual ridges
2. Labial and buccal vestibules
3. Lingual, labial and buccal frena
4. Buccal shelf areas
5. External oblique ridges
6. Sublingual space and lingual frenum
7. Retromylohyoid fossa
8. Retromolar pads.

Common Faults in Mandibular Impressions

1. Underextended in posterior lingual pouch (Fig. 5.12).

   Causes
   a. Tray flange is underextended in the region.
   b. Insufficient compound in the tray.
   c. Insufficient force in seating the tray.
   d. Tongue trapped under the tray due to failure of the patient to raise the tongue during the seating of tray.
2. Underextended in labial, lingual and buccal sulcus.

   Causes
   a. Lack of impression compound.
   b. Insufficient force to seat the tray.
3. Presence of void in the distobuccal border.

   Causes
   The check trapped beneath the border.
4. The edge of the tray show through the impression.

   Causes
   a. Tray not centered during seating.
   b. Use of too large tray or too small size tray.

Maxillary Impression

1. The cake compound is heated in a water bath at 55°C and sufficient amount is kneaded into a ball free of folds.

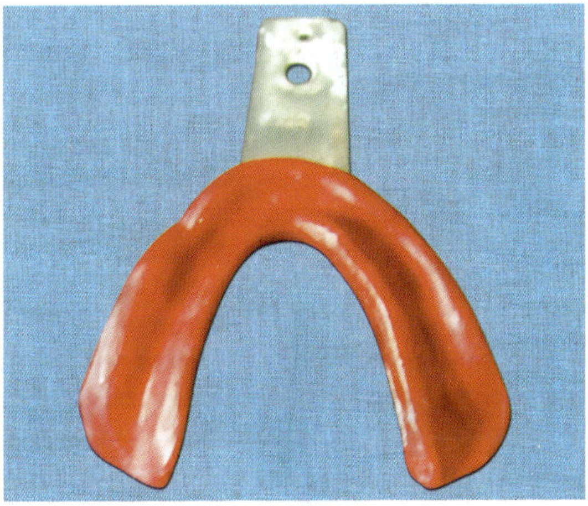

Fig. 5.11: Completed mandibular impression

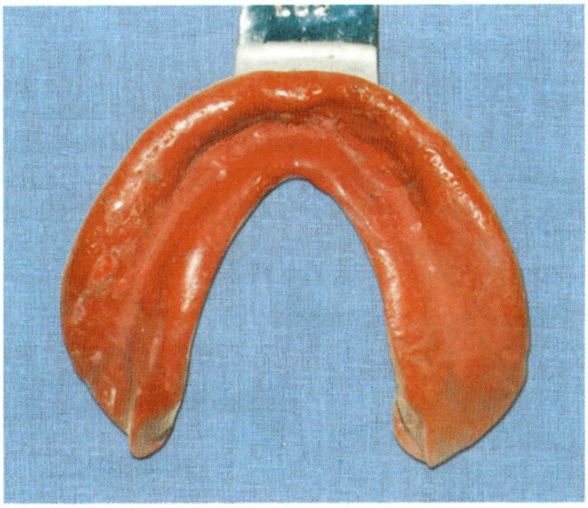

Fig. 5.12: Mandibular impression shows underextended lingual pouch

2. The tray is passed over the flame to dry it so that the compound will stick to it. The ball of compound is placed over the center of the tray (Fig. 5.13).
3. The compound is spread over the entire tray and a shallow trough is formed corresponding to the alveolar ridge crest (Fig. 5.14).
4. The surface of compound is flamed and tempered in the water bath.
5. The loaded tray is rotated into the half open mouth, positioned and centered relative to the maxillary ridge; the upper lip is lifted upwards to expose the whole labial surface of the residual ridge.

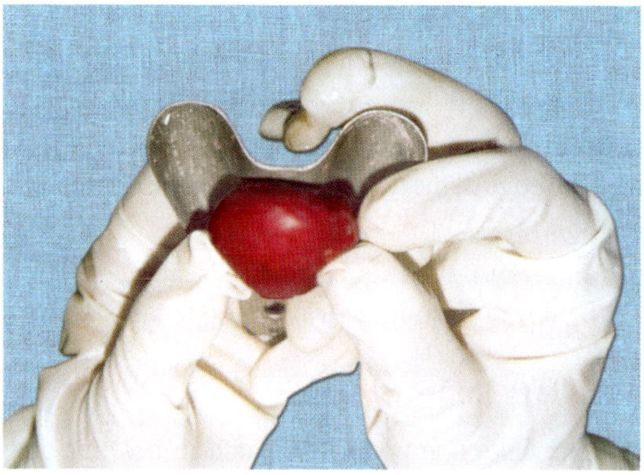

Fig. 5.13: The softened compound is moulded into a fall and placed in upper impression tray

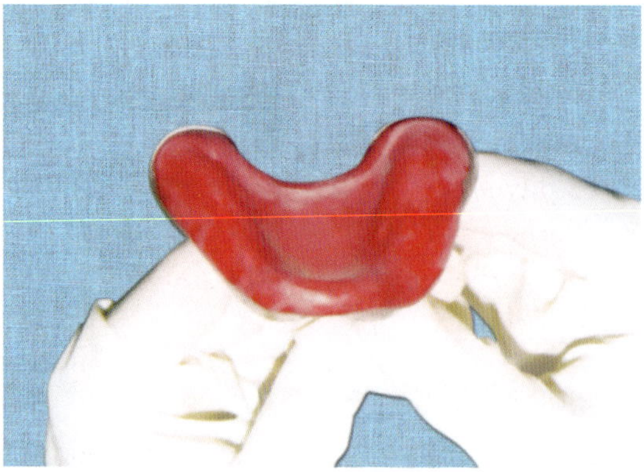

Fig. 5.14: The softened ball of compound is adapted to the ridge form

6. The impression tray should be seated gently in place while the patient sucks in the cheeks, pulls down the lip, and moves the mandible from side-to-side and then open wide. Alternately producing the "woo" and "eee" sounds molds the width of labial sulcus, the buccal frenum, and the height and width of the buccal sulcus. If the patient fails to assist, this may require to be manipulated gently by the operator.
7. These actions mold the border of the impression so as to record the functional sulcus. The tray is held stationary while the compound cools.
8. The cheeks are raised and pushed downward to break the seal and the impression is removed by forward pull on the handle of the tray.
9. The impressions are checked for necessary landmarks. If the impressions are satisfactory, they are dipped in 1 in 20 aqueous solution of chlorhexidine for disinfection and poured with plaster within an hour as the modeling compound flows at room temperature.

Maxillary Impression for Checking the Six Following Landmarks (Fig. 5.15)

1. Residual ridge
2. Palate

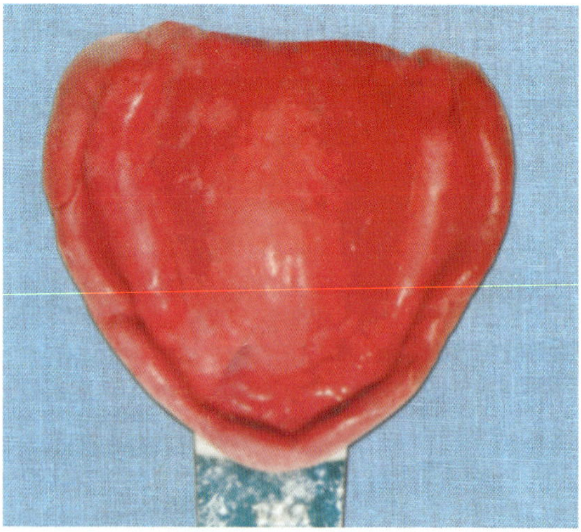

Fig. 5.15: Upper compound impression showing six important landmarks

3. Labial and buccal frena
4. Fovea palatinae and vibrating line
5. Tuberosities
6. Hamular notch

Common Faults in Maxillary Impressions

1. A large fold in the midline of posterior third of palate (Fig. 5.16).

    Causes

    a. Insufficient compound in the posterior area
    b. Insufficient pressure in seating of tray.
2. Excess compound flowing beyond the posterior border of tray (Fig. 5.17).

    Causes

    a. Excessive pressure during seating of tray.
    b. Excess of compound in the palatal area.
3. Impression with an underextended periphery. An underextended periphery can be identified in one of two forms.
4. A sharp periphery in the sulcus.

    Causes

    a. Mouth is widely opened and the lips become too tight.
    b. Failure to pull the upper lip outwards and upwards to allow the compound to flow into the labial sulcus.
    c. Selected tray is too narrow in the buccal region.
    d. Anterior portion of the tray is placed too far back into the mouth. The impression should be made again with proper degree of mouth opening, tray positioning, or tray selection.
    e. Insufficient compound.
    f. Inadequate pressure.
5. A flat and glazed periphery usually occurs in the tuberosity region.

It is better to rectify the area by adding green stick compound after drying, flaming, tempering, and reinserting rather remaking the impression.

Alginate Preliminary Impressions

The material of choice for ridges with undercut is a highly viscous alginate.

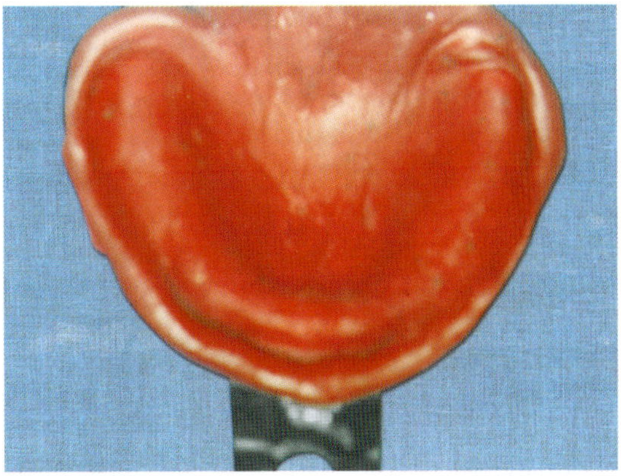

Fig. 5.16: A large fold in the midline of posterior third of palate

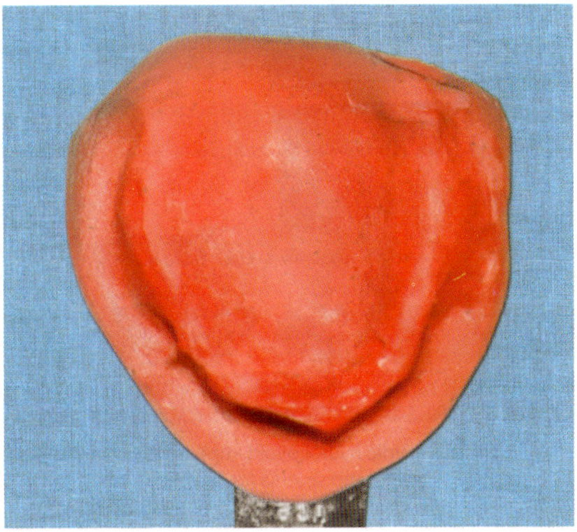

Fig. 5.17: Excess compound beyond posterior border of tray

Equipments and Material

1. Impression trays (Fig. 5.18)
2. Utility wax
3. Tissue clock
4. Irreversible hydrocolloid (Fig. 5.19)
5. Spatula

Mandibular Impression

The mandibular impression should be made first so that patient becomes accustomed with the procedures and materials before the more difficult maxillary impression is attempted.

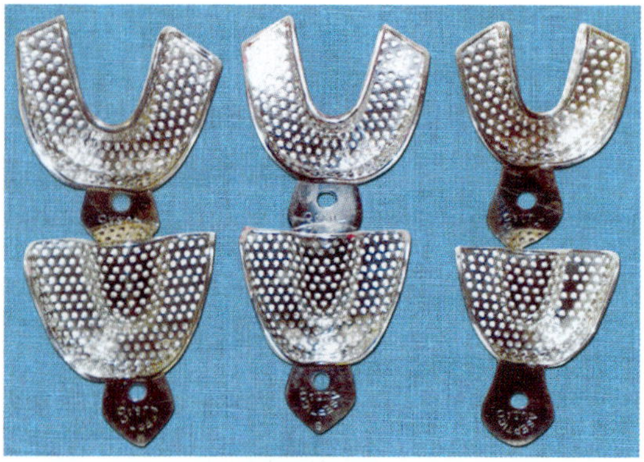

Fig. 5.18: Perforated upper and lower impression trays of different sizes

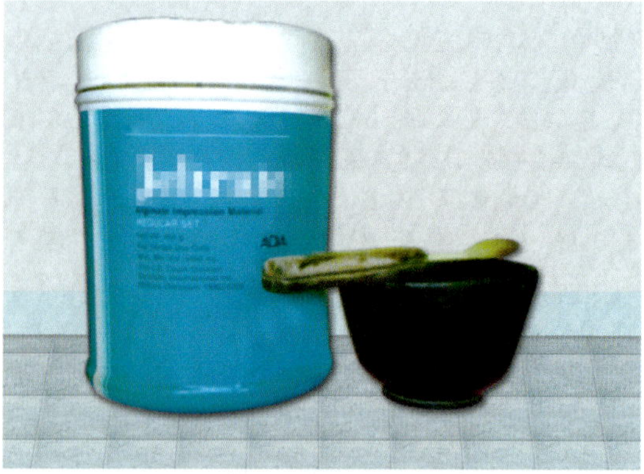

Fig. 5.19: Irreversible hydrocolloid impression material with bowl and spatula for mixing

1. The dental chair is adjusted so that the mandibular arch is parallel to the floor when the mouth is opened.
2. The border of the tray can be adjusted with utility wax where needed. The labial and lingual posterior borders usually require adjustment.
3. The alginate is mixed according the manufacturer's instructions and loaded in the tray. Some alginate can be placed in the retromylohyoid spaces, and labial and buccal vestibule.
4. The tray is inserted in the mouth and partially seated on the ridge and the patient is instructed to protrude the tongue slightly. The tray is gently vibrated downward.
5. The lower lip is gently pulled forward to prevent trapping of air in the labial vestibule.
6. The patient is instructed to close the mouth as far as possible without touching the tray with the upper ridge.
7. The tray is held to allow the material to set. The impression after setting is removed, washed under tap water and inspected for defects. The gross excess is removed with a sharp Bard Parker knife. If the impression is acceptable, cast is poured immediately.

Maxillary Impression

The patient is seated in the dental chair which is adjusted so that the maxillary arch is parallel to the floor. The impression is recorded from behind and side of the patient.

1. The tray borders are modified with wax if required. The posterior borders along the distobuccal area need often modification. If the palatal vault is high wax should be added to the palatal vault area of the tray. The mouth should be washed and dried with a gauge piece just before the impression is recorded.
2. The impression material is mixed according to the manufacturer's instructions and loaded into the tray. A small amount of material is placed in the palate and the buccal and labial vestibule.
3. Tray is inserted into the mouth and seated posterior first by centering on ridge until the impression material flows into the sulcus.
4. The lips and cheeks are pulled outward to prevent trapping of air. The patient is directed to close the mouth as far as possible without touching the mandibular ridge.
5. The impression is removed after setting, rinsed with tap water and excess is cut with a sharp Bard Parker knife. If acceptable, it is poured immediately.

Patient Instructions

The patient must be instructed to keep the existing dentures out of the mouth for at least 48–72 hours prior to the final impression. If it is not possible due to social or business obligations, tissue conditioning material should be placed in the existing dentures and repeated several times till optimum health of the tissue is restored before the final impression.

FINAL IMPRESSIONS

Definition

"The impression that represents the completion of the registration of the surface or object" (GPD-7). The final impressions are commonly recorded in special trays using a two-stage technique. This is done first making a record of the functional sulcus, using greenstick compound traced on the tray periphery. The final overall impressions are recorded in the modified tray with zinc oxide-eugenol paste. Elastic or elastomeric material can be used in case of large undercuts and in a very dry mouth.

CUSTOM/SPECIAL TRAY

Definition

A special tray is defined as; "A custom-made device prepared for a particular patient which is used to carry, confine and control an impression material while making an impression". The design of these trays varies with the impression technique. They should be rigid, evenly spaced from the tissues, and capable of adjustment to proper extension.

The method fabrication is described in details in Chapter 6.

Instruments and Materials (Fig. 5.20)

1. Handpiece and acrylic trimmer.
2. Mirror and spatula
3. Greenstick compound
4. Alcohol torch
5. Hot water bowl
6. Bard Parker knife
7. Scissors
8. Bunsen burner

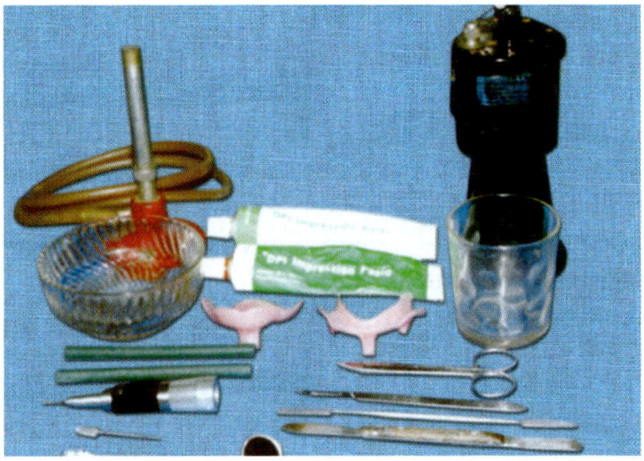

Fig. 5.20: Instruments and materials for the final impressions

Impression Materials

The following impression materials are now used for complete denture final impressions:

Border Moulding Materials

1. Low fusing greenstick compound
2. Polyether

Final/Wash Impression Materials

1. Zinc oxide eugenol paste
2. Silicone elastomers
3. Impression plaster (rarely used now)

Zinc Oxide Eugenol Pastes (Tray: Acrylic, Spacer 0.5 mm)

These are the most commonly used final impression material now. It is rigid material and cannot be used in presence of bony undercuts. It is useful in highly resorbed ridges in closed fitted tray as wash impression.

Silicone Elastomers (Tray: Acrylic, Spacer 1.5 mm)

These materials and alginate materials are used in spaced custom trays in presence of undercuts. A low-viscous alginate or silicone elastomers may be used for this purpose. The high-viscous materials are used for preliminary impression.

Impression Plaster
(Tray: Acrylic, Spacer 2 mm)

It was one time used frequently as a final impression material but it is not used now due to messy handling characteristic.

Border Moulding

Border moulding is defined as "The shaping of an impression material by the manipulation or action of the tissues adjacent to the borders of the impression" (GPT-7).

Importance of Border Moulding

Border moulding records the three-dimensional form of the peripheral sulcus by functional means. The border or periphery of the denture provides ample opportunity for the ingress of air. Correct adaptation of the denture border to the gingival sulcus and the inside of cheeks and lips ensures border seal. The soft tissues of the lips and cheeks move inwards due to atmospheric pressure and maintain contact with the dentures. This prevents ingress of air through the border to break the seal.

Methods of Border Moulding

1. One step border moulding
2. Sectional border moulding.

One Step Border Moulding

The whole border is recorded simultaneously in one step. It has some advantages—(i) number of insertion of tray is reduced to one, (ii) prevents the effect of error from one area to the other. Polyether is the material of choice for this method.

Sectional Border Moulding

This method utilizes the border moulding of custom tray section by section using stick compound.

The stick compound, also known as low fusing compound, is the most common material used for border moulding. It is available in several colors like green, gray and white.

Accurate border moulding depends upon the fit of the tray. It should be 2 mm short of the reflections. A pointed flame should be used preferable from an alcohol torch to soften the compound so that it is softened properly to adhere to the tray and has sufficient flow during moulding against the tissues. It should be tempered in warm water bath before inserting in the mouth to prevent burn. The compound should be dried when reheated to ensure uniform heating of the material. Border moulding is completed in two stages. First a slight overextension is allowed. Then the excess is removed by trimming from the inside of the tray and excess from outside. The final moulding should represent an accurate impression of the peripheral tissues. A knife trimming around the frena and retromolar pads is required after the refinement is completed as compound will be distorting these very displaceable tissues. Irrespective of which method is used, the same border moulding movements are to be carried out by the operator and the patient.

Mandibular Custom Tray Border Moulding

1. **The buccal extension of the lower tray is checked** in patient's mouth to ensure that it is 2 mm short of the functional sulcus. If overextended, the tray should be reduced until it has the correct extension. It should extend across the retromolar pad until it lies just anterior to the ascending ramus of the mandible. It should not extend beyond external oblique ridges.
2. **The lingual extension of the tray is checked** by asking the patient to protrude the tongue, to wipe across the vermilion border of the upper lip without noticeable displacement of the tray. If the tray lifts, this indicates overextension. It should be reduced until only slight finger pressure is needed to hold the tray in position.
3. **Border moulding (buccal and labial flanges) (Section 1–2):** Greenstick compound is then traced along a section of the dry lower impression tray, tempered in water bath for 3–5 seconds, and the tray is inserted into the

mouth. The impression of the functional buccal sulcus is made by asking the patient to suck in the cheeks.

4. **Distobuccal area and retromolar pad (Section 3–4):** The patient is asked to open and close the mouth when a downward pressure is exerted by the operator over the posterior aspect of the tray causes the masseter muscle to contract. This forces the buccinator muscle to push the softened modeling compound medially, creating the masseteric notch on the distobuccal border of the mandibular impression.
5. **Anterior lingual flange (premolar to premolar) (Section 5–6):** This area is moulded by asking the patient to move the tongue from one corner to other corner of the mouth to use the mylohyoid muscle and genioglossus muscle to determine the lingual border extension and anterior lingual border extension, respectively.
6. **Distolingual flange (premolar to retromylohyoid fossa) (Section 7–8):** This area is moulded by moving the tongue from one corner of the mouth to the opposite corner of the mouth which activates the palatoglossus muscle. The tray should be kept in position with two fingers placed on finger rests. The thumb is used to support the mandible during these procedures. Completed border moulded tray is checked for retention (Fig. 5.21).

Maxillary Custom Tray Border Moulding

1. The final impression trays are examined in the mouth to verify that trays should be 2 mm short of the functional sulcus. If the tray is overextended it should be reduced until it has correct extension. The posterior border of the upper tray should extend up to the vibrating line, the fixed and movable parts of the palate. It should be demarcated with an indelible pencil when the patient is asked to say 'ah'. The pencil mark is transferred to the fitting surface of the tray when seated in the mouth. The posterior border of the tray is then trimmed to the line.
2. **Labial and buccal flanges (Fig. 5.22):** Greenstick compound is warmed above a flame until it is soft. It is then traced quickly on the dried tray along the labial and buccal flange periphery up to tuberosity to a height of 3 mm. The material is adapted with the fingers to the tray border. The compound is resoftened with alcohol torch, gently to prevent burning.

   It is tempered in the water bath for 3–5 seconds, and the tray is seated in the patient's

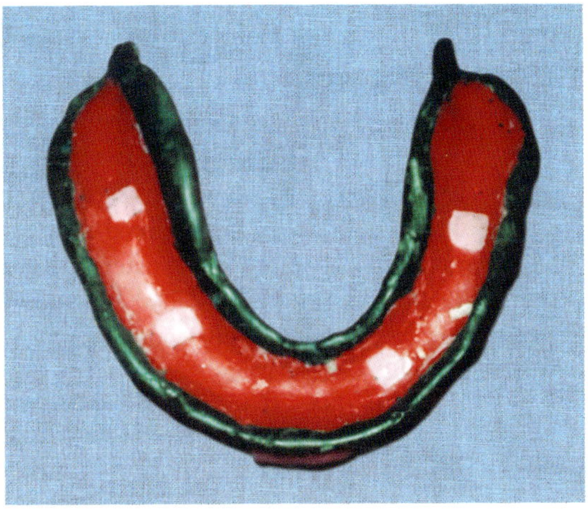

Fig. 5.21: Border moulded mandibular custom tray

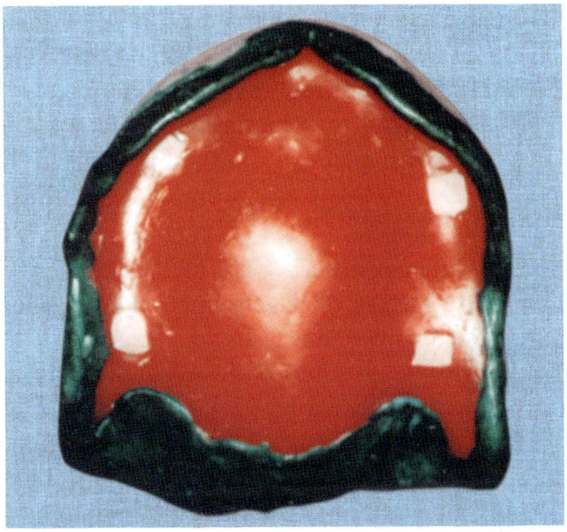

Fig. 5.22: Border moulded maxillary custom tray

mouth and the patient is asked to suck in the cheeks, pull down the lip, and move the jaw from side-to-side so as to mould the distobuccal flange by the action of the coronoid process. This should be repeated until the warm compound no longer turns downward. The same procedure is then followed on the opposite side of the tray.

3. **Tubersosity and posterior border:** Additional compound finally traced across the hamular notches along the posterior border of the tray on the fitting surface. The compound is heated with alcohol torch, tempered in water bath and the tray is placed into the mouth under pressure, so as to produce displacement of the soft tissues in the postdam area. The patient is instructed to swallow several times in order to mould the material in the hamular notches to its functional position. The posterior limit of the denture is now established by asking the patient to open the mouth wide and repeat the ward "ah" several times.

   The peripheral seal is tested. If require further addition may be made before tempering and reseating the impression.

   The compound that has been molded by the tissues will have a matt surface. If the compound is hard when inserted, or does not come in contact with the tissues, it will have a glossy appearance. Excessive compound on the fitting surface of the tray should be removed with a scalpel to approximately 3 mm from the buccal border.

Final Impression (Fig. 5.23)

Several different materials are used to refine the tissue-fitting areas of which zinc oxide eugenol paste is seldom used due to its advantages.

1. A thin mix of zinc oxide eugenol paste is smeared on the greenstick compound. The impression tray is then placed in the mouth, seated with positive pressure and the functional movement used to mold the compound is repeated, so that any minor errors can be corrected. Areas of heavy contact will be visible

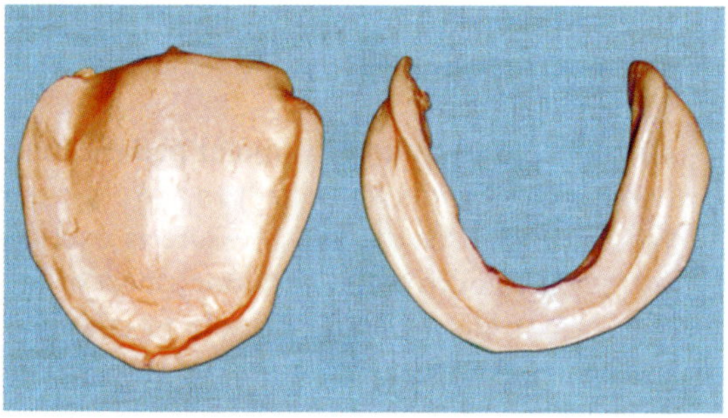

Fig. 5.23: Final mandibular and maxillary impression

   by piercing of the paste by the underlying compound.
2. The underlying compound should be cut back gently in these areas before the final impression is made.
3. Some dentists prefer to place holes over the medial palatal raphe and over the ridges specially over the displaceable soft tissues in the maxillary impression tray and along the crest of the ridge in case of mandibular tray with a # 8 round bur to provide escape ways for the final impression material. The reason for it is not to displace the denture-bearing tissues during recording.
4. Some dentists prefer to remove 0.5 mm of greenstick material from the inner, outer and top surfaces of the border and some are not in favor of this.
5. The entire impression tray is loaded with a fresh mix of zinc oxide eugenol paste. It is seated firmly in the mouth, anteriorly first and then posterior, and the patient opens his mouth wide. The mucous secretion in the posterior palatal seal area should be wiped dry with gauge just before the insertion of the loaded tray. The paste is allowed to set. The impression is removed by lifting the lip and cheek to break the seal and checked for defects. Small defects may be corrected by the local addition of pink wax. Large bubbles may be corrected by placing small amount of zinc oxide eugenol paste in the deficient areas and reseating the impression. Only essential

amount of paste should be used, otherwise a step will be produced.

6. All impression paste that has flowed past the posterior border should be cut back to the compound edge with a slight warm scalpel. A thin layer of impression paste in the postdam area indicates a proper sitting; a thick layer of paste in that area indicates failure to seat the tray fully. An adequate postdam seal will have to be produced by trimming the master cast at the latter stage.
7. An impression of the edentulous ridge must be compared with the structures of the mouth. Unless this is done, the whole procedure will be useless and fruitless.
8. Impression making may give rise to gagging in susceptible patient both for upper and lower jaws.

The simplest method is to divert the patient's attention from the mouth by asking to breath through nose several times during impression procedures. The patient's head should be brought forward and a bowl will be held by the patient under the chin to collect saliva. This will reduce the fear of chocking and gagging. If these measures fail, spraying of topical anesthetic over the soft palate and retromolar pads may be tried. If the above method fails and gagging prevents impression making impossible, the following behavioral techniques have been found to be helpful:

a. A discussion with the patient of fear related to dental procedures with advice to relaxation procedures several times a week preferable 'yoga' or 'meditation' methods.
b. Advise the patient to stimulate the palatal and ridge mucosa with a toothbrush or spoon or mouthwash.

Special Impression Techniques

The oral conditions particular to the patient have an influence upon the selection of the impression material and technique. There are several special impression techniques that are used in different clinical situations:

a. Impression of fibrous (unemployed) posterior mandibular ridge.
b. Impression of displaceable (flabby) anterior maxillary ridge.
c. Impression of flat/extremely resorbed ridge.

Impression of Fibrous (Unemployed) Posterior Mandibular Ridge

The preliminary impression is recorded in a stock metal tray with periphery adapted with impression compound. The impression is recorded with alginate or in severe painful case with plaster. The cast is poured and a custom tray is fabricated in self-cure acrylic resin with 2 mm wax spacer. The holes of 2 mm are cut at one-centimeter intervals on the ridge crest area of the tray. The impression of the cast is taken with that tray loading in impression compound. It is chilled in cold water. The impression is border moulded with greenstick compound in the patient's mouth. The retention is tested if alright the compound at the ridge crest area is cut with a sharp knife to expose the tray and the holes. The edges of rough compound should be smoothened and tried in the mouth till it is comfortable to the patient. The final impression is made with the modified tray in zinc oxide paste. The paste expels out the holes preventing pressure on the ridge crest. The peripheral tissues are loaded should show through the very thin impression paste. The cast is prepared and denture fabricated on this cast can be worn without pain.

Impression of Displaceable (Flabby) Anterior Maxillary Ridge

1. The preliminary impression is made with plaster with antiexpansion solution.
2. The cast is poured and a special tray is made of acrylic tray material with an opening surrounding the flabby tissue.
3. The extension of the special tray is checked in the patient's mouth and corrected in the mouth with greenstick compound.
4. A zinc oxide wash/medium bodied polyvinyl siloxane impression is made.

5. The impression is removed, checked and the excess around the opening is trimmed away.
6. The tray is reinserted in the mouth and a mix of impression plaster/light bodied polyvinyl siloxane if medium bodied was used is applied over the flabby tissue in the window.
7. The impression is removed when the plaster is set. This composite impression avoids distortion of displaceable tissue. The completed impression is sent for cast preparation (Figs 5.24A to D).

Impression of Flat Ridges/Atrophic Mandibular Residual Ridge

1. The primary impression is recorded with impression compound and a custom tray is fabricated with cold cure acrylic resin.
2. The final impression is recorded with an admix of 3 parts by weight of red compound and 7 parts by weight of greenstick compound made by placing the ingredients in a water bath.
3. The material is loaded in the custom tray and impression is recorded with border moulding. The setting time of the admix is 1 to 2 minutes.
4. The impression is chilled in cold water after removal from the mouth.
5. The impression is reinserted in the mouth and operator apply pressure alternately on the stub handles of the tray in the premolar regions.
6. If any discomfort is noticed, the area is relieved with a heated wax knife and the tray is reseated again and again until no further discomfort is felt. The impression is sent for pouring the final cast.

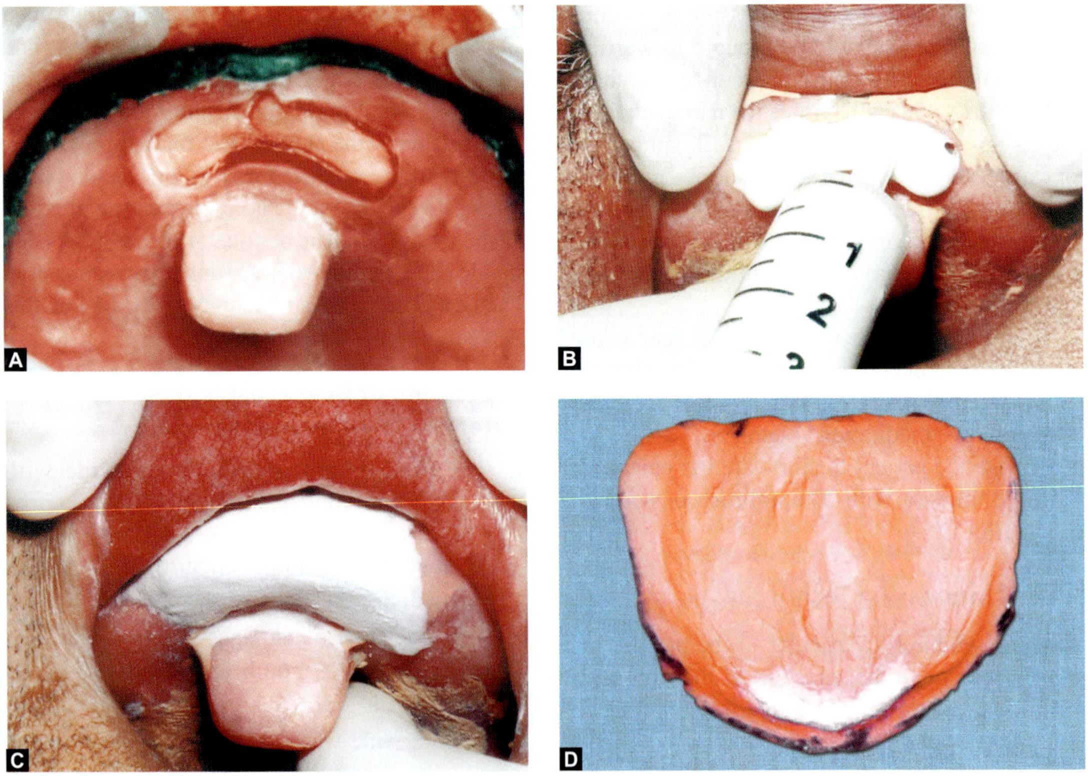

Figs 5.24A to D: Impression of flabby maxillary anterior ridge

CONCLUSION

The selective pressure impression technique can be applied to all varieties of residual ridges as it is customized to mucosal conditions, whereas the functional impression technique has limited application to a uniformly given ridge consistency.

BIBLIOGRAPHY

1. Boucher CO. Complete denture impression based upon the anatomy of the mouth. Jada 1944;31:1174.
2. Dunean JP, Sangeetha Raghavendra, Tylor TD. A selective-pressure impression technique for the edentulous maxilla. J Prosthet Dent 2004;92:299-301.
3. Ellinger CW. Minimizing problems in making a complete lower impression. J Prosth Dent 1973;30: 553.
4. Fisher RD. Fundamental rules for making full denture impressions. J Prosth Dent. 1951;1:1135.
5. Freeman SP. Impressions for complete dentures. JADA. 1970;80:1173.
6. Heartwell CM Jr. Complete denture failures related to improper interpretation and improper preparation of the anatomy of the mouth. Dent Clin N Amer. 1970;14:139.
7. Jogleker AP, Sinkford JC. Impression procedures for problem mandibular complete denture. JADA. 1968;77: 1303.
8. Luthra SP. Measurement of the area of the maxillary basal seat for dentures. J Prosth Dent. 1973;30:25.
9. Lye TL. The significance of the fovea palatini in complete denture prosthodontics. J Prosth Dent. 1975;33:504-10.
10. Maison WG. Denture outline form. JADA. 1976;59:938.
11. Neufeld JO. Dentures and their supporting oral tissues. Dent Clin N Amer. 1970;14:559.
12. Stock House JA. A comparison of elastic impression materials. J Prosth Dent. 1975;34:305.
13. Walsh JF, Walsh J. Muscle formed complete mandibular dentures. J Prosth Dent. 1976;35:254.
14. Young JM. Surface characterization of dental stone. Impression Orientation. J Prosth Dent. 1975;33:336.

Chapter 6

Preparation of Casts, Special Trays, Denture Bases and Occlusal Rims (Laboratory Procedures Involved with Impression Making and Jaw Relations)

INTRODUCTION

Most dental laboratory procedures are carried out on a cast. The words model and cast are frequently misused.

MODEL

A model is a reproduction for demonstration, accuracy is not important.

CAST

It is an accurate and positive reproduction of a maxillary or mandibular dental arch made from an impression of that arch.

Types of Cast

It is of various types according to the purpose for which it is made, e.g. preliminary cast, diagnostic cast, master cast, refractory investment cast, remount cast.

Diagnostic Cast

It is life size reproduction of a part or parts of a part or parts of oral cavity and/or facial structures for the purpose of study and treatment planning. It is also known as study cast.

Master Cast

It is a replica of the tooth surfaces, residual ridge areas, and/or other parts of the dental arch and/or final structures used to fabricate a dental restoration or a prosthesis.

Refractory/Investment Cast

It is a cast made of a material that will withstand high temperatures without disintegrating and incidentally, to perform certain functions relative to the burnout and depends on of the mould.

Remount Cast

It is a cast formed of prosthesis for the purpose of mounting the prosthesis on an articulator.

Preliminary Cast

A cast formed from a preliminary impression for use in diagnosis or fabrication of an impression tray (GPT-8).

Uses

1. Analysis of possibility of various forms of treatment.
2. Analysis of the relationship between maxilla and mandible when casts are mounted on articulator.
3. Analysis of static and dynamic relationship of the occlusal surfaces of opposing teeth.
4. Communication between the dental surgeon and patient or laboratory technician.
5. Construction of special trays.
6. Making records of various anatomical structures.
7. Survey of oral structures.

LABORATORY PREPARATION

Pouring the Cast

The preliminary impression may be poured in one of three ways as follows:

I. Mounding method: It is a two stage pour technique which is ecceptable for preliminary edentulous impression.

II. Boxing method: It is the enclosure of an impression to produce the desired size and form of the base of the cast and to preserve desired details. Strips of soft boxing wax are wrapped around the impression to form a mold for the gypsum. Generally, wax is extended 1 cm beyond the tissue side of the impression to form a base for the cast. The mixed gypsum is vibrated into the impression to enhance the flow of the material into the impression and avoid the entrapment of air bubbles. It is usually recomended for final or master impression.

III. Model former method: The pouring a cast is using a container called model former to form the base for the impression.

A double pour mounding method is acceptable for preliminary edentulous impressions and boxing method is require for final impressions.

Mounding Method

Steps

1. The impression is washed under cold running water to remove traces of blood or mucosa from its surface by shaking and dried with compressed air or a piece of gauze.
2. The impression is placed on the plaster bench in such a way that the posterior end does not contact the bench. This will prevent distortion of the impression and placing the tray parallel to the bench make it easy for pouring.
3. The cast may be poured in plaster of Paris or a mixture 50:50 plaster of Paris and dental stone or only dental stone. Usually 150 G of gypsum is adequate for single cast.
4. Water is poured and measured in a calibrated glass according to the plaster or dental stone mix used and placed in a plaster bowl. The plaster or dental stone is weighed and sifted slowly into the water (dental plaster of 100 gm is required to shift in 50 mL of water).
5. The gentle taps on the side of the bowl helps to prevent air inclusions.
6. The mixing is done with hand held spatula or a mechanical spatulator with a vibrator. The procedure is known as spatulation.
7. The impression tray is held in one hand with its handle touching the vibrator and small increments of plaster may be introduced with a spatula into the impression from the posterior region.
8. The vibrations continued until the impression has been filled to its periphery and it is placed with the tray parallel to the bench again.
9. The remaining plaster or stone is added to a height of 5 mm above the highest part of impression. Rough protrusions of gypsum are added to the surface to provide locking undercuts for the second stage of pour.
10. After the initial set, the impression is socked in a bowl of clear slurry water for 4 to 5 minutes to thoroughly wet the first pour gypsum.
11. A second mix of gypsum mixed with same water powder ratio and placed in a 12 mm thick mound on a glass slab and formed into the shape of the impression.
12. The filled impression is inverted and seated into the mass. The excess of plaster is drawn up over the outer periphery of the impression with sufficient bulk to allow for trimming later. Excess plaster is removed from the tongue space and allow the cast to harden (Figs 6.1A and B). Care should be taken to avoid locking the impression tray into the stone or plaster.

Separation of Impression

Compound Impression

1. When the cast material has reached its initial set, excess is cleaned from the tray.
2. After the final set of plaster (minimum 30 minutes) excess compound is removed from the outer surface of the tray by a plaster knife.

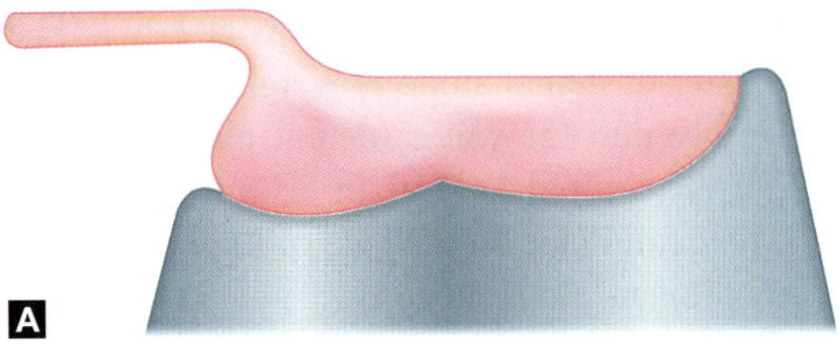

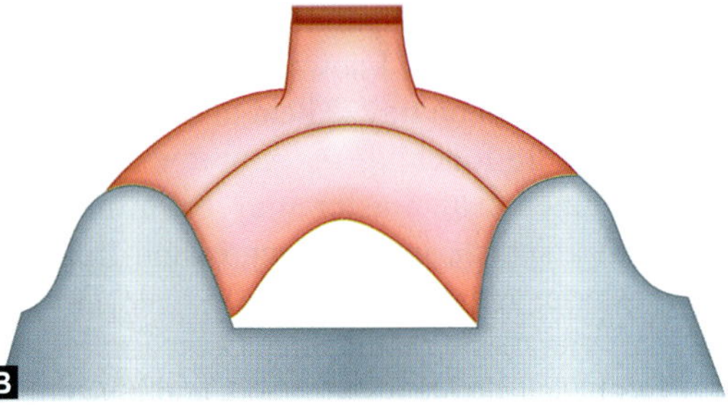

Figs 6.1A and B: (A) Pouring maxillary cast by mounting method; (B) Pouring mandibular cast by mounting method

3. The cast is held firmly with the fingers supporting the tray, and the thumb on the base of the cast.
4. The metal tray is removed by tapping it sharply at the base of the handle with a wooden mallet or by handle of knife.
5. If it not separated easily the cast is immersed in hot water of 65 degree centigrade for 5 minutes and the tray may be removed easily by lifting up the buccal area all rounds and then the palatal or lingual area. It should not be placed in too hot water to prevent sticking of melt compound to the cast. The compound overheated and adhering to the cast may be removed by pressing a ball of softened compound over the area and then removing it.

Alginate Impression

Alignate impression should be poured within 12 minutes after removal from the month.

Alignate impression if taken in perforated tray, material extended through the holes is first cut away before attempt to separate the cast from impression material. The alginate is then lifted from the cast on the buccal and labial sides with fingers. The cast should be separated from impression after 45–60 minutes of pouring and is allowed for final set.

Trimming Casts

It is the procedure of shaping the cast. It is normally carried out on a model trimmer in the following ways:

1. The wet cast is placed on its base on the platform of the model trimmer with posterior surface moved gently through the opening against the rotating carborundum or diamond wheel. The wheel is lubricated with water which disposes of the removed cast material. It should be trimmed about 5 mm from the hamular notch and retromolar pad.
2. The cast is then placed upright on its posterior surface and the base is trimmed so that the edentulous ridge lies approximately in the same plane as it would in the mouth. The base of the cast should be at least 10 mm thick for adequate strength.
3. The outer surface is trimmed 3 mm from maximum depth of the sulcus by placing the base on platform. The sharp corner produced are removed by knife to from a 45 degree chamfer about 1.5 mm wide.
4. The excess plaster on the lingual space of a lower cast is removed with a flat blade sculptor to leave a 2 mm deep lingual sulcus.

Disinfection

To prevent cross infection impressions should be thoroughly rinsed in water and then socked in 0.5% sodium hypochlorite solution diluted 1:10 for 10 minutes before pouring the cast.

Impression Trays

It is a device that is used to carry, confine, and control impression material while making an impression.

Parts of an Impression Tray

The stock tray consists of a body and handle. The body consists of a floor and flanges. The maxillary tray has a vault.

Functions of Impression Tray

1. To support an impression material in planed contact with oral tissues.
2. To allow placement of additional stress in selected regions of the residual ridge while recording other regions in a displaced state.
3. To support the set impression material when removed from the mouth so that a cast can be poured.

Requirements of Impression Trays

1. The tray should be rigid but not abnormally thick.
2. They should be clean and smooth.
3. To support the impression material when removed from the mouth so that a cast can be poured.
4. They should allow the correct thickness of impression material to be used.
5. The shape of the handle should not displace the lip during impression making.
6. They must hold the impression material against the whole areas to be recorded.
7. They should support the lips and cheeks in their pre-extracted position so that the recording of the sulcus is in its original shape and size.
8. They should be capable of modification by trimming and binding.
9. They should retain their original shape during construction and pouring of cast.
10. It should be easy to construct and require minimum time and cast.

Types of Trays

According to the Patients Status

1. Dentulous (box tray)
2. Edentulous (anatomical).

According to Design

1. Perforated
2. Nonperforated.

According to Material of Construction

1. Metallic
2. Nonmetallic.

According to Method Fabrication

1. Stock trays
2. Custom/special trays.

Advantages of Special Trays

1. Accurate peripheral extension is assured.
2. The border of the tray can be so adjusted that the movement of soft tissues around the impression remains undistorted.
3. The space provided inside the tray may be varied according to the nature of the impression material.
4. A uniform space may be created for impression material for dimensional accuracy.
5. There is less discomfort to the patient while making impression due to proper size of tray and reduced mass of impression material.
6. There is economy in impression material.

Fabrication of Special Tray (Laboratory Procedures)

An individual impression tray provides a support for obtaining a wash impression which accurately records tissue details and peripheral extension. These trays can be made best from tray material or from cold-cure acrylic resin. These can be made either by adapting a sheet of dough over the cast or by preparing a wax pattern on the cast, investing, boiling out, and packing the mould with cold-cure acrylic resin.

Outline: The outline of the tray should be marked on the primary casts by the dentist. The line is placed 2 to 3 mm short of the vestibular sulcus and all frena. If the tray is shorter more than 3 mm it will be very difficult to control and manipulate the compound during border moulding. In the maxillary cast the outline should connect the hamular notches passing through just 2 mm posterior to the fovea palatinae. If fovea is not visible the line is drawn straight from one hamular notch to the other. In the mandibular cast it should cover the retromolar pads (Fig. 6.2).

Forming the tray:

1. A uniform spacer of one thickness of modeling wax is provided over the outlined areas. The use of wax as spacer enables 'stops' to be incorporated into the inner surface of the tray.
2. These stops contact the mucosa before the rest of the tray. These enable the proper placement of tray in the same position every time when placed on the ridge. These stops also help to maintain uniform 2 to 3 mm thick impression material. The stops are made by cutting holes in wax 2 to 3 mm wide extending from a point slightly palatal to the ridge across to the gingival sulcus. They are located over the molar and canine area on both sides (Figs 6.3A and B).
3. A coat of alginate-separating media is painted over the outlined areas and allowed to dry, and a second coat is applied. A sheet of self-cure acrylic resin dough of 2 mm thick is adapted over the modeling wax to cover the outlined area (Fig. 6.4).

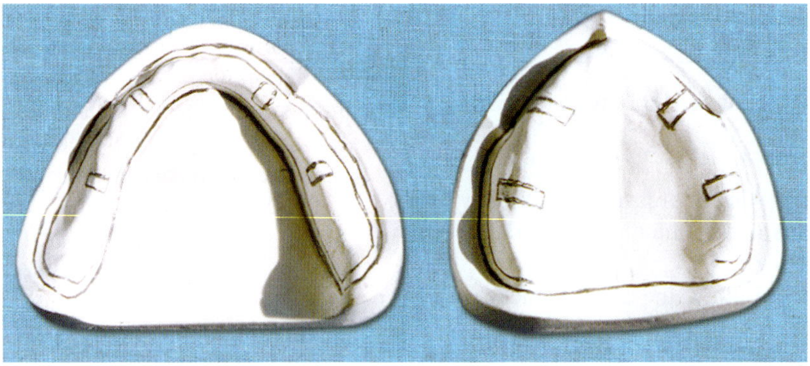

Fig. 6.2: The outline of the upper and lower special trays also bears marks of areas where steps are required

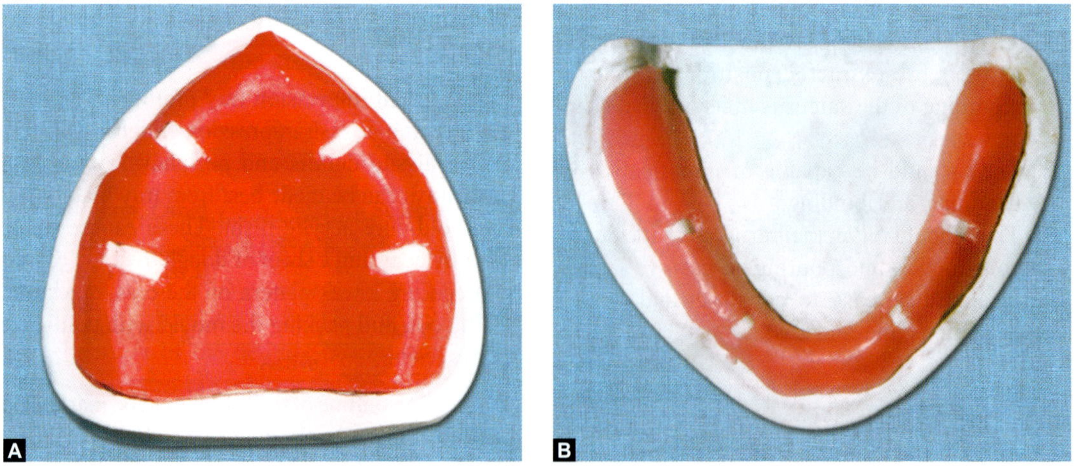

Figs 6.3A and B: A layer of base plate wax is adapted over the cast and wax is cut away in the areas where stops are desired. The acrylic tray when formed into these areas will serve as stops

4. An acrylic resin handle should be added in the midline of the crest of both upper and lower trays before the tray material has set. It should be joined by moistening with a small amount of monomer. Two narrow finger, rests (1 cm × 1 cm × 4 cm) are attached to the lower tray in the region of first molars (Fig. 6.5).

Separation of Tray and Cast

After the tray acrylic resin sets completely, the cast and tray is immersed in warm water to soften the spacer wax. The tray is removed from the cast by gently pulling by the handle.

Trimming the Tray

The borders of the tray are trimmed to round all corners and edges. They should have smooth border but not polished as the greenstick compound used for border moulding will adhere to a course surface.

The special tray can be prepared with shellac base, visible light cure material or vacuum formed thermoplastic sheets. Shellac trays need reinforcement to reduce distortion and improve strength. In the maxillary a wire is adapted across the palatal seal area. In the mandibular tray the wire is adapted along the lingual flange. The handles are made with self-cure acrylic resin.

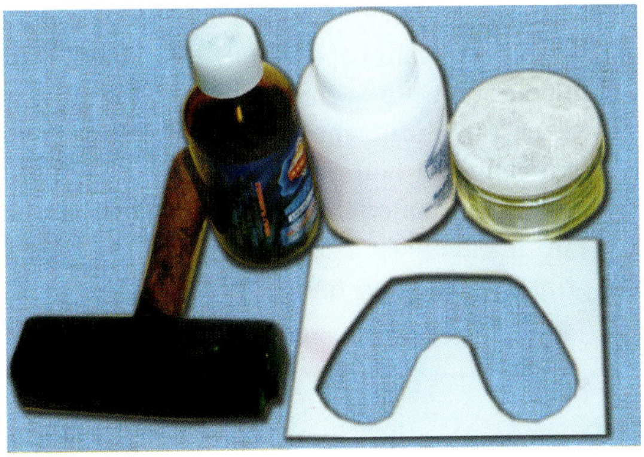

Fig. 6.4: Equipments and materials for preparation of acrylic trays

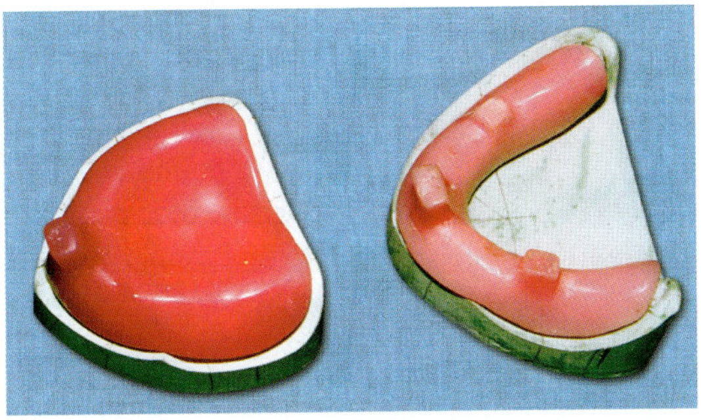

Fig. 6.5: The upper and lower tray on the casts

BOXING AND POURING OF MASTER CASTS

Introduction

Final impression should be poured with dental stone as soon as they are made. The use of dental stone is ideal as it provided sufficient strength without being very difficult to remove from the denture after processing.

Boxing Impression

It is the process of enclosure of an impression to produce the desired size and to form the base of the cast and to preserve desired details. It is usually utilized for pouring the master cast of edentulous ridges.

Wax Boxing

1. This boxing can be used for zinc oxide paste final impressions and also for rubber base as well as plaster impressions of edentulous ridges. A strip of beading wax or soft modeling wax may be used for beading. The wax is rolled into 5 mm diameter rod, long enough to encircle the impression tray.
2. It is wrapped around the tray 5 mm short of the depth of the sulcus and sealed to it by the use of a hot wax knife.
3. A sheet of modeling wax of 12 mm wide is adapted and sealed outside the beading wax to box the impression.

4. The lingual aspect of a mandibular impression is filled with a sheet of modeling wax cut into size and sealed to the wax roll.

Zinc oxide eugenol paste and rubber base impressions need no separating media and they are cast immediately. In case of plaster impression the liquid soap should be applied with a soft camel hair brush to form lather which is then washed off. This is repeated until sheen is visible on the surface of the impression. Soap forms an insoluble calcium deposit by reaction with the plaster which should be washed off.

Pouring of Cast

The cast is poured in dental stone mixed to a water power ratio of 30 cm sq/100 g. Small increments of stone is vibrated into the impression until the stone reaches the top of the box. The cast is allowed to harden for one hour. The cast on removal from the impression is trimmed in the manner similar to the primary cast.

Pumice-Plaster Boxing

1. This method can be utilized with most of impression materials especially for hydrocolloids where wax will not adhere to the impression surface.
2. A mix (1:1) of plaster and pumice is formed into a patty approximately 12 mm thick and the impression is seated into this mix with the tissue side up and horizontal to the table. The mix is then taken up to the level of 3 mm inferior to the buccal borders. For the mandibular impression the lingual side is flattened to form a platform 3 mm inferior to the lingual border. The mix when set is trimmed to form a 3 mm land area around the labial, buccal and lingual borders (Figs 6.6A and B).
3. A thin layer of plasticine (modeling clay) is applied on the whole land areas of the base around the impression (Figs 6.7A and B).
4. The impression is then boxed with boxing wax attached to the vertical wall of the plaster-pumice base with hot wax knife and sticky wax. Dental stone is mixed using appropriate water power ratio and vibrated into the boxed impression till it is filled up (Figs 6.8A to C).
5. After one hour the cast is separated by immersing in hot water to soften zinc oxide impression material.
6. The master cast is trimmed similar to the primary cast (Fig. 6.9).

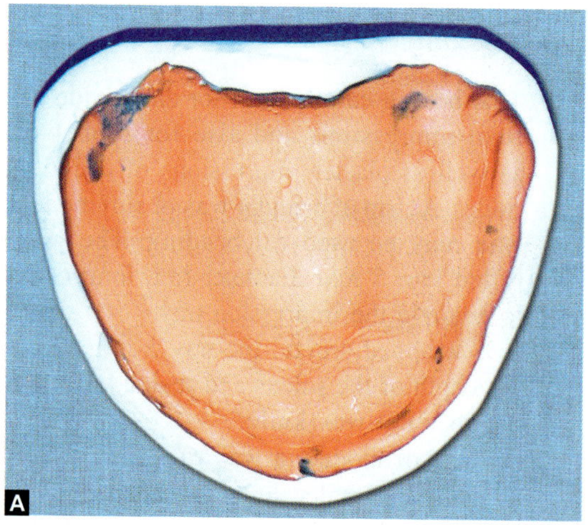

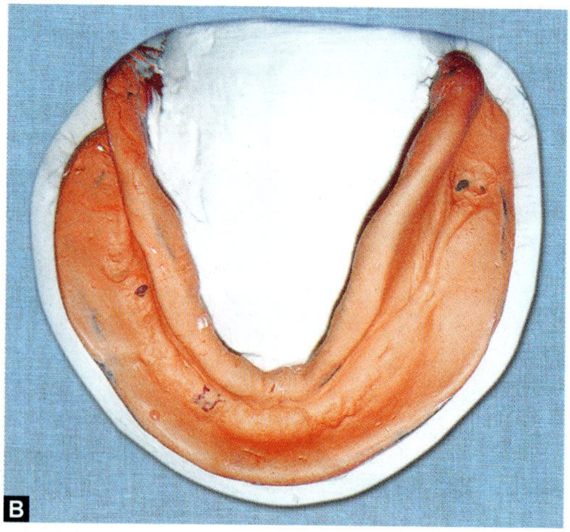

Figs 6.6A and B: (A) Maxillary impression set on plaster-pumice mix; (B) Mandibular impression set on plaster-pumice mix

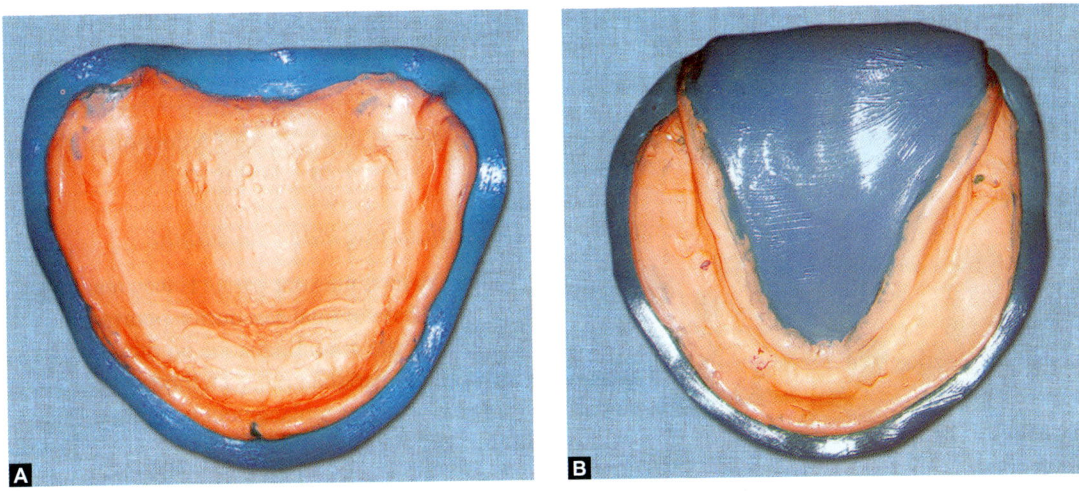

Figs 6.7A and B: (A) Application of modeling clay on plaster border of maxillary cast; (B) Application of modeling clay on plaster border of mandibular cast

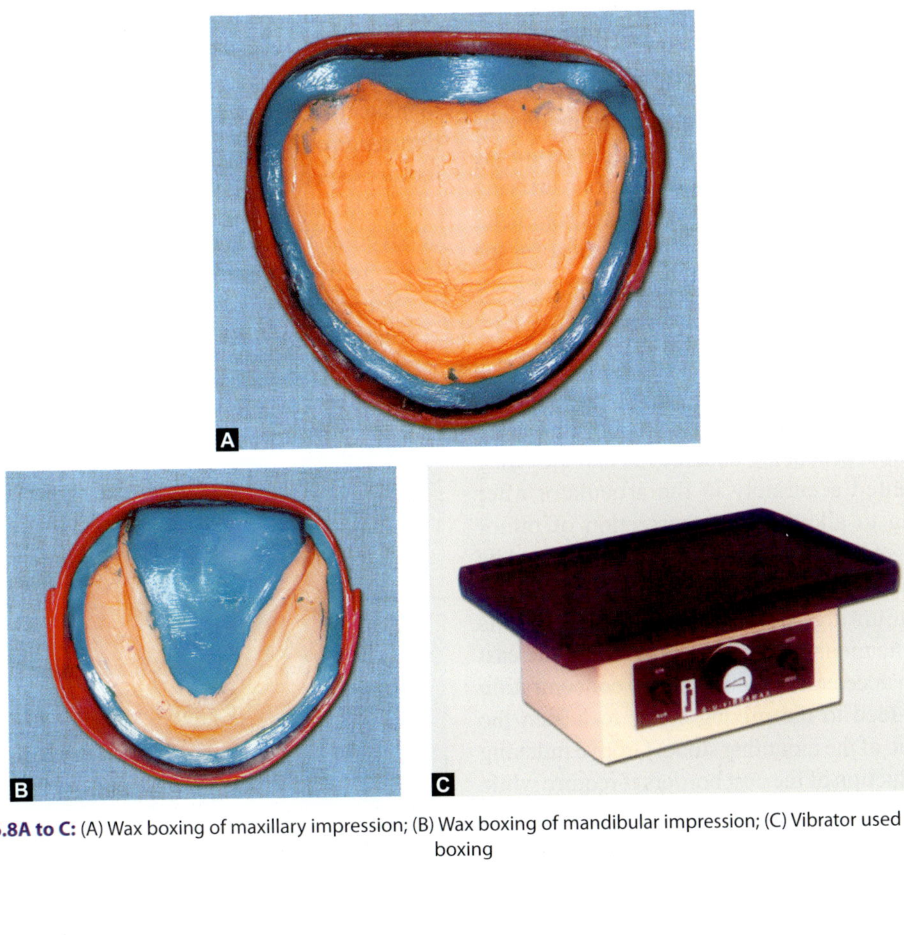

Figs 6.8A to C: (A) Wax boxing of maxillary impression; (B) Wax boxing of mandibular impression; (C) Vibrator used to fill up boxing

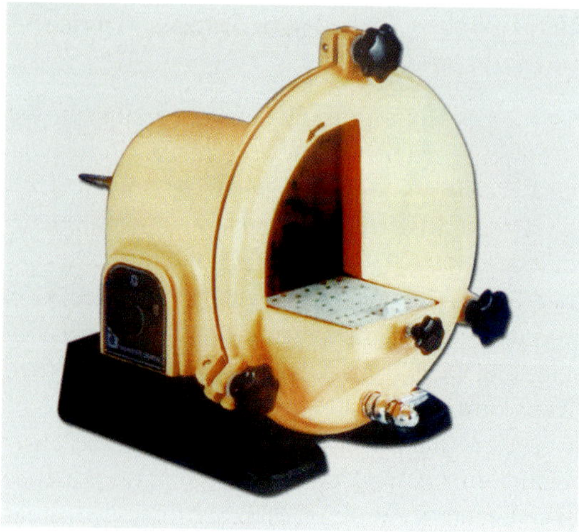

Fig. 6.9: Electric trimmer used to trim cast

Indexing the Cast

Indexing cast prior to mounting in articulator permit removal of the cast and accurate replacement in the articulator. It is helpful in remounting for removing processing errors of a denture and for verifying jaw relation records. Grooves, notches, or metal or plastic remounting plates may be placed in the cast for indexing.

Groove Indexing Method

The bases of the casts are indexed groove with a lathe mounted wheel. It will produce a smooth V-cut without producing undercut so that they may be remounted accurately in the articulator after processing to allow for the correction of minor processing errors. The bases of the casts should be lightly painted with petroleum jelly or soap solution before mounting them in an articulator. This prevents the mounting stone from sticking the cast firmly. An accelerator such as slurry concentration may be added to the mixing water to hasten the setting time of the mounting stone. Groove indexing allows reduction of the cast borders if require while retaining a positive index. It is also possible to avoid index notches in thin areas of the cast.

Notch Indexing Method

The notches are cut in the base of the cast at three or more points to provide positive index. The main disadvantage is that in case of reduction of cast to fit in a flask it will be lost (Fig. 6.10).

Split Remounting Indexing Method

It is done by mounting one part of Hanau remounting plate in the base of final cast during pouring and the other part in the mounting stone on the articulator. It is more precise than other methods and permits rapid removal and replacement of the cast on the articulator.

RECORD BASES AND OCCLUSION RIMS

Introduction

To obtain maximum benefit from a denture, it must be harmonize with the oral environment. Accurate record bases are necessary for correct jaw relation; to make the facebow transfer and record the vertical dimension of occlusion and the centric relation. This requires specific information from the mouth for use in the laboratory. The casts record the details of alveolar ridges but the following information is also required before dentures can be fabricated:

1. *Neutral zone is first determined on cast by anatomical landmarks (Mandibular canine and retromolar pad)*: It is the potential space where the forces between the tongue and cheeks

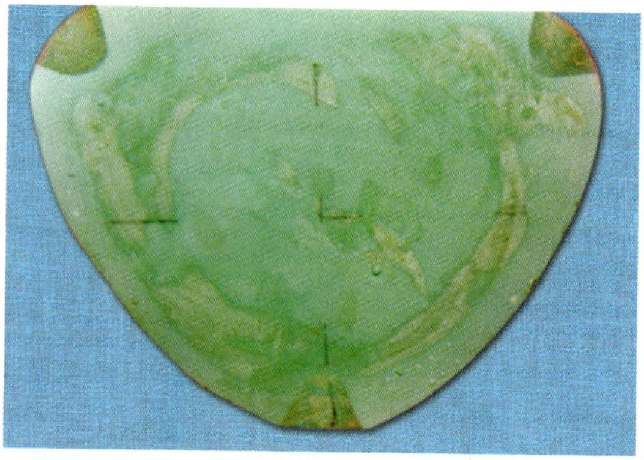

Fig. 6.10: Casts are notched at three widely separated areas

or lips are equal. A line is drawn from the buccal of the retromolar pad to the canine and another from the lingual of the retromolar pad to the canine. The occlusal rim should occupy this space only. The occlusal rim is the blue print for the denture construction within the neutral zone. Sir Wilfred Fish first describe it. He also describe a denture as having three surfaces—an impression, an occlusal and a polished surfaces. Each surface is developed separately within neutral zone.

2. *Centric relation*: The static relationship between maxilla and mandible when the condyles are in their most retruded position in the glenoid fossa at an established vertical dimension.
3. *Vertical dimension*: The distance between alveolar ridges of the maxilla and mandible when in centric relation.
4. *The occlusal plane*: The position and angle of a plane to which the occlusal surfaces of teeth meet.
5. *Labial contour*: The relation between the labial surface of the anterior teeth and lips.
6. *Normal or low lip line*: The rest position of the upper lip.
7. *High lip line*: The position of the upper lip when patient smiles.
8. *Canine or corner lines*: The lines drawn parallel with the pupils of the eyes.

The occlusal rim and base along with its associated information is the functional prescription. It accompanied with a written prescription, both of which are essential when denture is constructed in absence of the patient. The chair side time can be eliminated if the rim is constructed according to the size and shape of the natural dentition. Pre-extraction study casts are helpful for this.

When the correct jaw relations have been established, maxillary and mandibular casts can be correctly oriented on the articulator. The dentures fabricated at this position will function properly and esthetic becomes pleasing.

Record Bases (Base Plate, Temporary Base and Trial Base)

An interim denture base is used to support the record rim material for recording maxillomandibular records.

A record base or base plate is "a temporary form representing the base of a denture which is used for making maxillomandibular (Jaw) relation records and for the arrangement of teeth", for try-in stage and check the accuracy of previous recorded (Keyworth, 1929).

Before making the occlusal rims, the casts should be examined for the following: (a) presence of undercuts, (b) position of the periphery, (c) areas of relief.

a. The presence of undercuts when present will cause breakage of rigid materials as shellac or acrylic or break the cast during withdrawal. Such undercut areas, therefore, need to be blocked out before the base is adapted to the cast.
b. The periphery of the base is placed to fill the depth and width of the sulcus recorded in impression with freedom to the frena to move.
c. When impression is recorded with mucostatic impression material in a patient having prominent midpalatine raphe, the tissues is recorded in undisplaced state, denture made on the cast. When the denture is loaded occlusally in the mouth, the mucosa in the center of the palate will be displaced before the tissues over the ridge. This will cause pain and inflammation of mucosa, and rocking of denture causing loss of retention and fracture of the denture along the midline. The relief will be required.

Requirements of Record Base

When selecting a material for a record base, one should consider the following:

a. Strength and rigidity,
b. Dimensional stability,

c. Ease of fabrication,
d. Cost
e. Color.

a. **Strength and rigidity:** A record base should be rigid so that it is not affected by pressures while the jaw relation registration is made, and as a result a faulty recording transferred to the articulator. So, rigidity of the record base is essential for an accurate record to be registered and transferred.
b. **Dimensional stability:** During the whole course of treatment the record base will be subjected to heat during the laboratory procedures. So, the material selected should be one that will remain stable when subjected to difference of temperatures. Since variable time period is involved in making the dentures, a base material is required that will not distort with time.
c. **Ease of fabrication:** The relative ease of fabrication will reflect the cost of material, ease of manipulation and the final result.
d. **Cost:** A material should be selected for a good performance at a reasonable expense.
e. **Color:** The color of the base should be of the same pink color as the denture base material as it acts as a background when the teeth are seen during the try-in stage. The patient then will be able to see the teeth against their natural background to accept the denture esthetics.

Types of Bases

It is agreed that jaw relations are difficult to record accurately with poorly fitting bases made from material that is subject to distortion and dimensional change. Bases may be temporary or permanent.

Temporary Bases

These are made of shellac or cold-cure acrylic resin. Hard base plate wax is occasionally used but is unsatisfactory as got distorted when kept in the mouth for more than a few minutes. Vacuum formed vinyl or polystyrene are also used.

Permanent Bases

These are made of heat cure acrylic resin and chromium cobalt alloy made on the master cast. This usually causes destruction of the master cast during deflasking. The teeth are attached to them either with cold cure or heat-cure acrylic material. Many prosthodontists believe that it is only by the use of permanent bases that accurate intraoral records can be made and transfer to the articulator. Permanent bases ultimately become part of the complete denture.

Advantages of the Permanent Base

1. The errors in extension and adaptation of the base, due to faulty impression, can be detected and corrected before the denture fabrication is completed.
2. The mandibular movements are more likely to be normal due to better stability and retention making the horizontal relation record easier. This is particularly true in case of a nervous patient.
3. It gives an idea about the comfort, stability, and retention of final prosthetics.

Disadvantages of the Permanent Base

1. The setting of teeth may be difficult on the relatively thick base in case of limited interarch space.
2. It requires considerable time and more expensive.

Record bases are made from several different types of material such as shellac and acrylic resin.

Materials

Shellac

The most commonly used base material is available as flat sheets shaped as upper and lower arches.

The forms are heated in the open flame to soft pliable state after which they can be adapted to the cast with either the fingers or an instrument or a combination of both. The excess can be removed with either scissors or a knife. Shellac bases have the advantage of being inexpensive, uniform in thickness, and rigid. Their disadvantages are that the color is not the same as gingival, they are brittle and break easily, they are difficult to trim and make the periphery smooth. And future heating of the formed tray is likely to result in distortion.

It is a brittle material so reinforced with wires of 12 to 14 gauges. The wire is placed across the posterior edge in maxillary base. It is adapted with the lingual flange. The edges are readapted using pointed flame from Hanau alcohol torch and folded and burnished with No. 7 wax spatula.

Wax

Hard wax (Base plate) adapted on cast dusted with talcum powder and reinforced with ten gauge wire.

Acrylic Resin Base

Types

1. **Autopolymerizing acrylic resin base:** It is prepared by any of the following three methods:
   a. **Sprinkle-on method:** The coating the cast with tinfoil substitute. This is followed by shifting of polymer powder on the cast and saturating it with monomer liquid.
   b. **Adapting method:** The cast is coated with petroleum jelly, and acrylic resin is mixed in a pot. When it attains dough stage, it is rolled into a cigar shape. It is placed on a roller board and rolled to the desired thickness of 2 mm.
2. **Heat cure acrylic resin base:** A wax pattern of requisite thickness is prepared on the cast (3 mm). The flasking, dewaxing and packing with acrylic resin is done. Then curing, deflasking, finishing and polishing will produce a permanent base. In which teeth are attached with heat or cold cure acrylic resin. This base becomes part of the finished denture. The method requires more time and expenses but gives good clinical results and no dimensional changes occur after reprocessing the processed base.
3. **compressed air or vacuum-formed bases:** It can be used to form bases very quickly but it is very expensive and a machine is required for that.
4. **Light cure composite bases:** It can be used within short period but material is very expensive.

Stabilized Base Plate

A base plate lined with a plastic or other material, to improve its stability and adaptation. The materials used are:

a. Zinc oxide eugenol impression paste
b. Light-bodied rubber base impression material
c. Soft denture liner

Fabrication of Autopolymerizing Resin Base Plates

The autopolymerizing resin is the most frequently used material for base plates. It can be used by sprinkle-on method but the undercuts in the cast must be blocked by flowing minimal amount of wax before the resin is applied to the cast. The sprinkle-on method involves the application of a cold mould seal separating medium to the cast, and alternate application of cold-cure acrylic resin powder and monomer to the casts. The resin is applied gradually to build up to the required extent and thickness. It is desirable to keep excess polymer when applying the monomer and polymer, as excess monomer increases dimensional changes. To hasten polymerization and eliminate excess monomer, the cast and base is placed in hot water for 10 minutes. This causes rapid polymerization, and excess monomer is eliminated producing a nonporous base. If a pressure pot is available the cast should be placed in the pot under 30 lbs/sq inch of pressure. The initial separation of the record base and the master cast should be done avoiding damaging the cast. It is done usually by inserting an instrument between the cast and the base at the posterior border. If it cannot be separated with gentle pressure the cast should be placed in hot water to soften the block out wax.

All the peripheries of the record base is smoothened and rounded with a carbide acrylic bur. The areas of excessive thickness are reduced.

The base is polished with pumice slurry and a linen wheel on a dental lathe.

The block out wax is removed from the master cast and fitting surface of the base. The fit of the base is checked for stability.

A record base made by the sprinkle-on method is better than dough methods because they fit more accurately but require more time to fabricate.

Occlusion Rims

Synonyms: Record rim, bile rim.

Definition

An occluding surface built on temporary or permanent denture bases for making maxillomandibular records and teeth arrangement.

Objectives

Occlusion rims serve three purposes

1. To establish the vertical dimension of occlusion
2. To serve as record bases by which the jaw relation records are transferred to the articulator
3. To carry artificial teeth to the mouth for testing esthetics, accuracy of jaw relation records, and for arranging the posterior teeth for balanced occlusion.

Materials

The materials commonly used for fabrication of occlusion rims are base plate wax and modeling compound.

Rules for Fabrication

Record bases and occlusion rims (record blocks) are fabricated after the master casts have been poured and trimmed accurately. These are prepared by the dentist for the technician. Since the success and failure of the dentures is frequently related to the registration of jaw relations and construction of record blocks so, the record block should not be made haphazardly.

Since the accuracy of jaw relation record is essential for success of complete dentures the records should be obtained with processed record bases or temporary stabilized bases which do not allow movement when the records are being made. The wax rims are adapted in the stabilized bases. They should assume the position that the teeth will occupy. They are carried to the mouth and the rims are adjusted for correct lip length of the maxillary rim, and the midline is marked. The mandibular wax rim is adjusted until a tentative occlusal vertical dimension is established.

Laboratory Procedures

- Instruments
- Wax spatula
- Base plate wax
- Separating media
- Cold-cure acrylic resin monomer and polymer
- Carbide acrylic trimmer
- Rubber bowl/Pressure pot
- Lathe, felt wheel and pumice
- Plaster spatula
- Hot plate.

Fabrication of Occlusion Rims

1. A little moltened sticky wax is placed over the crest of the ridge of the base.
2. A half sheet of base plate wax is passed over the flame until soft and pliable throughout and rolled into a rod and its cross-section formed into a 12 mm square by pressing the

wax between finger and thumb of both hands simultaneously.

3. It is again softened and adapted to the alveolar area of the record base. The rim is sealed to the base using a hot spatula. The excess of length posterior is cut off. The labial surface is contoured to blend with the periphery of the base. The occlusion rims are trimmed to the dimensions as below:

Maxillary Rim (Fig. 6.11A)

1 Anteriorly, the occlusion rim should be 20 mm from the periphery of the base lateral to the labial frenum and posteriorly, at the molar area 16 to 18 mm high and 10 mm anterior to the hamular notch (Fig. 6.12). The buccal surface is contoured at the posterior part distal to the canine slightly, towards the palate to create space between the buccal surfaces of the posterior teeth and the cheeks. The space should also be provided over the alveolar tubercles which should not be occupied by a tooth.
2. The width of the rim anteriorly should be 6 mm (Fig. 6.13). The width of incisal edge seldom exceeds 3 mm but the relationship between the upper and lower anterior teeth can vary greatly. That is why the rim width is increased to allow upper and lower rims to contact during jaw relation recording.
3. The width of the posterior rim should be 8 to 10 mm to ensure contact with the lower rim.
4. The labial surface of the rim should be 10 mm anterior to the posterior end of the incisive papilla (Fig. 6.13).
5. The center of the occlusal rim in the posterior region should be 2–3 mm buccal to the center of the alveolar ridge.
6. The rim is tapered to the base at the distal part of tuberosity. This prevents the interference with the lower rim.
7. The side walls of the occlusal rim should be 90° angle with the occlusal surface up to the level of the crest of alveolar ridge, then gradually slopes towards the sulcus or palate. This allows spaces for tongue and buccal corridor.

Mandibular Rim (Fig. 6.11B)

1. The lower rim should be even with the center of the retromolar pad and parallel with the mean plane of the residual ridge.
2. The height of the mandibular occlusal rim in anterior region should be approximately 16 mm from the sulcus through the rim.

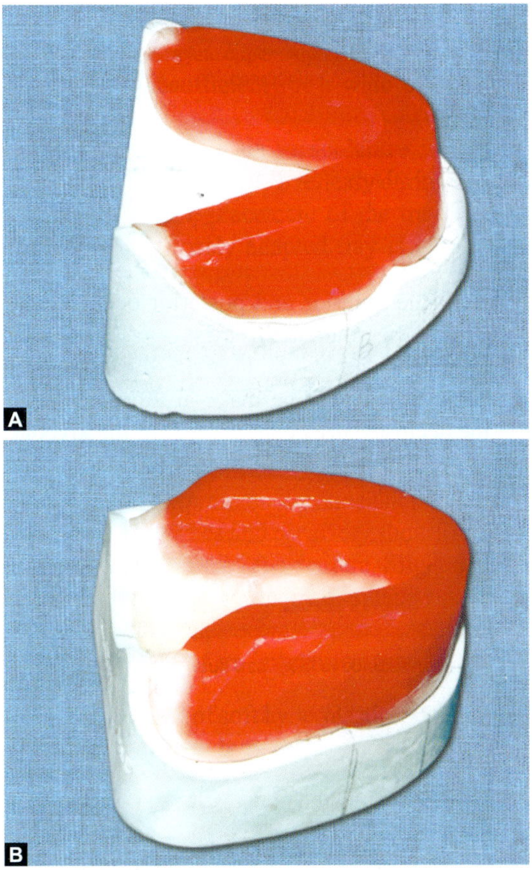

Figs 6.11A and B: Occlusion rims are constructed in the laboratory following general guidelines and then individualized as a chairside procedure

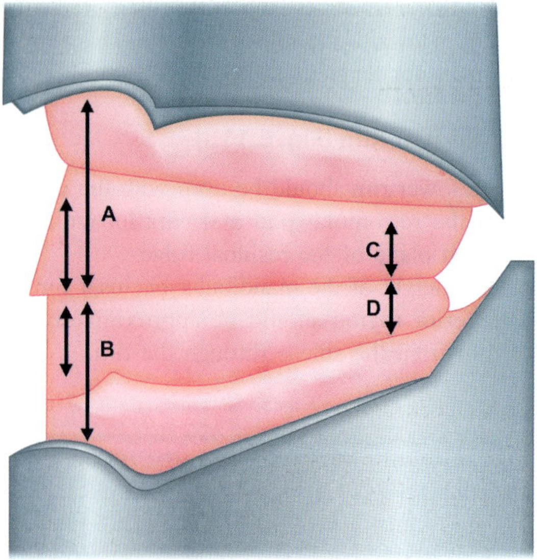

Fig. 6.12: Dimensions of maxillary and mandibular occlusal rims (A: 20–22 mm, B: 16–17 mm, C: 6–7 mm, D: 3–6 mm)

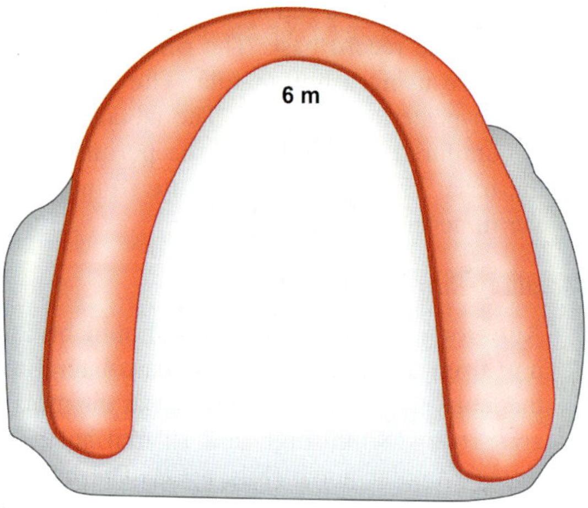

Fig. 6.13: Maxillary rim width

3. Both the anterior and posterior occlusal rim should be placed directly over the lower alveolar ridge.
4. The walls should be make at 90° angle with the occlusal surface up to level of the alveolar ridge, and then flare towards the buccal and lingual sulci.

BIBLIOGRAPHY

1. Academy of Prothodontics: Glossary of Prosthodontic Terms, 6th edn. J Prothet Dent. 1994;71:41-112.
2. Elinger CW, Rayson JH, Terry JM, Rahn AO. Synopsis of complete dentures, Lea and Febiger; 1975.
3. Heartwell CM Jr, Rahn AO. Textbook of Complete Dentures, 5th edn, BC Decker, inc; 2002.

Chapter 7

Articulators and Facebows

ARTICULATORS

Definition

The articulator is a mechanical instrument that represented the temporomandibular joints and jaws, to which maxillary and mandibular casts may be attached to simulate some or all mandibular movements.

Parts of Articulators

The following parts are usually found in an articulator (Fig. 7.1):

1. Upper member
2. Lower member
3. Condylar guidance
4. Incisal pin
5. Incisal guide

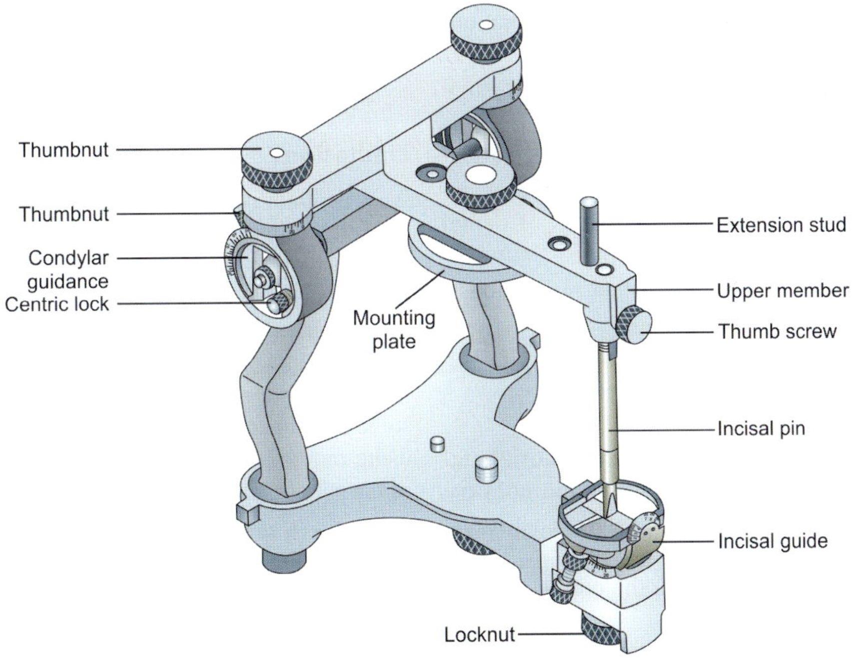

Fig. 7.1: The Hanau arc on H_2 articulator
(*Courtesy:* Teledyne Hanau, Buffalo, New York, USA)

6. Extension stud
7. Mounting plate.

Purpose of an Articulator

The purposes of an articulator are:

1. To orient the upper and lower casts in the same positional relationship as that of the human teeth and to reproduce the center-relation position.
2. To simulate mandibular movements. Three basic registrations are acquired from the patient and transferred to the articulator:
   a. Facebow, to relate the maxilla to the hinge axis.
   b. Maxillomandibular record to relate the mandibular cast to the maxillary cast.
   c. Eccentric registration to set the condylar controls of the articulator, e.g. protrusive, and left, right lateral records.

Uses of Articulators

1. The articulators are used in absence of the patient to facilitate fabrication of restorations outside the patient's mouth.
2. To diagnose occlusal conditions both in natural and artificial dentition.
3. To perform treatment planning, and patient presentation.
4. To fabricate the occlusal surfaces of dental appliances.
5. To correct and modify finished restorations.

Requirements of an Articulator

Minimum Requirements

1. The articulator should accept a horizontal axis transfer (facebow transfer) and hold the correct horizontal relationships, i.e. centric and eccentric relations.
2. It should hold the casts in the correct vertical relationships.
3. It should be able to perform open and close hinge movement.
4. It should be rigid in construction.
5. It should have an incisal guide pin and table.
6. It must have independent adjustable condylar paths and be able to accept protrusive record to set it.
7. The average person must be capable of handling it.
8. It should be reasonably priced.

Additional Requirements

1. The condylar elements should the part of the lower member and condylar guides as the part in upper member.
2. The condylar guides should be adjustable in three dimension.
3. There should be provisions for Bennett movements.
4. The incisal guide table should be adjustable in frontal and sagittal planes.
5. There should be a terminal hinge position locking device.
6. It should be provided with a third reference point relator.
7. It should have an adjustable intercondylar distance facility.

Limitations

An articulator is a mechanical instrument made up of metal with and plastic parts. It is subjected to error in tooling, and to error resulting from metal fatigue and wear. It is not possible for an articulator to duplicate all movements of temporomandibular joint. It is evident that articulator may not reproduce the intraborder and functional movements and some adjustments should be done in the mouth. But using mouth as an articulator also has limitations as the patients saliva, tongue and cheeks, and compressible tissues under the dentures will create problems in denture adjustments. So, a properly mounted casts on articulator is essential for better visualization of patient's occlusion especially from the lingual side which is essential for developing proper occlusion.

Classification

Articulators have been classified in the following ways:

Articulators Classification Based on Function (University of Michigan in 1972)

Class I: Simple holding instruments capable of accepting a single static registration with possible vertical motion, e.g. Barndoor articulator, Hinge articulator.

Class II: Instrument that permit horizontal as well as vertical motion but do not orient the motion to the temporomandibular joint (TMJ) via facebow transfer as:

1. Eccentric motion permitted is based on average or arbitrary values, e.g. Grittman articulator, Gysi adaptable articulator, Gysi simplex articulator (Figs 7.2 and 7.3).
2. Eccentric motion permitted is based on theories of arbitrary motion, e.g. Manson articulator (1914).
3. Eccentric motion permitted is determined by the patient using engraving methods, e.g. House articulator (1927).

Class III: Instruments that simulate condylar pathways by using mechanical equivalent for all or part of motion and allow facebow transfer.

1. Instruments that accept static lateral protrusive registration and use equivalents for the rest of motion, e.g. Hanau H_2, Dentatus.
2. Instruments that accept static lateral protrusive registrations and use equivalents for the rest of motion, e.g. Truebyte articulator, Stanberry articulator, Ney's articulator, Hanau 130-21. Teledyne articulator, Panadent articulator.

Class IV: Instruments that accept three-dimensional dynamic registrations with facebow, e.g. TMJ instrument of Kenneth Swanson.

1. The cams representing condylar paths are formed by registrations engraved by the patient.
2. The condylar paths can be angled and customized, e.g. Denar articulator, Staurt articulator.

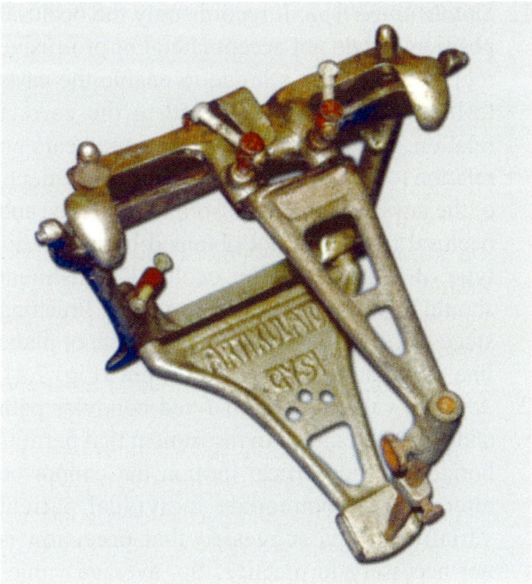

Fig. 7.2: The Gysi simplex articulator

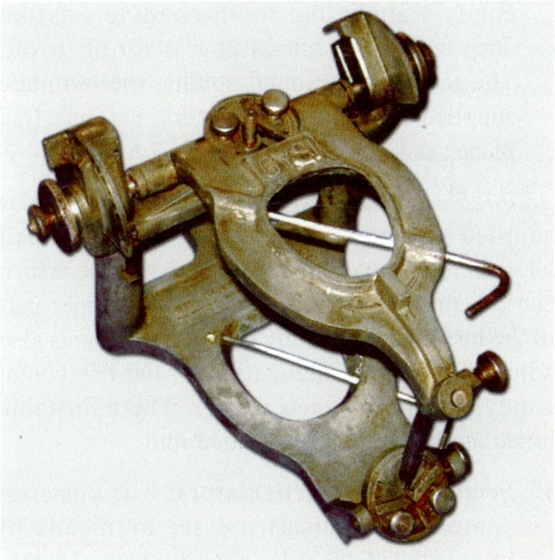

Fig. 7.3: The Gysi truebite articulator

Articulators Classification Based on Adjustability

Nonadjustable articulators: Articulators are divided into two classes based on their design as follows:

1. *Simple hinge type*: It records only the occlusal position and do not accept lateral or protrusive registration. It has a hinge to enable the casts to be separated and returned to the correct relation. The movement of the hinge bears no relation to the opening and closing movements of the jaws. The freedom from interference and occlusal balance is not obtained by using this type of articulator. The occlusal adjustment should be made either at the try-in or finishing stage in the patient's mouth, e.g. hinge or plane line articulator without incisal pin (Fig. 7.4).
2. Average value type with fixed condylar path and incisal inclines. An instrument that permits horizontal and vertical motion but cannot be altered to accommodate individual patient variations. It is suggested that precision is not necessary in practice. So, average values for condyle angle and tooth-condyle relations are used in these articulators. Using a fixed condyle angle and tooth-condyle relation cusp teeth must lateral curves for all cases. The teeth are arranged against the template supplied with such articulators, e.g. ash free plane, and Gysi simplex (Fig. 7.5).

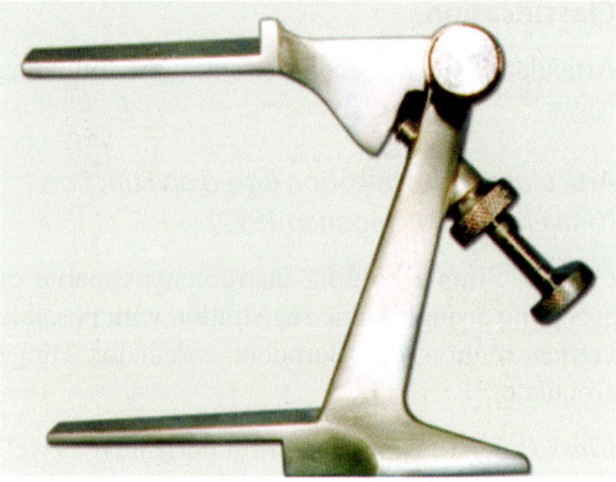

Fig. 7.4: The simple hinge a plane line articulator

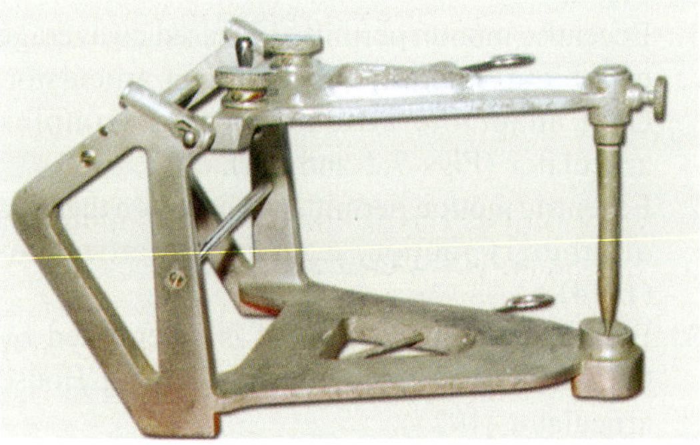

Fig. 7.5: The free plane average value articulator

Adjustable articulators: These instruments can be adjusted to accept records from the patient. All have an adjustable sagittal condylar guide which can be attached to either the lower or upper part of the instrument. In many the incisal guide is also adjustable and the inclination of the horizontal condylar path (Bennett angle). The adjustable articulators are further classified into:

1. **Semiadjustable articulators:** The posterior control mechanisms are set by means of interocclusal records, e.g Dentatus, Hanau, Whip-Mix articulators (Figs 7.6 to 7.8).
2. **Highly adjustable articulators:** The posterior condylar control mechanisms are set in three plane of motion and accept kinematic facebow transfer, e.g. Denar, Stuart articulators.
   These instruments simulate the movements of the mandible with the greatest accuracy both in the direction and form of movement from the

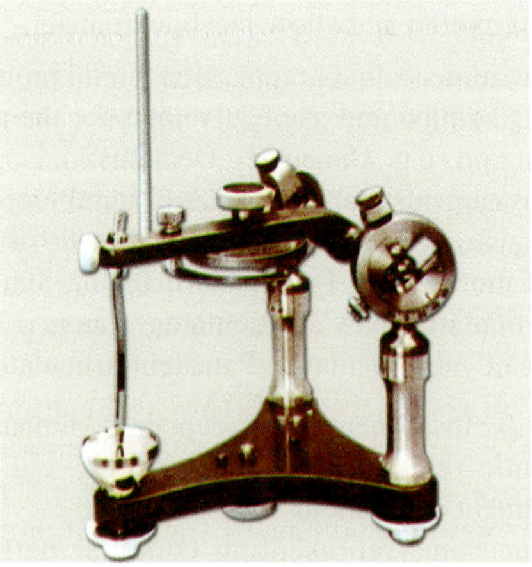

Fig. 7.6: The Dentatus AR series articulator

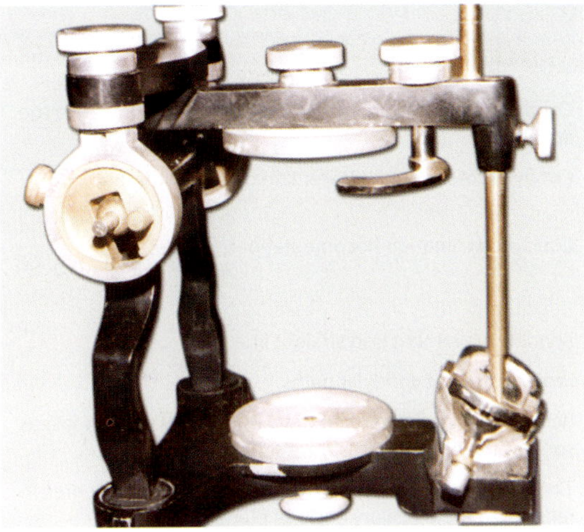

Fig. 7.7: Hanau H_2 articulator

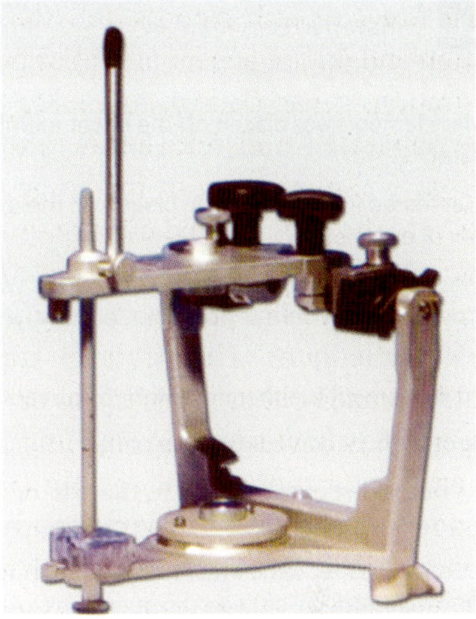

Fig. 7.8: The Whip-Mix articulator
(*Courtesy:* Whip-Mix Corp, Louisville, Kentucky, USA)

point of initiation to the point of termination, e.g. Stuart and Denar articulators.

Adjustable articulators are also classified according to the design of their posterior control mechanisms: Arcon and nonarcon (Table 7.1).

1. **Arcon articulators:** Articulators having the condylar path elements attached to the upper jaw member and condylar element in lower member. The word "arcon" is derived from the combined words "articulator" and "condyle", e.g. Hanau arcon H_2, Whip-Mix, Panadent. Arcon articulators are with either straight or curved condylar guidance pathway, e.g. Hanau and Whip-Mix has straight condylar guidance, hence, the use of the term condyle angle; Panadent' articulator has curved condylar guidance.
2. **Nonarcon articulators:** The nonarcon articulators have the condylar paths attached to the lower jaw member, and the condylar elements attached to the upper member. They are only available with straight condylar guidance pathways, e.g. Hanau H_2, Dentatus.

Description of Various Types of Articulators

Simple Hinge Articulator

It is the most simple form of articulator and consists of an upper and lower arm or bow to which casts are attached. The arms are capable of only opening and closing movements through a hinge, which bears no relation to the hinge axis of the patient. A stop and a screw, is used to fix the distance of the hinge movement so that, correct vertical relationship is maintained. Due to its limitations it is used in cases of where only a few occlusal surfaces are reproduced, like an inlay, a crown, a partial dentures with short span and when patient's jaw movement is only limited to chopping. It can be used in complete denture construction only when cuspless or inverted cusp teeth are used with template based on monsoon curve or when functionally generated path technique is utilized.

Average Value Articulator

The average value articulator is capable of lateral and protrusive movements in addition to its hinge

Table 7.1 Difference between arcon and nonarcon

Arcon	Nonarcon
1. Condylar elements are placed on the lower member of the articulator.	1. Condylar elements are placed on the upper member of the articulator.
2. Condylar fossae (mechanical) are placed on the upper arm/ member of articulator.	2. Condylar fossae on the lower arm of articulator.
3. Condylar inclination remains the same when wax wafers used to transfer terminal positions of condyles to the articulator.	3. Condylar inclination become steeper.
4. Bennett movement is either in straight or curved line.	4. Bennett movement is in straight line.
5. Provide straight or curved condylar paths.	5. Provide straight condylar paths.
6. Relationship of the maxillary cast to the axis orbital plane remains constant when the opposing casts are separated.	6. Relationship of the casts to the axis—orbital plane is lost as soon as the opposing casts are separated.
7. angulation of the mechanical fossa a is fixed in relation to the maxillary occlusal plane between an open and close position.	7. The angulation of the mechanical fossa changes 8 degree in relation to the maxillary occlusal plane.
8. Popular in fixed prosthodontics because the upper and lower member easily detachable for waxing and is more accurate.	8. Popular in complete denture prosthodontics because the upper and lower members are rigidly attached making the arrangement of the teeth easy.

movement. The lateral and protrusive movements are fixed at 30 degrees to the horizontal and incisal guidance is fixed to 10 to 15 degrees. So, it cannot be programmed to the individual patient's need. They are popular for their simplicity and low cost and less chair side time required. The denture fabricated on this articulator may not provide with the chewing efficiency and intraoral occlusal adjustment is required along with the development of patient's neuromuscular ability to control the denture during function.

Semiadjustable Articulator

Articulator of this type accepts a facebow transfer and the posterior control mechanisms are set by means of interocclusal positional records. Articulators of this class are the Hanau, the Dantatus, and the Whip-Mix:

1. **Hanau model H_2:** The Hanau H_2 articulator is a nonarcon type with the condylar guidance controls attached to the lower member of the articulator. It has a fixed intercondylar distance of 110 mm and does accept a facebow transfer. The horizontal condylar inclinations are set by protrusive interocclusal record.

   The amount of Bennett movement is calculated from the horizontal condylar inclinations and the vertical condylar posts are rotated accordingly to adjust lateral condylar inclinations.

   Bennett's angle (L) = (H/8) + 12 where his horizontal condylar inclination is 30 degree. l = 30/12 = 15.75 or 16°.

   The mechanical incisal guide table is adjustable both in sagittal and frontal planes. This articulator accepts facebow transfer.
2. **Dentatus:** The horizontal condylar inclination are set by protrusive interocclusal record. The Bennett angle on both sides are set by left and right lateral records. The incisal pin has an arc in it so that, closure can be made without changing the central position.
3. **Whip-Mix articulator:** This articulator use a ear-piece facebow so there is no measurement and marking of skin is needed. The horizontal condylar record are set by protrusive record. The Bennett angles on both sides are set

by left and right lateral records. The upper and lower members are separate because the condylar spheres are not fixed in the condylar housing by an axle.

Highly Adjustable Articulator

Denar Articulator

It is an arcon type and most popular highly adjustable articulator. As it has plastic guides in its condylar guidance instead of metal guide it can easily adjusted to follow precisely a pantographic tracing.

Selection of Articulator for Complete Dentures

The articulators available for complete denture fabrication vary from nonadjustable to highly adjustable articulator. The very simple articulators, the average value and simple plane line, do not locate any hinge axis from the patient and cannot receive precentric records effectively. At the other end the highly adjustable articulator will provide the nearest equivalent to the patient, with curved condylar guides, immediate and progressive side shifts, accurate intercondylar width and true hinge axis.

The highly adjustable articulator is not suitable for edentulous patients because the resiliency of the soft tissues; causes movement of the bases preventing accurate (pantographic) recording of the true path of movement of the bone. The movement of the dentures on their supporting tissues exceeds the fine adjustment capabilities of the articulator.

The most practical type of instrument is the semiadjustable articulator and its associated facebow. There are several excellent instruments available and the choice largely depends on personal choice. There is Dentatus ARH, Hanau H_2, and Whip-Mix 8300 articulator. The first two are nonarcon type and extensively used in complete denture fabrication, and later is used for fixed prosthesis. A highly adjust able articulator is usually used when extensive occlusal scheme is to be developed at one time in case of atypical mandibular movement.

Mounting of Casts on the Articulator

The ways in which casts are mounted on the articulator will affect the accuracy of the reproduction of the mandibular movement.

Hinge articulator: On a hinge articulator the casts are placed arbitrarily. The cast is mounted in the middle of the articulator with the occlusal plane parallel to the floor with plaster (10 mm) above and below the casts to hold them with upper and lower arms.

Fixed condylar path/fixed guide articulators: The occlusal rim is set on the plane indicated from the incisal pin to a cross bar at the back of the articulator. This orients the casts to the Bonewill's triangle.

Semiadjustable articulators: The correct location of the casts is effected by the use of a facebow. The maxillary cast is first mounted on the articulate with facebow record. The procedure is known as facebow transfer. The mandibular cast is mounted after recording the vertical dimension of occlusion and centric jaw relation. The methods are described in detail in chapter of Jaw Relations.

Highly adjustable articulators: It is done by locating the kinematic hinge axis, developing pantographic tracing and mounting the cast.

FACEBOWS

History

The history of facebow dates back to 1860, when Bonewil come out with his theory that 10 cm was a standard distance from the lower median incisal point to each condylar center. Snow (1899) was first to prove a facebow. He attempts to give the occlusal plane an individual positioning in the third dimension. He set the bite fork so that, the handle of the fork is parallel with a plane expanding from the bottom of the glenoid fossa to the anterior nasal spine (upper part of the tragus to the lower edge of the nostril). This is known as the Bromell or Camper's plane. Gysi used a similar plane which he called "the prosthetic plane". The most recent orientation has been to a plane that corresponds to the Frankfort plane with the help of infraorbital pointer which touches the lowest point of the infraorbital ridge. Snow introduced a facebow in 1907, which is known as Snow facebow. The most of the modern facebow are modified. Varities of Snows facebow.

Definitions

1. "The facebow is a caliper-like device used to record the relationship of the jaws to the temporomandibular joints or opening axis of the jaws and orient the casts in this same relationship to the opening axis of the articulator" (Boucher).
2. The facebow is defined in glossary of prosthodontic terms as "a caliper-like instrument used to record the spatial relationship of the maxillary arch to some anatomic reference point or points and then transfer this relationship to an articulator; it orients the dental cast in the same the relationship to the opening axis of the articulator. Customarily, the anatomical references are the mandibular condyles transverse axis and selected anterior point" (GPT-7). It is also known as hinge-bow.

Purpose of the Facebow

It is used to record the patient's maxilla and hinge axis relationship in three-dimensions, i.e. anteroposterior, lateral and vertical and to transfer the relationship to the articulator during the mounting of the maxillary cast. By accurately mounting the cast with the help of facebow, the mandibular movements of the patient can be simulated on the articulator.

The rotational axis of the mandible which are responsible for mandibular movements are:

1. Hinge axis: It is defined in the glossary of prosthodontic terms as "an imaginary line around which the mandible may rotate within the sagittal plane".

   When the mandible opens and closes, rotation occurs around a transverse axis it is commonly called *hinge axis*. This axis is called the' *terminal hinge axis* when the mandible rotates while in centric relation. The pure hinge like motion occurs only with 10 to 11° having a range of 18 to 25 mm.
2. Two vertical axis which passes through each condyle around which the mandible rotates in a lateral direction.

   Controversy exists regarding the presence of a single hinge axis, methods and validity of records which made the relation of the terminal hinge axis and centric relation.

Opinion of Different Schools of Thought on Hinge Axis

1. The first school of thought (McCollum, Stuart, Lucia) said that the hinge axis definitely exists and it should be located accurately.
2. The second school of thought says that the accurate location of the terminal hinge axis can be obtained but the benefits offered by doing so are not worth the extra effort required. Craddock stated that absolute location of the terminal hinge axis is of academic interest only and the true hinge axis is no more than a few millimeters away from the arbitrary one.
3. The third school of thought is the nonbeliever in hinge axists. They claimed that the axis exists in theory and not in reality. They argued that within a range of 2 mm many points exist and any one of them could be the point of rotation. So, a single hinge axis theory failed.
4. The fourth school came out with the concept of split axis theory. Trapozzan and Lazzan showed that the terminal hinge axis mark on one side of the face is higher than that on the other side. This fact was confirmed by Walker who said that very few people have the hinge

axis at the same point on both sides. So, each condyle rotates individually producing two axes, one for each condyle, both parallel to each other and perpendicular to the path of opening and closing of the mandible.

All controversies of hinge axis theories were put to rest by Aul and Stllart who on the basis of their work in 1963, disapproved the split axis theory and came to the conclusions that:

1. A horizontal imaginary line does exist connecting the two condyles at their horizontal rotational centers.
2. The terminal hinge axis exists in that position of the mandible when it is in its most posterior position and exists only for initial opening movement.
3. An arbitrary point of location of hinge axis fails to satisfy the requirements of path of closure.

These conclusions were further confirmed by Preston in 1979 who said that a single axis does exist and can be located.

Use of Facebow

The facebow transfer is a controversial issue which gives rise to two schools of thought. Some prosthodontists who believed in balanced occlusion use articulator and recommend facebow while others who do not believe in balanced occlusion and find facebow as unnecessary for complete denture fabrication. They recommend mounting of cast according to an average value technique by aligning the occlusal plane of the bite rim horizontally using a rubber band so that the apex of the Bonewill's triangle coincides with the middle point. They claimed that there is no proof of clinical superiority of facebow use over the simple average technique of cast mounting.

Some dentists think that the facebow is not necessary under the following conditions:

1. When cuspless teeth and monoplane occlusion scheme is selected.
2. Articulators used are not designed to accept a facebow transfer.
3. Balanced occlusion is not required.
4. Interocclusal check records to verify the jaw relation records are made with minimum thickness.

But many dentists recommended facebow because of following reasons:

1. An average location of hinge axis provides a more accurate placement of casts on the articulator than by simply placing them arbitrarily.
2. Facebow transfer allows for minor changes in the vertical dimension at the wax try-in without making a new centric registration.
3. The vertical dimension may change as a result of waxing, flasking, processing and mounting procedures.
4. The movements of the articulator simulate the patient's jaw movements.
5. The arranged teeth would function more accurately.
6. If the jaw relation record is made with increased vertical dimension, the articulator closes more accurately when the jaw relation record is removed.

Necessity of Facebow

1. The facebow transfer is required for analyzing and studying the occlusion of natural teeth.
2. It is an essential part of fabrication of complete dentures. A facebow transfer should be used when:
   a. Cusped posterior teeth are used.
   b. Balanced occlusion in eccentric positions is desired.
   c. Interocclusal check records are used for verification of jaw relations.
   d. The occlusal vertical dimension has to be changed. When hinge axis is determined by arbitrary method, the adjustment of vertical dimension can be done up to + or –3 mm.

3. It is also used in fabrication of fixed and partial denture when a definite cusp fossa or cusp tip to cusp incline relation is required.

   Although a correct centric occlusion position can be developed on an articulator without a facebow transfer record, when any adjustment of vertical dimension (decrease or increase common with complete dentures) or accuracy in lateral and protrusive movements (many patients do) is required then a facebow is a must.

Parts of Basic Facebow

A basic facebow consists of the following parts:

1. U-shaped metal (Duralium-Alloy of Aluminium) frame that fits around the face, keeping 2–3 inches away from it.
2. A bite-fork that is attached to the occlusal rim and acts as a support for bow, the occlusal rims and the casts during mounting procedures. It can be attached to the facebow by means of locknut.
3. Condylar rods are graduated rods on both sides of the bow and may be adjusted and fixed to it by means of thumb screws. The rods bear nylon ear pieces at the inner sides to location of posterior reference points.
4. An orbital pointer attaches to the facebow by means of thumb nut.

Types of Facebow

There are many facebows but mainly depending upon method of recording they are of two main types—arbitrary and kinematic (Table 7.2).

Arbitrary Facebow

They are based on an average location of the hinge axis and produce an error of 2 mm or less in majority of patients, e.g. Hanau facebow. The arbitrary facebow although not accurate as the kinematic facebow, is more commonly used and considered to be adequate for complete denture fabrication. It is due to the movement of the maxillary denture on its soft tissue foundation which causes changes in its relation to the hinge axis. Moreover, the use of the arbitrary facebow is simple and requires less time. The difficulty in attaching the lower occlusal rim to the edentulous mandible prevents the use of kinematical face for edentulous cases. The arbitrary facebows are of two types: facia type and earpiece type.

Facia type: The facia type arbitrary facebow recording can be made by placing the condylar rods on the marked arbitrary location of terminal hinge axis on face. Arbitrary rotational centers are generally located 13 cm anterior to the distal edge of tragus on a line drawn from the outer canthus of the eye to the superoinferior center of the tragus of the ear in both sides of the face, e.g. Hanau H_2, dentatus (Fig. 7.9).

Earpiece type: This type uses external auditory meatus for locating the arbitrary rotational center by placing earpiece attached to the condylar rod in it in both sides of the mouth. This position is 6 mm posterior to the condyles and compensated for attaching the facebow 6 mm anterior to the condyles on the articulator during mounting procedure. The

Table 7.2 Difference between arbitrary and kinematic facebow

Arbitrary	Kinematic
Approximate recording	Precise recording
Condylar rods placed near its rotational axis	Condylar rods placed accurately over its rotational axis
Bite fork attached to maxillary occlusal rim	Bite fork is attached to mandibular occlusal rim
Used for complete denture fabrication	Used for fixed or removable partial dentures and occlusal reconstruction
Can be used with semiadjustable articulator without extendible shafts	Can be used with semiadjustable articulator with extendible shafts only

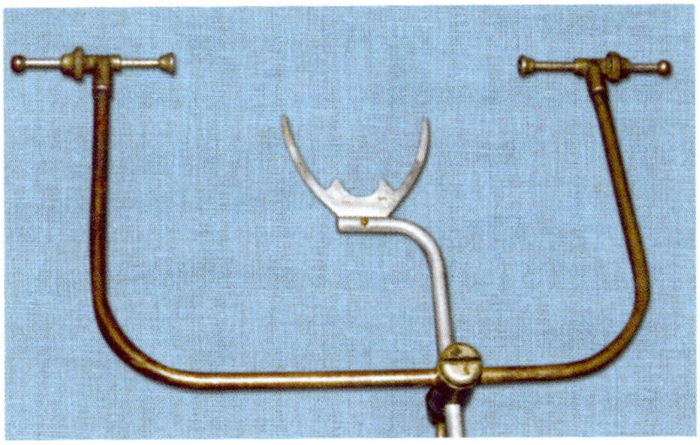

Fig. 7.9: The Hanau arbitrary facebow

plane of orientation is established for both types using a third anatomical reference point either infraorbital notch or the nasion. Most modern facebows are usually ear-piece type. Instead of arbitrary determining the position of the condyles and placing the facebow condylar pins over these points, the external auditory meatus is used to position the condylar pins. Locating pins are present on the articulator behind the condylar balls which correspond to the position of the external auditory meatus. The ear-bows are easier to use than facia bow and can be used single handed, e.g. Hanau earpiece, Whip-Mix, and Denar Slidematic facebows (Fig. 7.10).

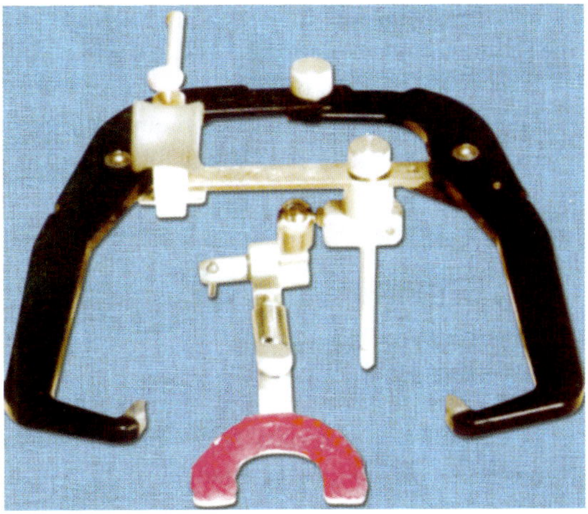

Fig. 7.10: Whip-Mix ear pet nasion relator and the quick mouth facebow with scale to determine the intercondylar width (*Courtesy:* Whip-Mix Corp, Louisville, Kentucky, USA)

Kinematic or Hinge Axis Facebow

The kinematic facebow or hinge axis bow is designed to locate the center of rotation at the true hinge axis points of the patient during opening and closing movements of the mandible and transfer the cast to the articulator in accurate relation to these points.

When the condylar styli move in an arc it is attached to a clutch, which in turn attaches to the mandibular teeth. The fork of the kinematic face is attached to the mandibular occlusal rim. The patient opens and closes the jaws, and dentist observes the movement of the condylar rods. When the points of the condylar rods rotate only and do not translate, these points are on the opening axis of the jaw. The points are marked on the skin as true hinge axis.

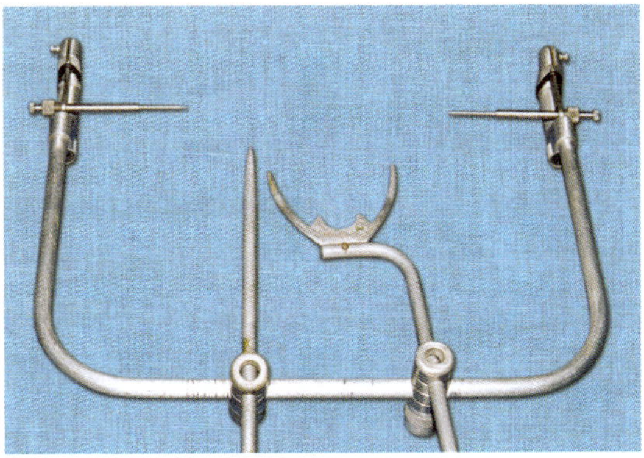

Fig. 7.11: The Hanau kinematic facebow

The mandibular clutch is detached and the facebow is attached to the maxillary rim. The maxillary cast can be related to this axis and transferred to the same axis of the articulator. This type of facebow works properly in presence of natural mandibular teeth to stabilize the clutch. This type of facebow is not used for complete denture fabrication due to the resiliency of soft tissues that causes instability of the mandibular base to locate the hinge axis almost impossible (Fig. 7.11).

The facebow record is not considered as a maxillomandibular relation record, as this record is made for orientation of cast to the articulator.

Different types of articulator require different types of facebow but the philosophy for use is same.

CONCLUSION

1. Due to the presence of soft tissue "realff" arbitrary facebow is sufficient for complete denture fabrication.
2. For most of the complete denture patient facebow transfer results better than arbitrary mounting in Bonewill's triangle.
3. An average value articulator may also be used with a transfer facebow for routine complete denture construction due to "realff".
4. A semiadjustable articulator should be used for analysis of a patients' natural occlusion. It should also be used for building occlusal surfaces of a fixed or removable partial denture prosthesis to harmonize with the natural dentition exhibiting canine guidance or group function. Kinematic facebow produces better results than arbitrary facebow in these situations.
5. If a patient had consistent problems with complete dentures or had a gross skeletal abnormality, the facebow registration of the maxillary rim allow for a more accurate location of the cast on the articulator.

BIBLIOGRAPHY

1. Bergstrom B. On reproduction of dental articulation by means of adjustable articulators. Acta Otodont. Canal. 1950;9:671.
2. Christiansen RL. Rationale of the facebow in maxillary cast mounting. J Prosthet Dent. 1959;9(3):388-98.
3. Rohn HO, Heartwell CM. Textbook of Complete Dentures, Philadelphia, Lea and Febriger; 1993.
4. Weinberg LA. An Evaluation of Base Articulator. J Prosthet Dent. 1963;19:622-64.
5. Weinberg LA. An Evaluation of Facebow Mounting. J Prosthet Dent. 1961;11:32-42.
6. Zarb GA, Bolender CL, Carlsson EG. Boucher's prosthodontic treatment for edentulous patients (11th edn). Mosby, St Louis; 1997.

Chapter 8

Jaw Relations and Methods of Registration

JAW RELATIONSHIP

- Synonyms
- Maxillomandibular relationship.

Definition

Any spatial relationship of the maxillae to the mandible is maxillomandibular relation; any one of the infinite relationships of the mandible to the maxillae (GPT-9).

Any one of many relations of the mandible to the maxillae is one maxillomandibular relation, such as centric maxillomandibular relation, eccentric maxillomandibular relation.

The term 'maxillomandibular relations' would be more appropriate than the term 'jaw relationship'.

JAW RELATIONSHIP RECORD

Definition

A registration of any positional relationship of the mandible relative to the maxillae is known as maxillomandibular record. These records may be made at any vertical, horizontal or orientation relations (GPT-9).

The jaw relation record is more commonly known as "Recording the Bite". The mandible is capable of three-dimensional (directional) movements. The mandible could move in more than one or two directions at the same moment. So, the recording any spatial relationship of mandible to maxillae is difficult. But to restore occlusion, the maxillomandibular relationship record is necessary. The habitual mandibular movements are always intraborder type. To obtain a fixed, reproducible record for mandibular movements, it is necessary to move the mandible to one or more of its border locations. This requires transferable occlusal records. These transferable records are utilized in fabrication of the prosthesis (indirect method) in the laboratory.

Objectives

The objective of the jaw relationship record is to position the casts of the dental arches on an articulator so that casts have the same relationship as the mandible and maxilla in the patient's cranium.

IMPORTANCE OF MAXILLOMANDIBULAR RELATIONS

The accurate recording of the jaw relationship is a very important step in complete denture fabrication. Correct vertical dimension and horizontal relations are equally important for this. An error at this stage may result in denture failure. The dentures are uncomfortable, or unusable, and may cause lasting damage to the health of the supporting bone, mucosa, the muscles of mastication and the temporomandibular joints. A study of Lawson (1959) as stated by Sharry on 200 disappointed patients has shown that 60% of dentures had decreased vertical dimension, 45% had increased vertical dimension and 30% had incorrect centric relation.

Common Errors in Maxillomandibular Relation Records

1. Incorrect vertical jaw relation
2. Incorrect centric relation
3. Uneven contact in both sides
4. Premature contact at the heels of occlusal rims
5. Premature contact at the heels of casts.

Recording Jaw Relations

There are three distinct phases to the procedures:
1. Facebow record
2. Vertical dimension record
3. Centric relation record.

Facebow Record

It is the record of the relationship of the of the jaws to the opening axis and to orient the casts in this same relationship to the opening axis of the articulator. This is a relationship between the jaws and the axis of movement and not an anatomical relationship between the jaws and the temporomandibular joints (TMJs), except to some extent it is near the TMJs. By recording that relationship, the arc of closure in the articulator simulates the arc of closure of the patient. The small movement (20–25 mm at incisor) of mandible from rest position to occlusal contact position occurs as a hinge-like movement and the axis is called hinge axis.

Hinge axis is defined as "an imaginary line through or near two mandibular condyles around which the mandible may rotate without any translatory movement". This axis can be recorded by means of a kinematic facebow or approximated by use of an arbitrary facebow. The facebow transfer is not a maxillomandibular record. It is a record used to orient the maxillary cast to the hinge axis of the articulator. The facebow recording can be made using selected anatomic references with an arbitrary facebow or by locating the true hinge axis with a kinematic facebow. The latter is more accurate. However, the kinematic facebow is not used in complete denture fabrication because of the resiliency of the soft tissue causing instability of the mandibular record base and difficulty in locating the rotational center precisely. The arbitrary facebow record is generally considered to be satisfactory for complete denture fabrication.

Vertical Dimension

It refers to the amount of separation of the mandible to the maxillae under some specific conditions. They are of following types:
1. Vertical dimension of occlusion (VDO)
2. Vertical dimension of rest (VDR).

The purpose of establishing the vertical dimension of occlusion is to determine the vertical dimension prior to the tooth loss so that the dentures should have the same vertical separation for proper function.

Centric Relation

It is the horizontal anteroposterior and mediolateral relationships of the mandible to the maxilla. There are many horizontal relations out of which the basic horizontal relation important in developing is occlusion in complete dentures—the **centric relation.** The other horizontal jaw relations are the eccentric relations. These include protrusive or forward relations and the right and left lateral relations. These three relationships are recorded and transferred to the articulator to develop an effective occlusion and articulation.

VERTICAL DIMENSION

Definition

A vertical measurement of face between any two arbitrarily selected points conveniently located, one above and one below the mouth, usually in the midline.

Vertical Dimension of Occlusion

The vertical dimension of the face when the teeth or occlusion rims are in contact in centric occlusion. The vertical dimension of occlusion is established by the occlusal contact of the maxillary and mandibular teeth when natural teeth are present and in occlusion. When the natural teeth are lost the vertical dimension of occlusion is also lost. It is re-established by the vertical height of the two dentures with the teeth in contact. The vertical dimension of rest is not affected by the loss of natural teeth. It can be utilized for re-establishing the vertical dimension of occlusion in edentulous mouths.

Vertical Dimension of Rest

The vertical dimension of rest is defined as **the vertical dimension of the face with the jaws in rest relation.**

The vertical dimension of rest depends upon the physiologic rest position of the mandible. The physiologic rest position is a postural position maintained by the muscles of opening, closing and protruding the mandible. The physiologic rest position remains constant throughout life and is repeatable within a range and, therefore, useful for establishing vertical dimension of occlusion.

Significance of Vertical Dimension

The vertical dimension of rest position is a valuable guide used to determine the lost vertical dimension of occlusion in denture construction. This is because the difference between the occlusal vertical dimension and the rest vertical dimension is the interocclusal distance. The interocclusal distance or freeway space is defined as the distance that exists between the upper and lower teeth when the mandible is in the physiological rest position. It is usually 2 to 4 mm in the premolar region.

The equation of this concept is:

Vertical dimension of occlusion = Vertical dimension of rest – Interocclusal distance.

Interocclusal distance is **the distance between the occluding surfaces of the maxillary and the mandibular teeth, or the occlusal rims when the mandible is in its physiologic rest position.**

The interocclusal distance is very important for both patient's comfort and the function of his denture.

If the interocclusal distance is too much, the vertical dimension of occlusion is insufficient (closed).

If the interocclusal distance is insufficient, the vertical dimension of occlusion is too much (open).

There are many theories of measurement of the vertical dimension of occlusion for edentulous patients but there are few precise practical methods for measuring the vertical dimension. Fortunately, the patients adapt to the denture after fabrication without the accurate measurement of the vertical dimension.

Incorrect Vertical Dimension of Occlusion

These errors in vertical dimension may cause difficulties with the dentures in some patients but well tolerated by others.

EFFECTS OF EXCESSIVE OCCLUSAL VERTICAL DIMENSION

1. The increased risk of trauma to the tissues underlying the dentures due to absence of freeway space causing continuous clenching of the teeth.
2. Denture sore mouth particularly under lower denture due to trauma from constant contacts of teeth and may cause temporomandibular joint dysfunction.
3. There is alteration of the cortical pattern that automatically controls the mandibular movements during functions. This will cause considerable discomfort to the patient until a new cortical pattern has been established.
4. Muscular fatigue due to absence of rest for muscles of mandibular movements.
5. Clicking of dentures during speech and problems of speech as the space between the upper lower teeth is reduced, e.g. 'p', 'b', and 'm'.
6. It must cause elongation of the face with poor esthetics when the amount is more but may go unnoticed when only slight.
7. It may cause residual ridge resorption (RRR).

EFFECTS OF REDUCED OCCLUSAL VERTICAL DIMENSION

1. Aged appearance due to closure approximation of the nose to chin.
2. Creases at the corner of the mouth and angular cheilitis.
3. Reduction of masticatory efficiency due to decrease in pressure exerted between the teeth in contact.
4. Check biting during mastication due to loss of muscle tone and trapping of cheeks between the teeth during mastication.
5. Pain of temporomandibular joint due to strain.
6. Cons ten's syndrome (eustachian tube blockage, deafness, tinnitus, burning sensation of tongue, tenderness on palpation on the temporomandibular joint and dryness of the mouth).

METHODS OF DETERMINING VERTICAL DIMENSION OF OCCLUSION

The methods of recording the vertical maxillo-mandibular relations can be classified into two groups (Table 8.1):

The ideal method of recording the correct vertical dimension is the pre-extraction method. In absence of pre-extraction records, facial measurements after swallowing and relaxing, tactile sense, phonetics and facial expression are methods of recording the vertical dimension of rest position.

Table 8.1 Methods of determining vertical dimension

Pre-extraction record methods	Post-extraction methods
1. Profile photographs	1. Physiological rest position
2. Profile radiographs	2. Phonetics
3. Diagnostic casts in	3. Aesthetic occlusion
4. Dakometer—facial	4. Swallowing threshold measurement
5. Ridge parallelism	5. Proprioception
6. Measurement of former denture	6. Boos biometer/ gnathodynamometer

The pre-extraction records may not always be the reliable method in determination of vertical dimension. But pre-extraction measurements or previous dentures should not be ignored, because it is better than not having any record at all in a totally edentulous patient. Changes can be done to the pre-extraction records when indicated.

Pre-extraction Records

The mechanical method of recording the vertical dimension of edentulous patient is done by using pre-extraction records. The dental surgeon either extracts the teeth and fabricates the dentures, or replaces existing dentures. It is often the patients present themselves for treatment with either natural or artificial teeth. When patient's teeth are extracted by the dental surgeon he has the opportunity to record the vertical dimension and position and shape of the teeth before the extraction. There are several methods to obtain those information beforehand as follows:

Profile Photographs

The photograph of the patient's facial profile with the teeth in occlusion are taken and enlarged to life size (i.e. 1:1 ratio). A camera with close focusing can be used to make the photograph of the profile of the patient. A 6-inch ruler is held at the center of the face by attaching with a pair of spectacle. The image of the ruler along with the patient's profile is enlarged to its actual size. The printed picture of the patient face is cut out leaving the background to serve as a template of the profile. The template is used when the jaw relation records are made and again in the try-in stage to check the vertical dimension of occlusion.

Profile Radiographs

The profile cephalometric radiograph with 1:1 ratio of the patient may be used to determine the vertical dimension of occlusion, but not recommended for radiation hazards.

Diagnostic Cast

Plaster cast of dental arches obtained with natural teeth mounted on articulator in occlusion can be used for determination of vertical dimension by measurement between two relatively stable points such as incisive papillae and the crest of the lower ridge. Incisive papilla to the maxillary incisal edge is 6 mm and mandibular incisal edge is 4 mm.

Facial Measurements

Dakometer

This is an instrument which is used to record the vertical dimension and the position of upper central incisors. The recording of the vertical dimension and the position of the maxillary central incisors are done before extraction of teeth. These records can be used during determination of vertical dimension in edentulous state. There may be an error of ± 1 mm.

Willis Bite Gauge

Willis designed the bite gauge to measure the distances between the chin and nose and between the hairline and the eyebrows which are considered to be equal with the mandible in rest position. He utilized the "equal-thirds" concept used by the famous artist Leonardo da Vinci (1452–1519) and named as "divine proportions". But these methods of Willis and Wright are of little practical value as the points of measurements are too vague, e.g. top or bottom of eyebrows to be measured.

Ridge Parallelism

Sears suggests that the correct vertical dimension is obtained by paralleling the maxillary and mandibular ridges plus a 5° opening in the posterior region. The mounted casts on articulator showing excessive divergent indicates an increased vertical dimension and should be rechecked.

Disadvantages

i. Not effective in case of loss of teeth at different times leaving the ridges unparalleled.
ii. The edentulous ridges due to resorption developed discrepancy in height. Parallelism of the posterior ridge on mounted cast may not be used to determine the vertical dimension of occlusion as the amount of ridge resorption is not uniform due to extraction of the natural teeth at different times, this method is not reliable.

Measurement of Former Denture

The dentures used by the patient can be measured with a figure of 8-shaped calipers (Fig. 8.1) between the ridge crest and occlusal plane. These measurements can be utilized in new dentures. The changes can be made if required by observing the dentures in the patient's mouth.

Post-extraction Methods

Physiologic Rest Position

The physiologic rest position of mandible is determined first and from that the occlusion position is established 2–4 mm less than rest position. Niswonger (1934) suggested this method and stated that facial height, the vertical dimension and subsequently, the interocclusal distance, are constant throughout life. He also noted an average interocclusal distance of 2 to 4 mm in rest position.

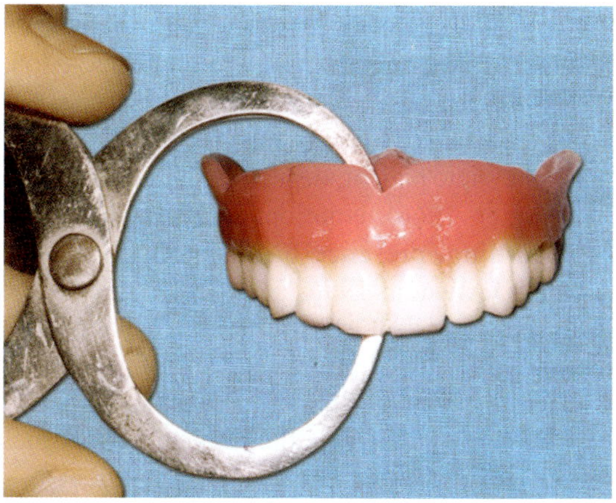

Fig. 8.1: Measurement of former denture with 8-shaped calipers

This distance between the two vertical relations is important for comfort, efficiency, speech and esthetics of complete dentures. This method is most commonly used now in determining the vertical dimension. But works of Moller (1966), Atwood (1956), and Tallgren (1957), questioned the theory of constancy of the vertical dimension of rest. However, it is still a useful method when combined with other methods.

The facial measurement is done by placing two reference points, one at the base of the nose and the other on the chin and then measuring the distance between them when the patient swallows and relaxes. It provides the measurement of approximate vertical dimension of rest. The same method is repeated several times until the measurements are consistent (within a small range). This measurement is then used to establish the vertical dimension of occlusion by reducing the interocclusal space (distance) of 2 to 4 mm in most individuals. A millimeter ruler is convenient and not alarming to the patient.

The determination of rest position by **electromyography** is based on the theory that the muscles display the least amount of electrical activity at the rest position. Electromyography may be used to determine the rest position, but it cannot be routinely used in dental clinic.

Disadvantages

The physiologic rest position is not a reliable method of determination of vertical dimension, due to two reasons:

a. The amount of freeway space is highly variable in the same patient, depending on head posture (Moller, 1966), emotional state, and time of recording, presence or absence of natural teeth (Atwood, 1956; Tall Green, 1957), the insertion of dentures (Berry and Wilkie, 1961; Carlson and Eriction,1967), environmental factors (Perry et al, 1960; Yemm, 1968).
b. The marks move with the skin, and sometimes difficult to obtain constant measurement.

Silverman's Phonetic Methods (1955)

The phonetic methods are widely used to determine the correct vertical dimension of occlusion. When the patient pronounces the letter "S" as pronounced in 'six', sixty, six or Mississippi, the anterior teeth come very close to touching end-to-end. It is known as ***Silverman's closest speaking space***. It is space between the teeth that, according to Dr Earl Pound, should have 1–2 mm clearance between the incisal edges of anterior teeth when the patient is unconsciously repeating the latter "S". If the distance is more than 2 mm a small vertical dimension of occlusion is established. If the distance is very small, the anterior teeth touch when these sounds are made; the vertical dimension is probably large. The mandibular posture in making the sibilants depends upon the position of the teeth and, unless the occlusion rims have been trimmed to the final tooth positions, the mandible will not be in right position to produce the speech sounds. So, this method is perhaps more meaningful at the try-in stage after the teeth are arranged than with wax rims at the jaw relation stage. Silverman's closest speaking space which measures the vertical dimension in phonetic method is not to be confused with the freeway space of the physiological method of Niswonger's (1934) and Thompson (1946).

The freeway space establishes vertical dimension when the mandible is in rest position. The closest speaking space measures vertical dimension when the mandible is physiologic function. One method is static method and the other method is dynamic or functional method.

Disadvantages (Table 8.2)

a. This method is not applicable in the patients having 8 to 10 mm "closest speaking space". They will require other method for determination of vertical dimension.
b. It does not correlate to the original occlusal vertical dimension of the patient as denture patients wearing the same denture for more than 14 years and loose 10 mm or more of

Table 8.2 Difference between closest speaking space and freeway space

Closest speaking space	Freeway space
1. Measures the vertical dimension when the muscles are at complete rest, or in physiologic function of speech	1. Measures the vertical dimension when the mandible and muscles involved are in tonus and the mandible in rest position
2. Dynamic or functional position	2. Static position
3. 2 mm in incisor region	3. 2 to 4 mm in first premolar region

the original occlusal vertical dimension yet are able to say "Mississippi" with the same dentures.

Esthetics

The vertical dimension also affects appearance. The occlusal rim is trimmed until the patient's appearance looks satisfactory. The lips come together comfortably. The face does not look stretched and too long, or too short with averted lips and nose too near the chin. This method most likely produces an increased vertical dimension because the occlusal rims do not provide sufficient lip support and the jaw relations are recorded with greater height in order to provide a satisfactory appearance. Both the patient and the dentist determine esthetics by observing the appearance of the patient with the occlusal rims in the mouth.

Swallowing

Swallowing can be used to determine the vertical dimension of occlusion and rest position. The maxillary and mandibular teeth make light contact during swallowing, and after the completion of the swallowing; the mandible assumes its rest position. Soft wax cones are made on the lower denture base with a height more than the assumed vertical dimension of occlusion. The patient is given a piece of candy or sips of water and asked to swallow repeatedly. The wax cones are reduced to the correct vertical dimension of occlusion. The softness or hardness of the wax will influence the final position and this method gives inaccurate results.

Proprioception

A method using patient's proprioceptive ability can be used as a guide to establish the occlusal vertical dimension (Tactile sense). The patient with the bite rim can sense when the jaws assume the same position of the vertical separation as in the dentulous state. A central bearing screw may be used with the central bearing plate. The central bearing plate is attached to the maxillary occlusal rim and the central bearing screw is fixed to the mandibular occlusal rim. Adjustment of pin height is done with patients perception. In fact, patient's perception varies a great deal and it is time consuming and produces uncertain result.

Biometer

Boos biometer or gnathodynamometer is an instrument that records biting force at varying degree of jaw separation. A person can exert maximum biting force at the vertical dimension of rest or maximum force, minus 2 mm. It can be measured with a biometer or dynamometer placed between the jaws and the patient is asked to bite. The vertical dimension is then adjusted with the screw until the maximum biting force is exerted. Men average 60 to 65 lbs of biting force and women produce 25 to 30 lbs.

Although these methods give satisfactory results individually, it is advisable to combine two or more methods to establish the vertical dimension of rest. The registration of vertical dimension mostly depends upon clinical judgment and the accuracy of the record varies within a range rather than a point.

Centric Relation

Centric relation is the most important maxillo-mandibular relation on horizontal path of movement, from which the excursive movements of occlusion start. Centric relation was defined in the Glossary of Prosthodontic Terms, as "The most posterior position of the mandible relative to the maxillae at the established vertical dimension. It coincides with a reproducible posterior hinge position of the mandible and it may be recorded as a very useful reference or starting point for establishing jaw relationships in any prosthetic treatment, particularly in complete denture fabrication. In the natural dentition most functional tooth contacts occur in an area slightly anterior to centric relation, i.e. centric occlusion. In edentolous patient lack of centric occlusion, centric relation is recoded which is independent of teeth and centric occlusion is establish using preferred vertical dimension of occlusion. Centric relation and centric occlusion thus coincide." A tentative centric relation record is made with the record rims during the jaw relation record. Again a new record is made at the try-in stage that must prove it correct. New centric relation records are again made at delivery. They are most accurate as the permanent denture base fits the basal tissues more accurately than the temporary record bases.

SIGNIFICANCE OR IMPORTANCE OF CENTRIC RELATION

The most important maxillomandibular relation is the centric relation irrespective of its method of determination. An accurate centric relation record at the proper vertical of occlusion is absolutely essential to satisfactory complete denture fabrication because of the following reasons:

1. It remains constant for any patient during the denture fabrication (though may change slightly in patient's life time) and therefore, serves as a definite reference point.
2. It is not affected by the presence of teeth or by the posture of the head.
3. It is the starting point for developing occlusion.
4. It is reproducible and so can be verified.
5. It is a functional position but fleeting in nature.

Centric Occlusion

In natural dentition, centric occlusion is defined as, "the occlusion of opposing teeth when the mandible is in centric relation. This may or may not coincide with the maximum intercuspation position". Maximum intercuspation is defined as "the complete intercuspation of the opposing teeth independent of condylar position".

So, by definition, the tooth contacts in these two situations could be different in natural teeth. Normally, this is not the case with complete denture occlusion. In complete denture occlusion, maximum intercuspation is the preferred term instead of centric occlusion.

Centric occlusion is almost always 0.5 mm anterior to the centric relation. Centric occlusion is a tooth-to-tooth relationship with no consideration of the relation of the mandible to maxilla whereas centric relation is a maxillomandibular relationship. In complete denture, centric occlusion should coincide with centric relation. Neuromuscular reflexes set up by the proprioceptive elements in the periodontium enable the patient to develop a consistent closure in centric occlusion with natural teeth. When all the natural teeth are lost, centric occlusion is lost. Centric occlusion, therefore, cannot be determined accurately in edentulous patients. Centric relation being a bone-to-bone relation can be determined accurately in an edentulous patient and often used in complete denture fabrication.

Difference between centric relation and centric occlusion is given in Table 8.3.

DIFFICULTIES IN RECORDING CENTRIC RELATION

Biological Reasons

1. The structure of temporomandibular joint causes displacement of condyles downward by uneven pressure between the jaws when records are made for most retruded position. This can never occur on articulator. It results in a deflecting contact, instability, soreness, and

resorption of bone. The denture bases made from the best impressions will not withstand the ill effects of an incorrect centric relation.

2. The registration is further complicated due to varying thickness of soft tissues. The undue pressure in recording the relation should be avoided by using soft materials. Ideally, the same pressure and same material is to be used as in impression making. To record centric relation with minimum pressure, the soft plaster, zinc oxide eugenol paste, or soft wax may be used.
3. The patient may not be able to perform mandibular movements due to either neuromuscular problems or TMJ problems.

Mechanical Reasons

1. The poorly fitting denture bases are difficult to stabilize in the mouth. It makes the recording of centric relation difficult.
2. It is very difficult to secure centric relation record with minimum pressure to prevent soft tissue displacement.

Psychological Reasons

Sometimes, it becomes difficult to make the patient relaxed, and unstrained closing of the mouth. Moreover the operator may be in a hurry or not have a calm state of mind to perform the recording successfully.

Methods of Recording Centric Relation

There are various methods for making centric relation records. These may be classified in three general classes as: (1) Graphic recordings, (2) Functional recordings, and (3) Interocclusal recordings. These records are used for transferring maxillomandibular relationships from the patient to the articulator.

Graphic Recordings

These records use tracings of mandibular movements in horizontal plane to record the centric relation. It also records the protrusive and lateral movements of the mandible; which can be used in setting the horizontal and lateral inclinations of the articulator. The tracing obtained by this method is known as Gothic arch tracing or arrow point tracing. The apex of tracing represents centric relation, with two arms of the tracings originating from the apex, being the lateral movements, and the protrusive movement of the mandible produces the straight line in the middle (Fig. 8.2). This is the basis of graphic methods of recording centric relation. It should not be confused with pantographic tracings made in three planes. It is apparent that terminal hinge position and the apex of the Gothic arch tracing are identical retruded border position of the mandible.

The tracing can be made with intra oral or extra oral tracer (Figs 8.3A to D). In both

Table 8.3 Differences between centric relation and centric occlusion

Centric relation	Centric occlusion
1. Centric relation is a condylar-determined relation of jaws	1. Centric occlusion is tooth-to-tooth contact determined relation of the jaws
2. Centric relation is the starting point for developing denture occlusion	2. Centric occlusion is present in natural dentition
3. Centric relation coincides with centric occlusion in complete denture	3. Centric occlusion may or may not coincide with the maximum intercuspal position in natural dentition
4. Centric relation is located posterior to centric occlusion in natural dentition	4. Centric occlusion is located anterior to centric relation (0.5–1 mm) in natural dentition
5. It can be determined, verified and repeatable. It is a position of rest and relaxation	5. It cannot be determined when teeth are lost as proprioceptive impulses are lost. It is habitual and unguided closure
6. It is the position from which movements start and end	6. It is a functional or working position, but fleeting in nature

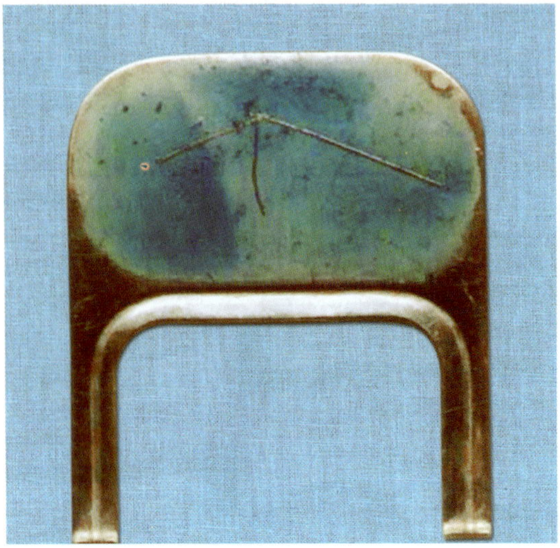

Fig. 8.2: The Gothic arch tracing showing sharp apex

methods, the patient's jaws are moved through excursive movements, making sure that the most retruded position of the mandible is recorded. In extraoral tracer a stylus is attached to one jaw and a recording plate is mounted on the other jaw. The jaws are separated by a central bearing point, which maintains the vertical dimension. The central bearing point acts as the stylus in the intraoral tracer. An advantage of extraoral method is that the tracing is large and is visible while recording, thus making it easier to instruct the patient and evaluate the record. The advantage of the intraoral tracer is the tracing point is stout enough to resist biting pressures and can be held in any chosen position (centric, lateral, or protrusive). In intraoral tracer, the position of the tracer and the tracing plate can be interchanged between the jaws.

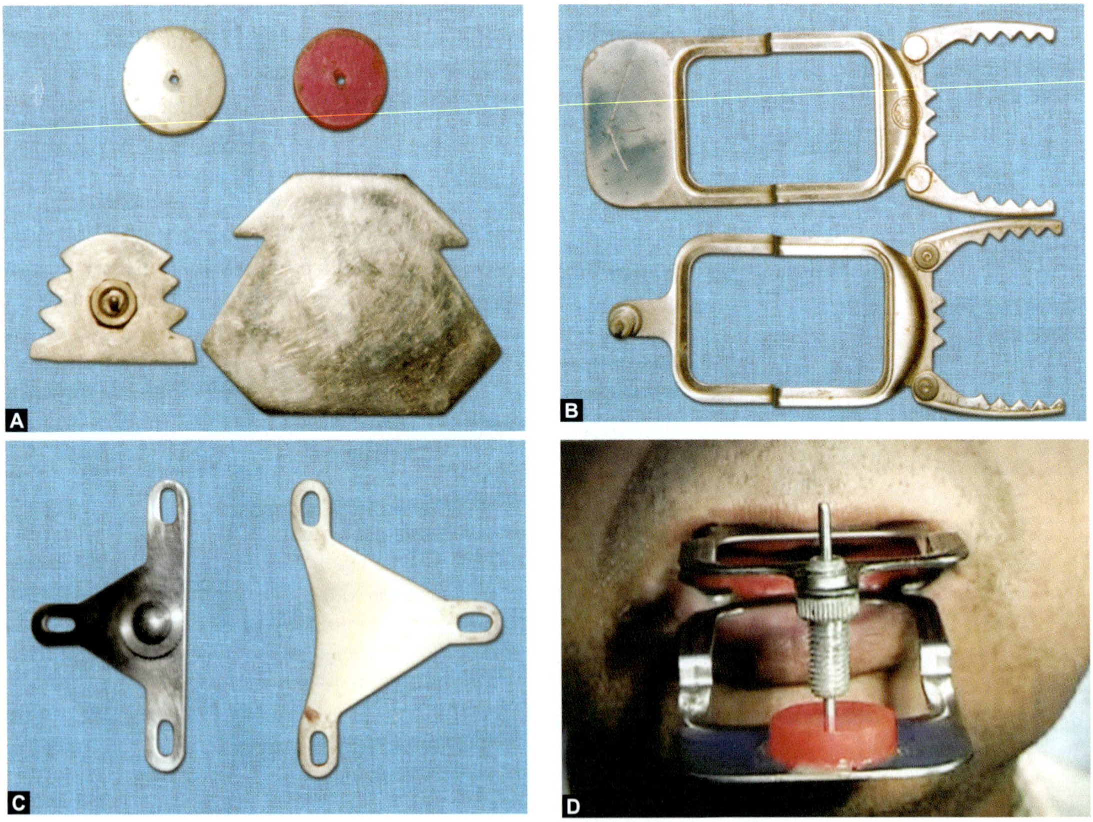

Figs 8.3A to D: (A) Intraoral Gothic arch tracer parts; (B and C) Extraoral Gothic arch tracer parts; (D) Extraoral Gothic tracing up in patients mouth

CONTRAINDICATIONS OF GOTHIC ARCH TRACING METHOD

The Gothic arch tracing (both intraoral and extraoral) is contraindicated in the following situations:

1. This method is not suitable for class II and class III jaw relations due to difficulty to stabilize the bases and centralize the biting force. It is difficult to locate the center of the true arches to centralize the forces with the tracing device.
2. It is contraindicated in flabby or easily displaceable tissues on the residual ridges. It is difficult to stabilize the record base against horizontal forces on flabby or otherwise easily displaceable tissues.
3. Patients having no voluntary control of jaw movements.
4. Patients having large awkward tongues. It is difficult to stabilize bite rim carrying the tracing device.
5. In flat ridges, it is difficult to stabilize the bite rim during tracing.
6. This method cannot be utilized in reduced interarch space, due to inadequate space available to accommodate the tracing device.

Functional Recordings

These methods of recording centric relation utilize functional movement of the mandible during recording. These methods are also known as "chew-in" methods. In House's method (1918), the vertical dimension of occlusion is first determined with the occlusal rims fabricated with a rigid material like modeling compound which serves as a recording medium. The recording is done with four metal studs that cut tracings into an opposing occlusal rim in the form of four diamond-shaped tracings incorporating the movements in three planes. The studs are placed at the apex of the tracing and the record bases are joined by plaster for transfer to the articulator. It can also be done by using Meyers (1934) 'Functionally generated path' method using soft wax on the occlusal rim and performing functional movements. Paterson (1923) used plaster on bite rims and carborundum paste to grind it down in mouth. All these methods are difficult and time consuming.

Another method is the swallowing technique which is based on the theory that patient swallows in centric relation.

Interocclusal Recordings (Clinical Method)

These are static methods which include the direct intraoral check bite where the centric relation is recorded by placing a recording medium (wax, compound, zinc oxide and eugenol, or plaster) between the record bases when the jaws are positioned at centric relation. The common recording materials are wax, plaster, and zinc oxide paste. It is the commonly used method in clinical practice because this method is simple, requires no special instrument, and can be done and verified in a short period of time. All articulators will accept the interocclusal record. The shortcoming of interocclusal recording is that they provide accurate recording only in one vertical dimension only. However, in graphic recording the instruments must be fixed to the jaws otherwise inaccurate results will be obtained, therefore, offer no advantage over the more arbitrary interocclusal records.

Although all the above methods are capable of recording the accurate position, several factors that complicate the recording are:

1. Resiliency of the tissues supporting the denture bases.
2. Stability and retention of the record bases.
3. The state of health of muscles, ligaments, temporomandibular joint and its neuromuscular mechanism of the patient.
4. Amount of pressure applied in making the record.
5. Technique employed in making the record.
6. Ability of the dentist.

Eccentric Jaw Relation

Definition: Any relation of mandible to the maxilla other than centric relation.

Objectives of eccentric relations: The primary purpose for making eccentric records is to record the horizontal and lateral condylar inclinations on an articulator to arrange the tooth in balanced occlusion in complete dentures.

The question of necessity for eccentric records is controversial, because accuracy is a problem in the recording methods and the capabilities of the articulator to receive and reproduce the record. The inaccuracies are due to instability of records, resiliency and displaceability of denture-bearing areas, materials used, equipments and lack of coordination of muscle. From this controversy arises the different concepts of occlusion and tooth form required for complete dentures. There is no scientific data to support superiorly of one concept over the other.

Types of Eccentric Relations

Protrusive Relation

It is the jaw relation resulting from a protrusion of the mandible. When the mandible is protruded, the condyles move forward and downward on to the articular eminences. The drop of the condyles results in similar drop of the lower posterior teeth creating space between occlusal surfaces. This occurrence of space is known as Christensen's phenomenon. The purpose of protrusive record is to measure the amount of drop. This could be recorded by soft wax placed between the bite rims, and the record is transferred to an adjustable articulator. The articulator's horizontal condylar guidance is so set that a similar drop will take place when same amount of protrusion occurs during setting of teeth. This is known as protrusive balance.

Methods of Recording

1. *Graphic recording*: Gothic arch tracing using a 6 mm protrusive position from the centric relation can be used.
2. Functional recording by House needles chew in records.
3. Interocclusal check bite recording.

Lateral Relations

It is the relationship of the mandible to the maxilla in left or right of the midsagittal plane. A separation occurs between the upper and lower occlusal rims on the opposite side of movement. This is due to downward and medial movement of the condyle along the medial slope of the articular fossa.

Methods of Recording

1. Interocclusal check bite of wax or plaster.
2. Graphic methods—pantographic tracing. A light pantograph by Denar with its simple clutch system can be used. This method is not suitable for complete denture fabrication.
3. Hanau's formula.

CLINICAL AND LABORATORY PROCEDURES

The procedure of recording jaw relations are carried out in three separate clinical steps for the sake of accuracy of each record:

1. The vertical dimension of occlusion
2. The facebow transfer record
3. The centric relation record

PRELIMINARY VERTICAL DIMENSION OF OCCLUSION

In the edentulous person, the fine directional guidance of the mandibular position are lost. It is advisable to remove the dentures the patient wearing for at least 24 hours prior to the maxillo-mandibular relation is recorded. In this way, it is possible to minimize the possibility of obtaining an eccentric position of the mandible instead of the centric relation position.

Instruments and Materials (Fig. 8.4)

1. Occlusal rim on bases and casts
2. Disclosing paste or wax

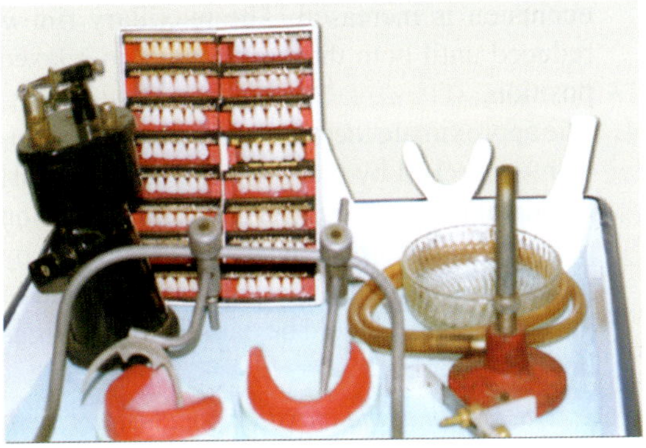

Fig. 8.4: Instruments and materials jaw relation records

3. Greenstick compound
4. Denture adhesive
5. Hanau torch
6. Fox plane
7. Willis gauge or calipers
8. Bunsen burner
9. Facebow
10. Water bowl
11. Indelible pencil
12. Tooth moulds

Checking the Retention of the Record Bases

The temporary bases will not have the positive retention as with permanent bases but no movement should be seen when the mouth is half open or during limited movement of the mouth.

The poor retention is evident when the bite block moves in an occlusal direction after the seating pressure is released. Poor retention arises from.

a. *Overextension of the periphery*: This is the most common cause of poor retention. This can be detected by applying disclosing paste or wax to the denture border and placing it in patient mouth and have the patient open the mouth wide in case of maxillary denture base. In case of mandibular base, patient has to open the mouth and protrude the tongue. The base on removal from the mouth will show the areas of overextended border as shown through the paste. The overextension should be removed by trimming the periphery of the base plate.
b. *Underextension of the periphery*: This may be the cause of poor retention. Border molding of the base with greenstick compound and remaking of the final impression with zinc oxide-eugenol paste is indicated.

Assessment of Lip Support

a. The maxillary rim only is inserted in the mouth of patient seated in an upright position. The patient's full face profile is checked with the lip at rest. With lip at rest, the occlusal rim should support the upper lip so that the lip appears to be slightly concave and a normal amount of vermilion border is visible showing a depression at philtrum. The face should have a relaxed appearance. When insufficient support has been given to the lip only a small amount of the vermilion border will be seen and the nasolabial groove may be deep, the philtrum is flattened, and the commissures drop. When oversupported, the grooves are shallow, the philtrum is obliterated, and the commissures are distorted laterally. When oversupported or undersupported, the labial contour may be increased or decreased by adding or removing wax from the outer surface of the occlusal rim. The facial surface of maxillary rim should be 8 to 10 mm anterior from the center of the incisive papilla.
b. The mandibular occlusal rim is then placed in the patient's mouth and the labial contour is built up by adding or removing wax from its outer surface till the lip appears to have adequate support (Figs 8.5A and B). A photograph of the patient with natural teeth is helpful.

Adjusting the Height and Orientation of the Occlusal Plane

1. The height of the mandibular rim is marked at the level of the corners of the mouth with lip relaxed.

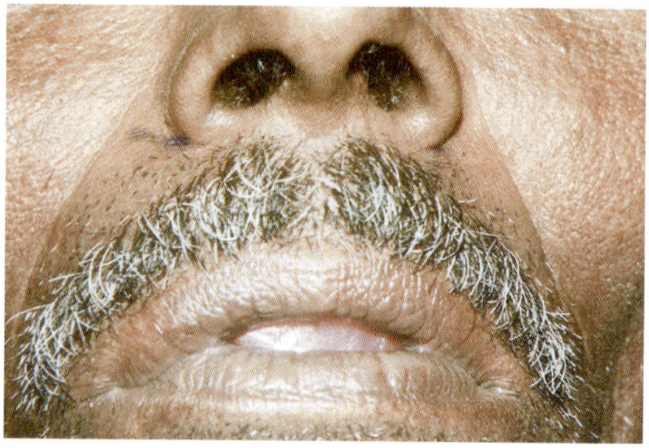

Fig. 8.5A: The upper lip is oversupported by the bite rim

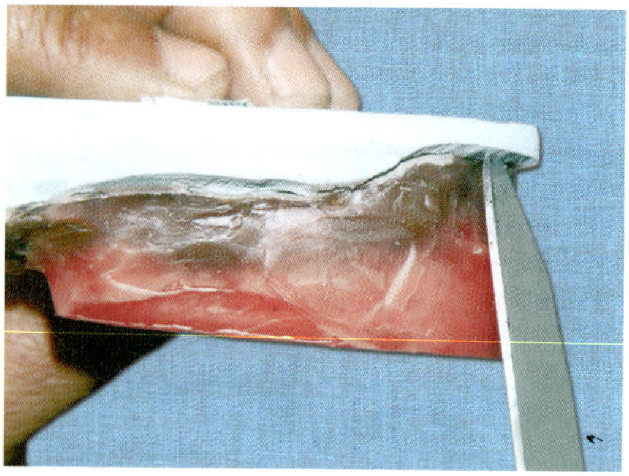

Fig. 8.5B: Decreasing oversupported rim using hot plate

2. The cast is marked at the level of two-thirds up to the retromolar pads. The height of the wax rim is marked at the level of the two-thirds as the retromolar pad. The mandibular rim is removed from the patient's mouth and placed on the cast. The mandibular wax rim is reduced up to these marks.
3. The mandibular occlusal rim is placed again in the patient's mouth and checked the tentative occlusal plane. If it is satisfactory the maxillary occlusal rim is placed in the patient's mouth and patient is asked to close the mouth until the rims contact evenly at rest position. If contact occurs in posterior region, the maxillary rim is contoured until both the rims contact evenly. In case the rims contact but lips are apart in relaxed position, the vertical dimension of occlusion is increased. The maxillary rim is reduced until both the rims contact in relaxed position.
4. The approximate location of the plane of occlusion is checked by placing a fox plane against the maxillary rim (Fig. 8.6A). In anterior region plane of orientation is usually determined by making it parallel to interpupillary line and in posterior region should be parallel to ala-tragus line (Fig. 8.6B).

Note: *The length of the maxillary occlusion rim in the anterior region should be visible by 1 to 2 mm at the physiologic rest position. It should be adjusted accordingly. Variations may occur in relation to the length of the upper lip. With a long lip the level of the rim may be so trimmed that no wax is visible. With short incompetent lip 4 to 6 mm of the rim may be visible under the lip at rest. A comparison with previous dentures may modify the incisal length as selected and a change of more than 3 to 4 mm is generally not recommended. With natural age related changes in the lips, older patients will display progressively less of the maxillary anterior teeth (Vig and Brundo 1978). Under 30 years of age group an average of 3 mm of maxillary anterior teeth will be displayed. In an over 60 years age group 0 mm of teeth will be displayed. The length of the upper lip increases from 10 to 35 mm, the amount of maxillary tooth displayed decreases from 4 to 0.25 mm, the amount of mandibular tooth exposed increases from 0.7 to 2.3 mm.*

In any age group of lip length, female exposes on an average twice as much of maxillary central incisor but only half of the mandibular central incisor than males. Caucasians display on an average of 2.4 mm of the maxillary central incisor and 0.98 mm of the mandibular central incisor. Negros and Asians display 1.5 to 1.8 mm of the maxillary central incisor and 1.4 to 1.5 mm of the mandibular central incisor (Cade, 1979; Vig and Brundo, 1978).

The maxillary rim only is placed in the mouth. The patient is asked to pronounce "five fifty-five", when the incisal edge of the maxillary rim contact

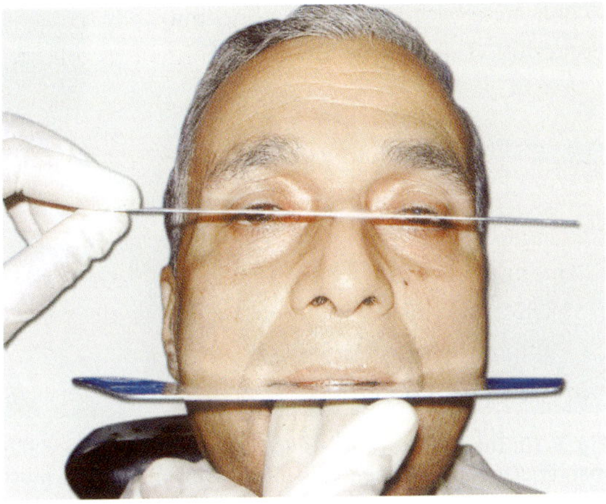

Fig. 8.6A: Anterior plane parallel to interpupillary line

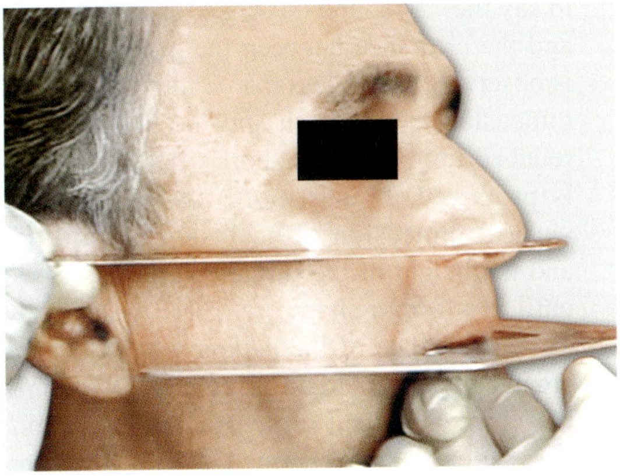

Fig. 8.6B: Posterior plane parallel to Camper's line

the vermilion border of the lower lip at the junction of the moist and dry mucosa. The maxillary occlusal rim is reduced in length until the inferior border makes similar contact with the lower lip.

Determination of the Rest Vertical Dimension

a. Only the maxillary base with occlusal rim is inserted in patient's mouth. The patient is seated in an upright position with his back unsupported by the chair so that the Frankfort plane (a plane passing through the lowest point in the margin of the orbit and the highest point in the margin of the external auditory meatus) is horizontal. A small dot or horizontal line is placed on the patient's tip of the nose and another on the immovable part of the chin (Fig. 8.7).
b. The measurement between the dots is taken when the patient: (i) says "M", "M"."M" repeatedly, (ii) licks the lips, swallows, and relaxes. The measurement gives the rest vertical dimension. A millimeter ruler or dividers is convenient for this (Fig. 8.8). The procedure is repeated several times until the measurements are consistent. This distance is recorded as rest position. An error may result using this method if the lower marker on chin moves. This is usually occurring when patient attempts to close on bite rims with a height excess of that of the rest position.

A Willis gauge may be used in measuring vertical dimension by holding its arms against the underside of the nasal septum and chin (Fig. 8.9).

Establishment of the Tentative Vertical Dimension of Occlusion

a. The mandibular base with occlusal rim is inserted in the patient's mouth and it is reduced until the upper and lower rims meet evenly at the vertical dimension of occlusion 3 mm less than the rest vertical dimension. The skeletal

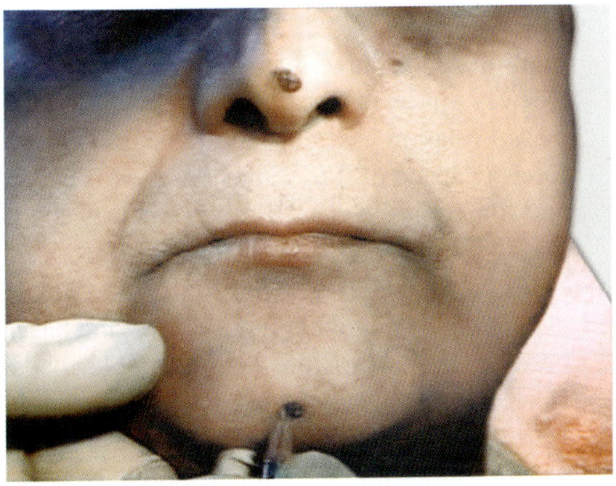

Fig. 8.7: A small dot is placed on its tips, nose and arc on chin

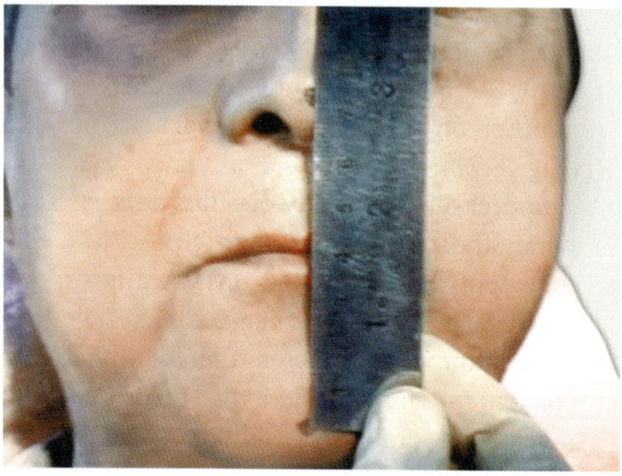

Fig. 8.8: With the patients jaw in the rest position the distance between the marks measured with a ruler

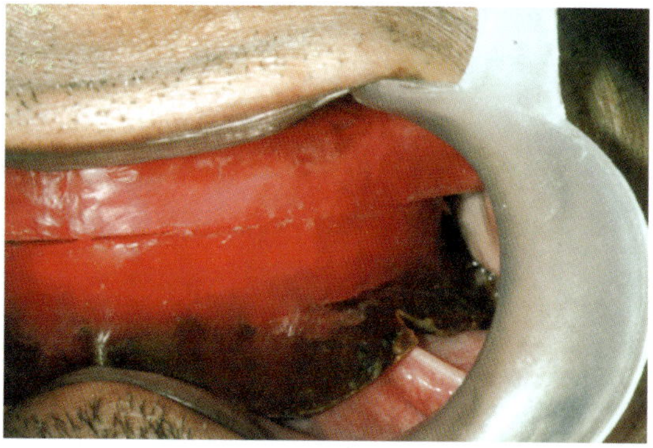

Fig. 8.10: The contact relationship between the maxillary and mandibular wax occlusion rims must be even. The rims must be contoured to provide support to the lips at the established occlusal vertical dimension

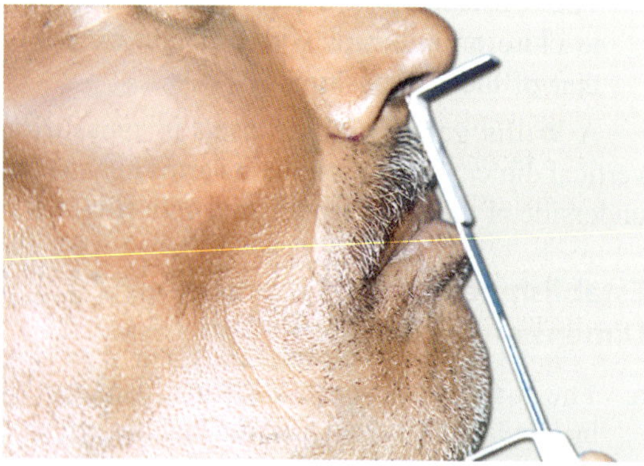

Fig. 8.9: The use of the Willis gauge is measuring the vertical dimension

relation of the jaws has some effect on the freeway space in complete dentures. Skeletal class I relation cases usually have an average freeway space of 2 to 4 mm. In class II cases, and sometimes in class III cases freeway space may be more than 4 mm (Fig. 8.10).

b. Both the base plate should fit the tissue evenly on closing without contact of the bases between the tuberosities and retromolar pads. If necessary, the base plates may be thin down.
c. If there is any doubt about the accuracy of the vertical dimension the patient should be asked to say the "S" sound (sixty-six or Mississippi) and the clearance between the occlusion rims is observed. If it is less than 2 mm the vertical dimension is too much and the lower rim is reduced until it 2 mm short when "S" sound is produced. If it is more than 2 mm the vertical dimension of occlusion is too little and the height of the rim should be increased until it is 2 mm short.
d. The appearance of the patient when the rims are in contact should be observed for assessing the correct vertical dimension of occlusion. The patient with decreased vertical dimension has a crumpled appearance with thin lips, and with nose chin approximation. The patient with increased vertical dimension will have a strained appearance with lengthening of face and lack of labial seal.

Useful Guidelines

The following guidelines are placed on the maxillary occlusal rim which is useful for arranging the teeth.

a. *Midline or central line*: It is the line bisecting the whole face in the midline. It should be recorded on the labial surface of the occlusal rim. The mesial surface of the upper central incisors will contact this line.

b. *Low lip line*: The low lip line relax lip line is the line which determine the vertical incisal length.
c. *High lip line/gum line/smile line*: It is almost straight line with a slight upward component. It is used as a guide in the arrangement of the teeth. The amount of teeth that revealed superiority and laterally will depend on the type of smile line of the individual have.
Some patient have broad smile, others have not so broad and still others have a rare smile depending upon the personality. The patient is requested to smile and the smile line is marked on the maxillary rim.
d. *Canine lines/corner lines*: The canine lines are marked on the occlusal rims in the mouth with a pointed instrument. This will pass on the occlusal rim at the corner of the mouth. Vertical lines recorded at this point will coincide with the tip of the cuspids and only accurate within 3 to 4 mm (Fig. 8.11).

Facebow Transfer and Mounting the Cast on Articulator

Hanau's earpiece facebow is used as follows:

1. The bite fork is warmed and attached to the maxillary occlusion rim so that the midline of the fork corresponds with the midline of the rim (Fig. 8.12)
2. The lower occlusion rim is inserted into the mouth and has the patient is instructed to close the jaws tightly into the previously obtained tentative vertical dimension of occlusion.
3. The facebow is carried over the patient's face and the facebow toggle assembly is slipped on to the stem of the bow fork.
4. The earpieces are inserted in the ears of the patient and the bow is centered so that both the scale of the condylar stylus has equal readings. The locknuts at the condylar rods are then tightened to suspend the facebow, and the bite fork is securely locked to the assembly.
5. The infraorbital pointer is directed at the infraorbital notch and locked in place (Fig. 8.13).
6. The condylar locknuts are then released, and the facebow and attached occlusion rims are transferred to the articulator (Fig. 8.14)
7. The articulator should be locked in centric with the incisal pin flush with the upper member.
8. The condylar rods are inserted over the condylar rod extensions and centered before being locked in position by tightening the lock nuts.

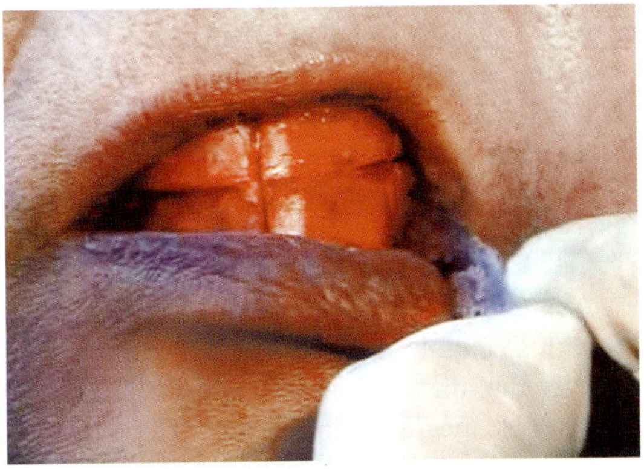

Fig. 8.11: Useful canine lines

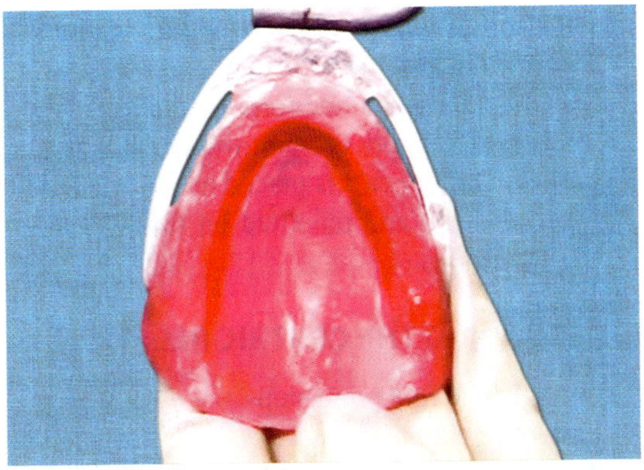

Fig. 8.12: Bike fork attached to the occlusal rim so that midline of the fork corresponds with midline of the rim

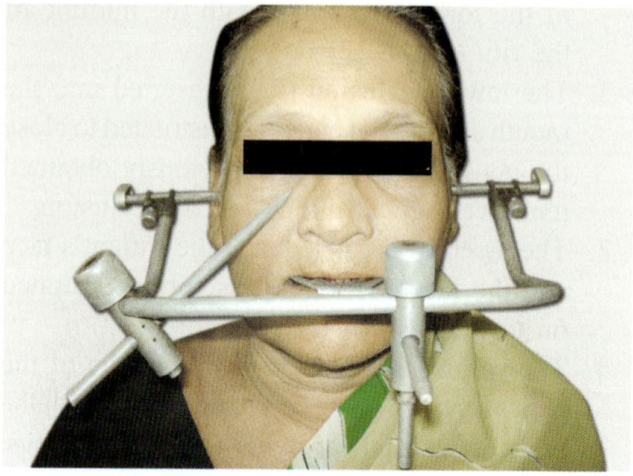

Fig. 8.13: Facebow carried over patient's face, centered and locked. Infraorbital pointer directed to infraorbital notch is locked

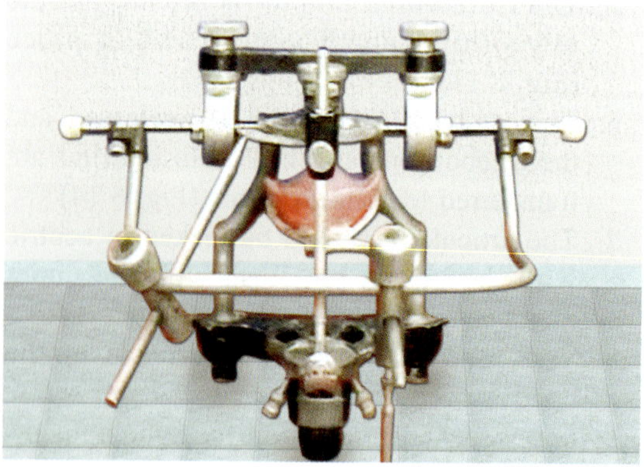

Fig. 8.14: Facebow is transferred to articulator

9. The facebow is raised or lowered to adjust the infraorbital pointer to touch the pointer plate attached to the articulator.
10. The facebow is secured in position with facebow support beneath the occlusion rim. The maxillary cast is placed accurately in the occlusal rim and mounted on the articulator with plaster.

RECORDING THE CENTRIC RELATION

It consist of the following steps:

a. *Recording tentative centric relation*: The facebow fork is removed from the occlusal rim. The maxillary and mandibular occlusal rims are inserted in the mouth and the patient is asked to swallow and close in retruded position. The occlusal rims are sealed together, removed as one unit and transferred to the articulator, where the lower cast is mounted with plaster. The incisal pin is locked in place so that it will maintain vertical dimension. The lower rim is reduced 2 to 3 mm in height. This is necessary to prevent contact between rims in eccentric movements with arrow point tracer is in position.
b. *Verifying the centric relation*: An intraoral tracer consists of a flat metal plate and a central bearing point are mounted on the rims as close as possible to the center of the lower arch. The screw of the tracing stylus is adjusted to contact the tracing plate at the correct vertical dimension and secured by means of the locking nut. The bases with attached tracer assembly are taken from the articulator to the mouth. When the patient closes the central bearing point touches the metal plate, the correct vertical dimension is transferred from the articulator to the mouth. The vertical dimension should be verified now. If the vertical dimension is satisfactory, tracing can be made. The tracing plate is painted lightly with a thin layer of blue inlay wax (Fig. 8.15).
   The patient made the tracing by moving the jaw from side to side and from protrusive to retrusive several times. The plate is removed to see if a clear apex indicating centric relation. The bases are returned to the articulator and with a piece of articulating paper over the point of the tracing the articulator is closed. The mark made by the pin should coincide with the apex of the tracing. If it does not coincide, the centric relation record is incorrect. A new correct record is required for remounting the lower cast.
c. *Remounting the lower cast*: A clear small disk with a central whole is mounted with the hole over the apex this is attached to the tracing plate by means of sticky wax. The bases are returned to the mouth and the patient retruded the lower jaw and closes till the pin falls into the hole (Fig. 8.16). The patient holds this

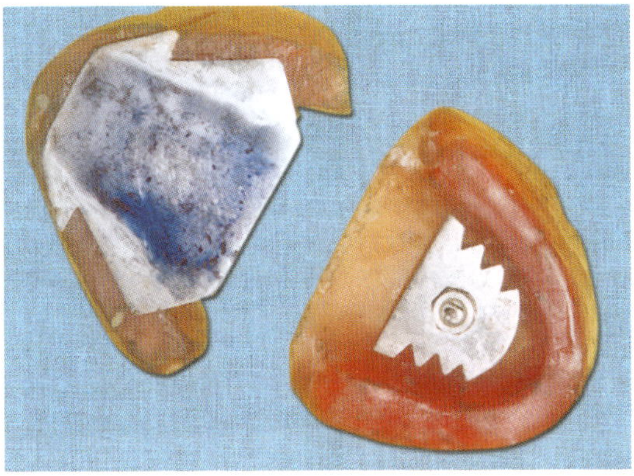

Fig. 8.15: Intraoral Gothic arch tracer mounted on occlusion rims

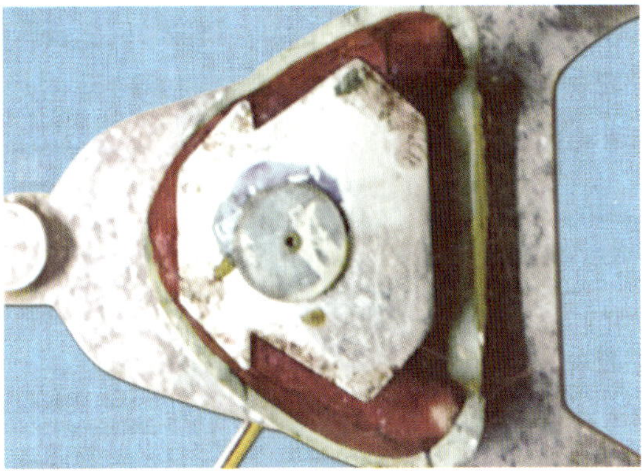

Fig. 8.16: A clear apex marked with a small disk with a central hole over centric point

position while quick setting plaster is inserted between the occlusion rims and allowed to set. When plaster is set the tracer assembly is removed as a single unit from the mouth to be used to mount the mandibular cast in centric relation. The mandibular cast is removed from the articulator and remounted with the new centric record.

Protrusive Interocclusal Record

After the mounting plaster sets a protrusive record can be obtained by moving the plastic disk back 6 mm from the apex of the Gothic arch tracing and sealed there with sticky wax. The assembly is placed in patient's mouth and asked the patient to

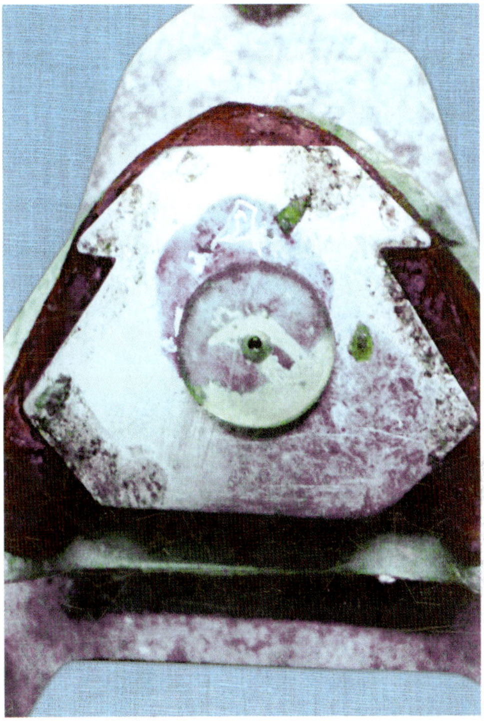

Fig. 8.17: A small disk with a central hole over protrusive point

move the jaw forward until the pin fall into the hole. Fresh plaster is injected with a syringe to obtain the protrusive record. The record is used to set the condylar guides of the articulator (Fig. 8.17).

Protrusive Record Setting into Articulator

The incisal pin is open wide and the condylar guides are loosened in all aspects. The protrusive record is set on the lower cast, and the condylar guides are rotated in such a way that the upper and lower occlusal rims fit the respective casts and the plaster wafer exactly.

Lateral Interocclusal Records

It is wise to set the lateral condylar guides before adjusting the instrument for protrusive record as because a change later will change the sagittal condylar angles. Hanau was of opinion that the

lateral condylar guidance can be set to an average of 15 degrees or by using Hanau formula as follows: L = H / 8 +12 or lateral equals horizontal divided by eight, plus twelve.
(Hanau's formula is embossed on the underside of the lower member of the Hanau's articulator)

L = Lateral condylar angle (Bennett angle)

H = Horizontal condylar angle.

The lateral condylar angle can be obtained using this formula, e.g.

Horizontal	Divided by	8 plus	12 equals	Lateral
0	"	" 8	" 12	" 12
8	"	" 8	" 12	" 12
16	"	" 8	" 12	" 12
24	"	" 8	" 12	" 12
32	"	" 8	" 12	" 12
64	"	" 8	" 12	" 12

As soon as the jaw relation have been transferred to the articulator the lower occlusal rim should be rebuilt for the teeth set up.

CONCLUSION

Establishment of jaw relations is an important step in the fabrication of complete dentures. Orienting the maxillary and mandibular dentures in correct horizontal and vertical relation to each other is important for the function, esthetics, health and comfort of the patient. The necessity of eccentric record is a course controversial, we do not know how much accuracy is required.

BIBLIOGRAPHY

1. Atwood AA. A critique of research of the posterior limit of the mandibular position. J Prosth Dent. 1968;20:21.
2. Becker CM, Kaiser DM. Evolution of occlusion and occlusion instruments, J Prosth Dent. 1993;2:33-43.
3. Cohn LA. Two techniques for interocclusal records. J Prosth Dent. 1963;13;438.
4. Downs B. The capture and use of centric relations. Dent Clin N Am. 1964;p.p611.
5. Gattozii JG. Nicol BR, Somes GW, Ellinger CW. Variations in mandibular rest positions with and without dentures in place. J Prosth Dent. 1976;36;159.
6. Hickey JC. Centric relation a must for complete denture. Dent Clin N Am. 1964.p.587.
7. Ismail YH, George WX. The consistency of the swallowing technique in determining occlusal vertical relations in edentulous patients. J Prosth Dent. 1968;19;230.
8. Joniot B. Physiologic Mandibular resting posture. J Prosth Dent. 1974;31:4.
9. Kapur KK, Yurkstas AA. An evaluation of centric relation records obtained by various techniques. J Prosth Dent. 1957;7:770.
10. Kapur, Yurkstas. Factors influencing Centric Relation Records in Edentulous Mouths. J Prosthet Dent. 1964;14;1054.
11. Mood GN. Centric occlusion, centric relation and the mandibular posture. J Prosth Dent. 1968;20:292.
12. Villa: Gothic Arch Tracing. J Prosthet Dent. 1959;9:624.

Chapter 9

Artificial Tooth Selection and Arrangement

ANTERIOR TOOTH SELECTION, ARRANGEMENT AND ESTHETICS

INTRODUCTION

After the jaw relation records have been obtained, suitable artificial teeth should be selected before the patient is dismissed. The selection and arrangement of anterior teeth for creating an esthetic denture is an art dominate the science. Denture esthetics is defined as "the cosmetic effect produced by a dental prosthesis which affects the desirable beauty, attractiveness, character, and dignity of the individual". There are guidelines for selection and arrangement of artificial teeth which serves as a starting point only. Tooth selection and final arrangement are the responsibility of the dentist. The preliminary arrangement can be done by the laboratory technician; it remains the dentist responsibility to select the mould, shade, and material and final arrangement of teeth.

OBJECTIVES

Artificial teeth should be placed in the complete denture to serve the following needs of the patient.

1. They are chosen for the fabrication of complete dentures that will function properly in the mouth.
2. They should allow the patient to speak properly.
3. They should appear esthetically pleasing.
4. They should be easy to set against the ridges.
5. They should not damage the residual ridges.

METHODS OF SELECTION OF TEETH

The selection of the anterior and posterior teeth should be done in two stages because function is the primary consideration for the posterior teeth, whereas esthetic is the primary consideration for the anterior teeth.

1. Selection of anterior teeth
2. Selection of posterior teeth.

Artificial teeth are available in various sizes for class I jaw relationship only for clases II and III mandibular anterior teeth are chosen from a different mould depending upon space.

Anterior Tooth Selection

Tooth selection is done in two different methods:

Direct Methods of Tooth Selection

This method is for patient present in the clinic with some remaining teeth so that information can be obtained from the patient regarding the form, size, and the position of the teeth.

a. *Patients own teeth*: The form and position of the natural teeth is the best guide for selection and arrangement of artificial tooth. If the natural teeth are not of proper size, shape and shade harmonious with the patient's face, they are not imitable, but will at least provide a basic guide for alteration and change from the natural teeth. Extracted teeth preserved at the time of extraction if available may be the best in producing natural result with less difficulty.

b. *Diagnostic casts*: Diagnostic casts of natural teeth provides the best record of the size, shape, and position of the natural teeth. It should be made for all patients where tooth loss is expected. These can be a valuable aid for choosing and positioning of artificial teeth if the patient is happy with the appearance of his teeth. If the patient does not like his own teeth it gives an idea of the patient's dislike.
c. *Previous dentures teeth*: If the patient had a previous set off denture, the easiest and most sensible approach is to converse with the patient. The denture made previously if found satisfactory is helpful in selection of artificial teeth.
d. *Photographs*: The close up photographs that show the patient happy and smiling help in assessing lip support. A photocopy of any relevant pictures should be taken with patient's permission to be used in the laboratory for setting of teeth. Such photographs should be measured for the ratio of patient's horizontal intercanine distance, and relate it to the inter-pupillary distance in the photograph. The width of the upper six anterior teeth can be established by applying the following formula:

$$\frac{\text{Width of six upper anterior teeth in a photograph}}{\text{Interpupillary width in photograph}} = \frac{\text{Width of six anterior teeth}}{\text{interpupillary width}}$$

e. *Radiographs*: The pre-extraction radiographs with no distortion can be used to determine the width, length, and shape of the natural teeth.

Indirect Methods of Tooth Selection

In absence of the natural teeth, and diagnostic casts, dentist will use indirect methods of selection and arrangement of artificial teeth. The dentist's judgment is the only means of selection of artificial teeth. The dentist should take the help of the patient to make tentative decisions about the shade, mould and position of teeth to be used. The tentatively selected teeth should not be given for inspection or comment, as the patient cannot at this stage judge the effect of the final arrangement. The patient's approval is to be obtained subsequently in the try-in stage. A selection should be made arranging the teeth on occlusion rim and viewing them in the patient's mouth before adequate judgment.

Selection of Upper Anterior Teeth

There are four main considerations when selecting anterior teeth:

1. Size
2. Shape
3. Color (shade)
4. Material

Selection of Size

The size and shape of the anterior teeth especially the maxillary central incisors are extremely important to the overall visual effect of the teeth. Teeth are judged to be too large or small, too narrow or wide, or of ethically disproportionate in shape when compared with the overall proportion of the other facial structures leading to esthetic disharmony. Sherry, Boucher, and Pound all condemned the practice of selecting teeth based on measurement of master cast. All advocated that the selection of size should be based on facial measurements and proportions.

To select the appropriate size of maxillary anterior teeth there are two dimensions to consider

a. Length and
b. Width.

a. *Length*: The length of the maxillary bite rim is first established by phonetics pronouncing the "F" and "V" sounds. The length of the maxillary central incisor is measured from the incisal edge of the maxillary rim up to the high lip line (smile line)—the position of the upper lip during smiling.

The second method of tooth length selection is based on the proportional size between the face and tooth. There is a harmony in the proportion of the maxillary anterior teeth and the face. The length of the maxillary central incisor is 1/16 of the length of the face from the hairline to the tip of the chin.

b. *Width*: Several anatomic guides are there to select correct width of maxillary anterior teeth. These are extreme variable guidelines. It is, therefore, suggested that several of these can be compared before coming to conclusion.
   1. *Intercommissural distance*: The corners of mouth can be marked on the correctly contoured maxillary occlusal rim. The combined width of the six upper anterior teeth represent the measurement between these marks.
   2. *The width of six maxillary anterior teeth* equals to the bizygomatic width divided by3.3. The facebow can be used to measure the bizygomatic width.
   3. *The width of the maxillary central incisor* is usually 1/16 of the bizygomatic width (Sears, 1941). The lateral incisors are 2 mm narrower and the canine 1 mm wider than the central incisors. The chart supplied by the manufacturer should be consulted to find the mould that possess the same width.

Levin observed that the widths of the maxillary teeth in frontal view lie within the "golden Proportion" of 1.681 (central incisor is 1.681 times wider than lateral incisor in frontal view).

The studies showed that the combined width of the six maxillary anterior teeth is normally 46 mm or more and anything less than 45 mm is unusual. The width of the most natural central incisors is over 8.5 mm and teeth less than 8 mm is unusual. Artificial teeth are usually smaller in size than natural teeth so slight larger mould should be chosen (Fig. 9.1A).

The dentist may have a collection of upper anterior tooth moulds set in acrylic resin on the arc of Bonwill's circle indicated by their mesiodistal width (Figs 9.1B to E).

Selection of Shape

Leon Williams (1914) and House and Loop (1939) popularized the geometric theory that the shape of the maxillary central incisor has the contour of the inverted face form (normal hairline to the chin). They classified faces into four types as square, tapering, and ovoid facial forms to determine the most pleasing size and shape of a maxillary central incisor (Fig. 9.2). However, Wright found that 60.7% of persons do not have natural maxillary

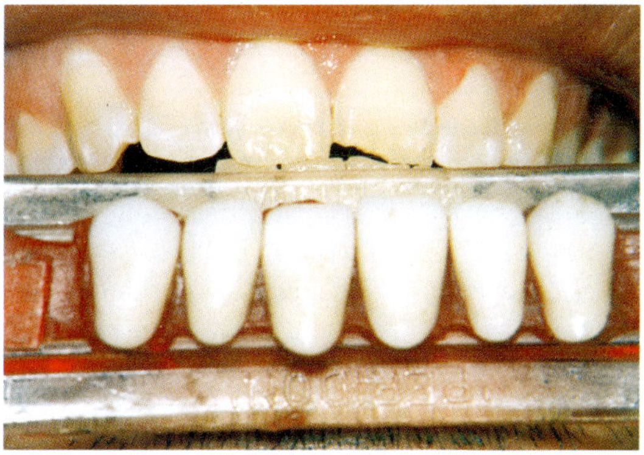

Fig. 9.1A: Artificial teeth are smaller in size than natural teeth so it is better to settle anterior teeth which are slightly larger in size

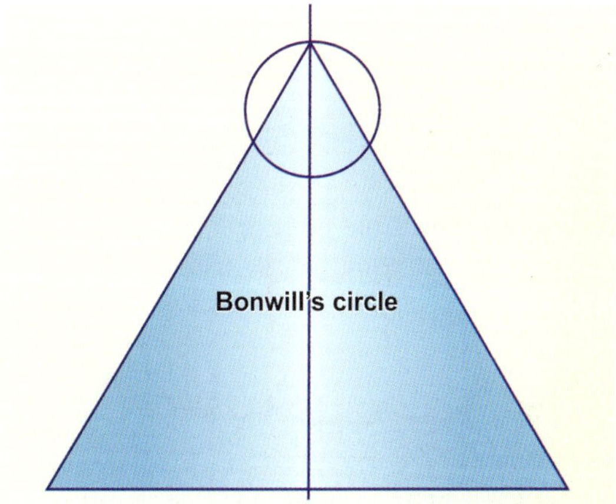

Fig. 9.1B: Bonwill's circle on Bonwill's triangle

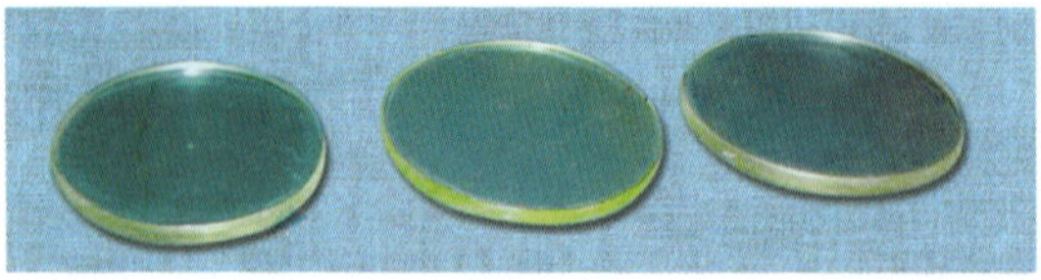

Fig. 9.1C: Bonwill's circles prepared for various moulds of anterior teeth

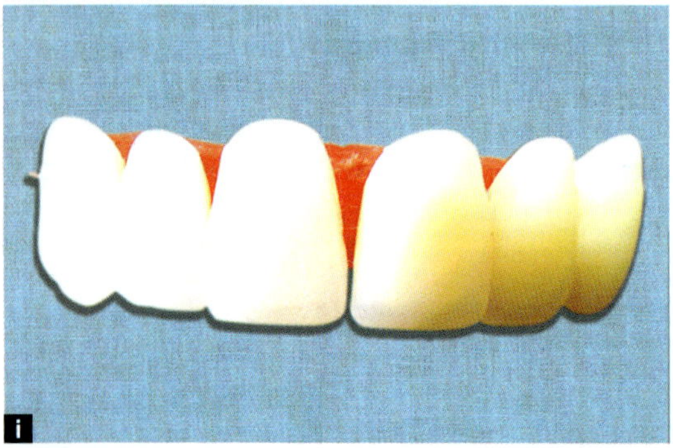

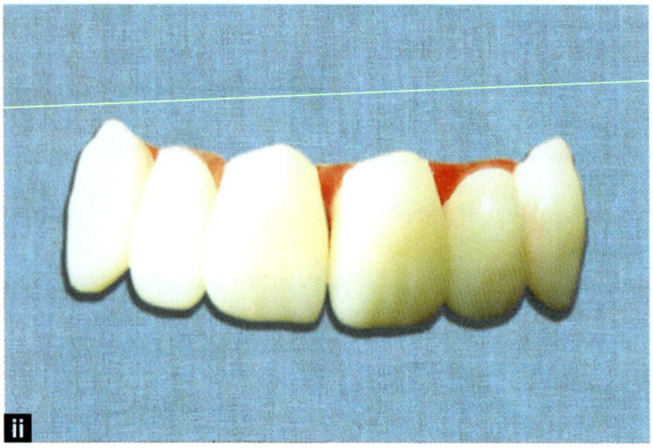

Figs 9.1D (i and ii): A collection of upper anterior teeth mould set on arch of Bonwill's circle

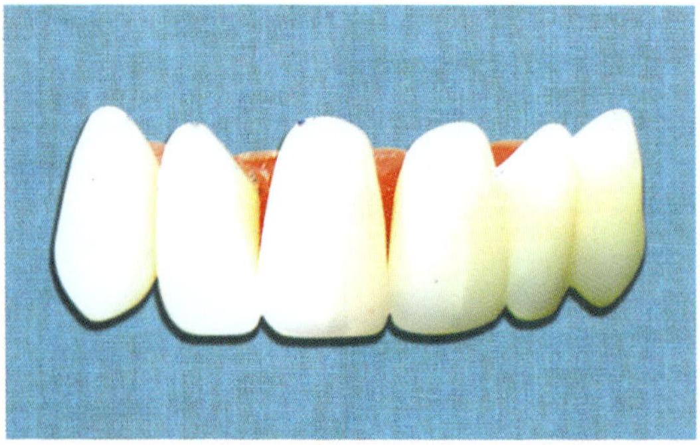

Fig. 9.1D (iii): A collection of upper anterior teeth moulds set in acrylic resin on arch of Bonwill's circle

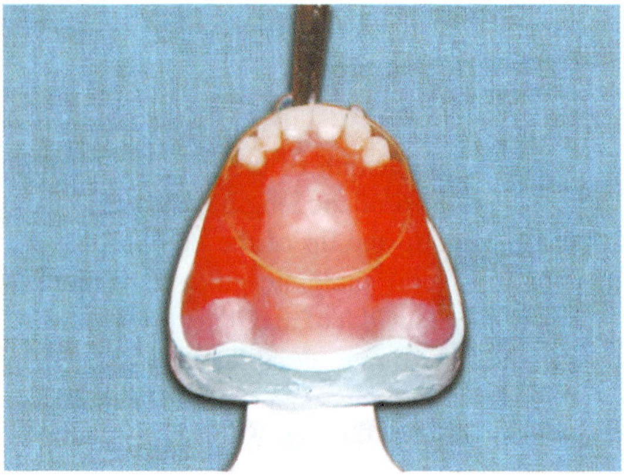

Fig. 9.1E: Anterior teeth set according to the arch of Bonwill's circle

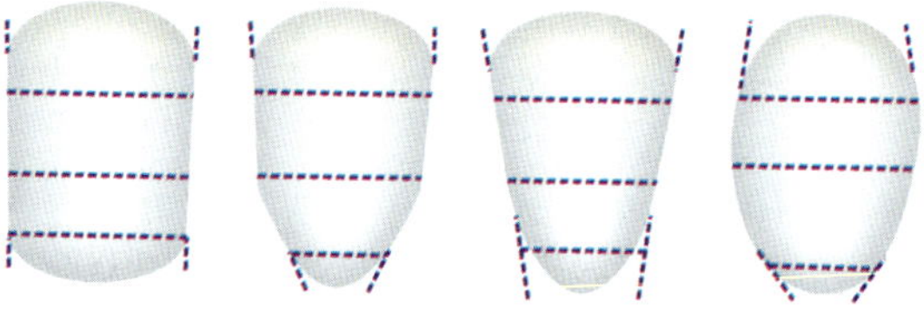

Fig. 9.2: Face form: square, square tapering, tapering and ovoid

central incisors of the inverted facial form. John Sherry remarked that natural tooth may not have the shape similar to the face form. Recent research of Mavroskoufis and Ritchie (1880) invalidates the work of Leon Williams' tooth selection method; it may be used as a starting point from which appropriate changes can be made.

Lee (1962) described an alternative method of tooth selection. He uses three facial measurements and relates the proportions of teeth to the proportions of face. He classified face in three forms based on their bizygomatic and biangular widths. The maxillary anterior teeth were selected according these forms as follows:

1. *Square*: The bizygomatic width, the width of forehead, and the biangular width are equal.
2. *Ovoid*: The bizygomatic width is wider than the biangular width and the width of forehead.
3. *Tapering*: The biangular width is less than the bizygomatic width and width of forehead.
4. *Square taper*: The bizygomatic width and width of forehead are wider than biangular width.

Tooth Curvature

The labial curvature of the anterior teeth should have the same curvature of the face in profile view both mesiodistally and incisogingivally. Some of the tooth manufacturers designed their tooth mould accordingly.

Dentogenics

As a general rule, the maxillary central incisor must be in general proportion to facial morphology. To be esthetically pleasing, it must be in general proportion to facial morphology. Proportion must be based on the character of the individual's facial features, whether weak/delicate or strong/vigorous. Frush and Fisher (1950, 1956, 1957, 1958, and 1959) developed the "Dentogenic" concept and their work characterizing denture teeth based on age, sex, and personality of the patient with the shape, shade, and form of his teeth. It is also known as SPA (sex, personality and age) factors for selection and arrangements of artificial teeth. Although these esthetic guidelines are not absolute, they are helpful in enhancing the esthetic result.

Dentogenic Concept

Age

The amount of anterior teeth visible in rest or in function often related to age. With increase in age, the amount of the maxillary central incisors showing with lip just parted will decrease, e.g. at 60 years no tooth will show whereas at 30 years and 3+ mm of tooth. The mandibular incisors will show opposite, e.g. 0.5 m at 30 years and 3 mm at 60 years of age. There are some exceptional cases.

Natural teeth wear with ages in most patient and the wear can be simulated by grinding the incisal edges of the denture teeth. With age there is exposure of roots and interdental papillary become blunt (Table 9.1).

Sex

The shape of anterior tooth differs in sex. The masculine characteristics are flat labial surfaces, square in shape, incisal edges are flat whereas the female characteristics are more curved in shape (Table 9.2).

Table 9.1 Age

Young	Old
• Lighter shade	• Darker shade
• Incisal translucency more	• Less
• Less wear	• More wear
• Smile line carved	• Smile less flat
• Cementoenamel junction not exposed	• Exposed makes of teeth

Table 9.2 Sex

Male	Female
Square	Tapering or oval
Flat and square labial surface	Curved labial surface
Square incisal edges and corners	Rounded incisal edges and corners
Large	Small
Darker shades	Lighter shades
Lateral incisors larger in comparison to the centrals	Curved arch form
Square arch form	
Mesial of lateral incisor rotated distally	Mesial of lateral incisor rotated mesially
Flat smiling line	Curved smiling line
Diastemas	Absent

Personality

The personality ranges from delicate to medium pleasing to vigorous. A delicate personality is very small in percentage of population. Larger group is vigorous and the vast majority is in the medium range (Table 9.3).

Selection of Lower Anterior Teeth

Lower anterior teeth may be chosen to match the selected uppers in reference to the manufacturer's charts. This is appropriate for a class I skeletal jaw relationship. With classes II or III jaw relationships, a small change in size can be made to match the space available. Gross difference of sizes of upper or lower anterior teeth are detrimental to esthetics. It is preferable to omit or add a tooth. The corresponding sizes of lower incisors provided by manufacturers are generally smaller than occur in life. To overcome this difficulty simply use of a much larger size of lower incisor teeth is advised. The size is decided correctly by using each lower incisor 0.6 times the width or, the lower four incisors should be 2.4 times the width of an upper central incisor.

Table 9.3: Personality

Vigorous	Medium	Delicate
Masculine	Masculine and Femine	Femine

Artificial teeth are available to the dentist on tooth cards designate tooth mould and shade. Six maxillary or mandibular teeth are available on tooth cards, with their mould identification number of each manufacturing unit. A mould guide is provided with. So, it is necessary to maintain appropriate mould guides in the clinic or laboratory for each manufacturer's teeth. There are three values allocated per mould (Figs 9.3A and B):

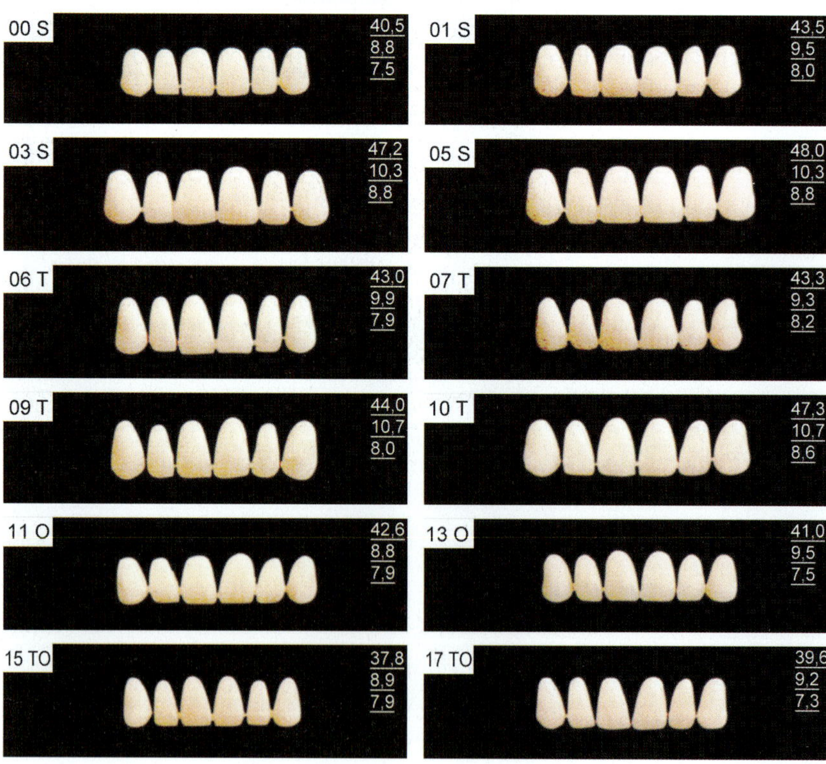

Fig. 9.3A: Acrylic denture teeth chart—upper anterior

recommended darker tooth for older patients, for men or patients with vigorous personality and lighter tooth for women and patients with delicate personality.

The natural teeth are polychromatic and consists of three distinct shades:

1. Cervical
2. Incisal
3. Transitional middle third. The shade possesses three qualities:
   - *Hue:* It is the specific color of the object, e.g. a tooth classed as red, yellow and grey.
   - *Value:* The relative brightness or darkness of the color. There is a transition of the shade from the central incisor to canines.
   - *Chroma:* The amount of concentration of color. In most of the shade guide, yellow is the prominent hue, chroma is the amount of yellow in each tooth. The canines have more chroma than the central incisor.

The following points are useful:

1. The shade selection should be done with the patient sitting upright position so that teeth can be seen in the clinic under the same conditions under which they are seen in public life.
2. Each manufacturer have its own shade guide with different shades, therefore, several shade guides should be used during shade selection.
3. Manufacturer's shade guide contains three basic shades or hues red, yellow and grey. The operator looks for the basic hue of teeth that is harmonious with the patient's complexion. Then the value or the corresponding lightness or darkness of the patient's skin is selected. Three values in each basic color/hue is sufficient.
4. The standard daylight should be used either in the form of natural northern sunlight in the middle of the day slightly overcast as well as suitable color corrected artificial light of same standard.
5. The shade guide should be moistened when used so that they have the an effect on the reflection and refraction of light and color.
6. The "Flash Perception Technique" is more preferable. Several shades of teeth are wetted and held under the upper lip in order to cheek the correct hue and value. The operator observes the shade that blends best with the surroundings to select proper shade. Two shades of teeth one light and one darker may be utilized first gradually merging of two extremes leads to a pleasant shade.
7. The "Squint Test" is helpful. In this technique, several shades of teeth are held under the patient's upper lip. The dentist looks at the teeth with the eyes nearly closed. The shade that fades most quickly is the most compatible.
8. The patient's relatives or friend may be useful if available in selecting shade.
9. The patients choice must be given preference as the patient will have to wear the dentures.

A standard shade guide (VITA Germany) is calibrated in shades A, B, C and D. Grouping of shades within the various color are as follows:

A1-A4	Reddish brown
B1-B4	Reddish yellow
C1-C4	Grayish shades
D2-D4	Reddish grey

Materials (Table 9.4)

A choice must be made between:

1. Conventional acrylic resin
2. Interpenetrating polymer network (IPN) acrylic resin,
3. Composite resin
4. Porcelain.

The choice depends on esthetics, wear resistance; hardness, noise in tooth contact, ease of setting; repair and processing. The older acrylic wore and discolored quickly. The newer cross-linked acrylics are more wear resistant than old acrylic resin teeth. The acrylic resin teeth can be ground very thin to fit into small spaces without losing of strength of bond to the denture base. The teeth can be reshaped for esthetics and can be polished easily. They do not cause much noise in function. They wear with time depending on the nature of cleaning. The IPN acrylic resin teeth are harder, more abrasion resistant than conventional acrylic resin teeth. They can be set up and used as

Table 9.4 Differences between acrylic and porcelain teeth

Porcelain	Acrylic
1. Wear is clinically insignificant over a long period of time.	1. Wear clinically significant.
2. No significant loss of vertical dimension.	2. Loss of vertical dimension of occlusion due to wear.
3. Maintain comminuting efficiency.	3. Loss of comminuting efficiency, due to wear.
4. Can be ground and polished and hold shape for years.	4. Self-adjusting and self-polishing.
5. Difficult to grind and fit into close inter-ridge space without loss of retentive element.	5. Easy to grind into close inter ridge space.
6. Allow for total rebasing procedures.	6. Rebasing allowed by replacing base material of palate without alter teeth.
7. The texture can be easily improved and stain and restoration can be added.	7. The texture cannot be changed nor staining easy
8. Appearance maintained indefinitely as resistance to abrasion.	8. Appearance not maintained indefinitely as no resistance to abrasion.
9. Make more noise when occluding.	9. Make less sound when occluding.
10. May cause severe abrasion to opposing gold crowns and natural teeth.	10. Minimal wear to opposing natural tooth and gold crowns.
11. It is costly than acrylic.	11. Resin teeth are cheaper than acrylic and so extensively used.
12. Mechanically retained to the base material.	12. Chemically bond to acrylic base material.
13. Modulus of elasticity is 9 times higher than acrylic resin so transmit greater proportion of masticatory force to the underlying mucosa.	13. Modulus of elasticity is very less than porcelain so transmit less masticatory force to the underlying mucosa.

conventional acrylic resin teeth. Porcelain teeth are more nature looking but easily fractured. They cannot be grounded to fit narrow space. They are the most wear and stain resistant. They produce more noise upon contact than acrylic resin teeth. They cannot be used due to presence of retentive pins where the teeth would have to be ground when interarch space is small. The porcelain anterior should not be used with acrylic posterior since wear of posterior will put pressure on porcelain anterior.

PRELIMINARY ARRANGEMENT OF ARTIFICIAL TEETH FOR TRIAL

Introduction

The arrangement of the anterior teeth to accomplish the desired esthetics helps to get acceptance by the patient. The use of a photograph is helpful. If not available, the patient should be asked about the size of teeth, presence of diastemas, or the lapping of anterior teeth.

The arrangement of the teeth for try-in is done by setting the teeth into basic positions, and these positions may be altered to meet the anatomic and physiologic variations found in different patients. The teeth are set in centric occlusion with the casts in centric relationship. Setting them in balance occlusion is useless until the jaw relation records have been verified and found correct in the try-in stage. The anterior teeth are arranged in basic positions mainly for esthetics. The posterior teeth are arranged in maximum planned intercuspation (cusped teeth) or occlusal contact (noncusp teeth) on a plane. But they are not inclined to meet any concept of balanced occlusion in eccentric positions until try-in have been satisfied. The proper preliminary arrangement of the artificial teeth minimizes rearrangement at the try-in appointment, when jaw relation records and esthetics are verified.

Order of Teeth Arrangement

It is customary to arrange the maxillary six anterior teeth first; then the mandibular anterior teeth, and finally the lower posterior teeth followed by upper posterior teeth. Alternatively, all the maxillary teeth may be set first and the mandibular first molars placed in position, followed by the second molars, the premolars, and finally the lower anterior teeth, omitting or grinding a lower incisor if there is insufficient space in the anterior region. The last method tends to produce accurate occlusion of the posterior teeth. Of course, the order to be followed is a matter of personal preference.

Arrangement of Anterior Teeth

When the jaw relation record is completed, the master casts are mounted on the articulator at the tentative vertical and horizontal relations the anterior teeth are set in the laboratory according the customized occlusal rims.

The arrangement of the anterior teeth is done to fulfill certain biomechanical needs viz. incision, phonetics as well as esthetic needs. Therefore, the placement of the anterior teeth is governed by certain rules to achieve the best mechanical advantage during function. There are four factors that govern the basic positions in arrangement of anterior teeth:

1. Horizontal position
2. Vertical position
3. Inclination
4. Esthetic arrangement and customization.

Horizontal Position

The horizontal positions of anterior teeth in edentulous arch usually follow the form and shape of the arch. Arch forms are classified as: (1) Square, (2) Tapering, or (3) Ovoid. The arrangement of the anterior teeth for the tapered arch places the central incisors further forward than the canines. The arrangement of the anterior teeth for the square arch places the central incisors more horizontally in relation to canines. The arrangement of anterior teeth for the ovoid arch places the six anterior teeth in a gentle curve (Figs 9.5A to C).

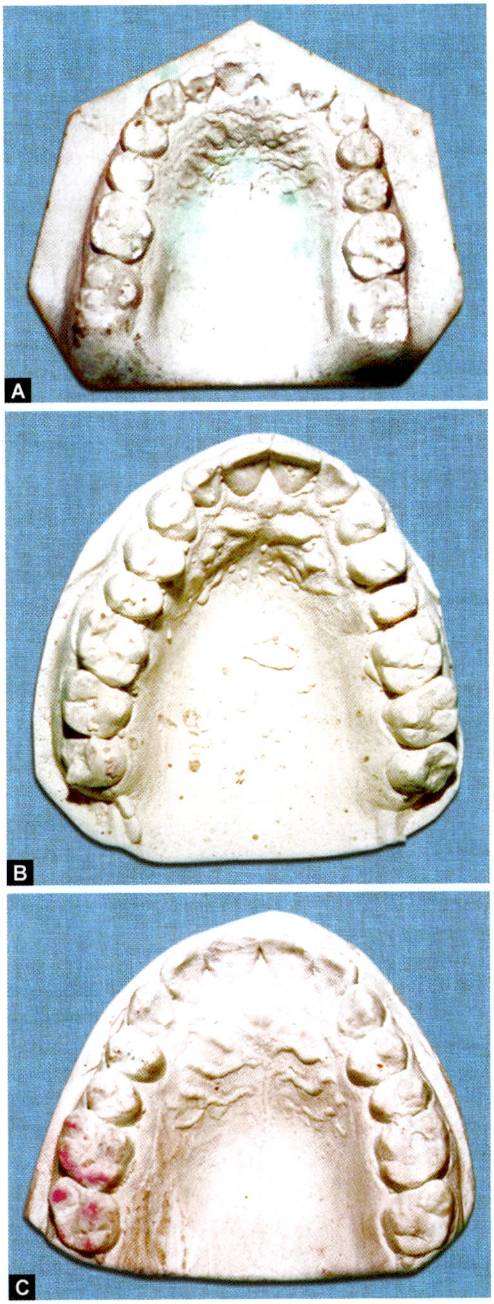

Figs 9.5A to C: (A) Class I sqare arch; (B) Class II tapering arch; (C) Class III oval arch

The anterior teeth, both maxillary and mandibular, are always set in front of the ridge, the amount depending on the degree of bone resorption which has occurred. The position of labial surfaces of the anterior teeth is determined in the patient mouth during jaw relation record with the bite rims. The information is utilized during the arrangements of the teeth. The incisive papilla is a relatively constant anatomical landmark that is not changed with age. The labial surface of the maxillary central incisors lies on a line 8 to 10 mm anterior to the center of the incisive papilla (Schiffman, 1964; Ortman and Tsao, 1979). The midline of the arch passes through the center of the papilla. A line drawn bisecting the incisive papilla and perpendicular to the midline will pass through the tip of the canines (Schiffman, 1964). In a typically square or modified square arch, the distance from the center of the incisive papilla forward to the labial surface of the maxillary central incisors was found to average 5 mm. In the ovoid arch, the maxillary central incisors are positioned average 6 mm anterior to the incisive papilla. In the tapered arch, the maxillary central incisors are usually appears to be 7 mm or more labial to the center of the papilla. These distances are average, but they serve as reasonable guides and starting point to set the central incisor. The labioincisal angle of incisor teeth should be placed such that the labial two-thirds of the incisors to support the incisal lip in a pleasing appearance. The most common error in tooth positioning is setting the teeth "over the ridge" with loss of esthetic appearance.

A perpendicular line to the midsagittal plane drawn through the center of the incisive papilla will pass through the tips of the canines in 78 percent cases and within 1 mm in 14 percent of cases (Fig. 9.6).

The final adjustment of the horizontal position of the teeth will be determined by the relationship of the ridges. Any adjustment of the position of these anterior teeth may be made at the try-in stage.

Adjustments for functional requirements are made depending upon the ridge relation are as follows:

- In class I relation the lower incisal edges should be no further anterior than mucobuccal fold.
- In class II relation the upper anterior have to be set slightly lingually.
- In class III relation the upper anterior have to be set on the upper ridge and inclined forward while lower anterior should be moved to ridge crest (Fig. 9.7).

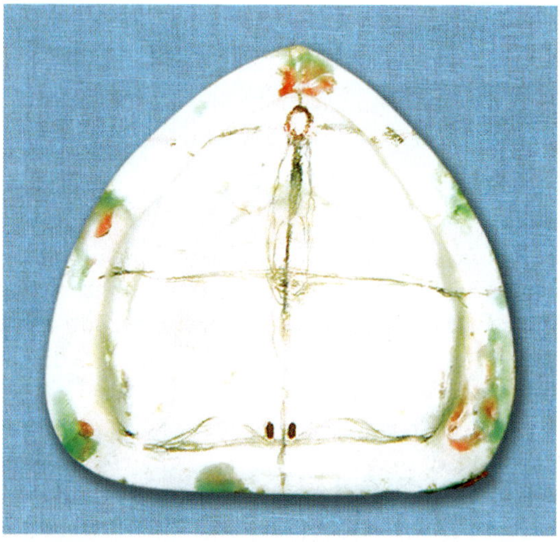

Fig. 9.6: Maxillary cast guidelines—lines on cast indicating cupid to the incisive papilla

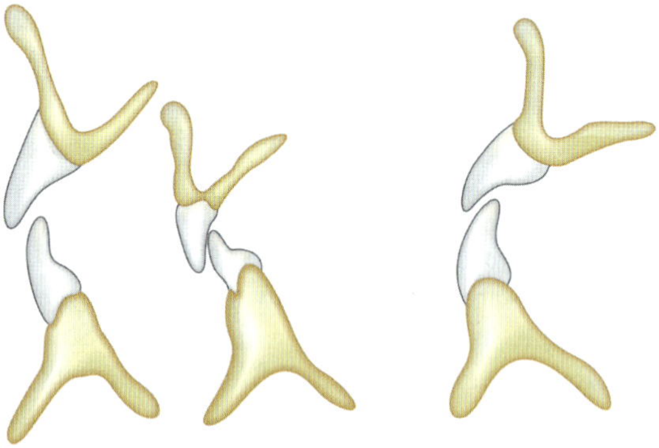

Fig. 9.7: In class I relations, lower incisors edge should not be forward than mucobuccal fold. This is also for class II relations, but the maxillary incisors may incline more lingually. In class III, lower incisors should be placed at ridge crest and the maxillary incisors inclined forward

Vertical Position

The correct vertical positioning of teeth should provide: (1) Denture stability, (2) Lip support, (3) Esthelic.

The length of the maxillary central incisors is established by esthetic and phonetics. The incisal edge may be visible below the relaxed upper lip in the range of 0 to several millimeters depending upon the lip length. The lip fullness is determined first followed by determination of the length by having the patient enunciate "F" and "V" sounds. The length is determined by the contact of incisal edge to the junction of the wet and dry line of the lower lip (Fig. 9.8).

The vertical position of incisal edges of the maxillary anterior teeth are done by using the low lip line and smile line of the upper lip. The lateral incisors should be slightly higher than the central incisors and canines should be somewhat higher than the lateral incisors. This arrangement establishes a curve known as smiling line. According to Frush and Fisher a pleasing smiling line should follow the curvature of the lower.

The vertical positioning of lower anterior depends on:

a. Phonetic and esthetic requirements
b. Ridge relations
c. Occlusal scheme
d. Interridge distance.

There should be no occlusal contact in centric relation. The amount of anterior overjet will be dictated by the relationship of the upper ridge to the lower ridge, i.e. normal, protrusive, or retrusive, or straight, concave, and convex respectively.

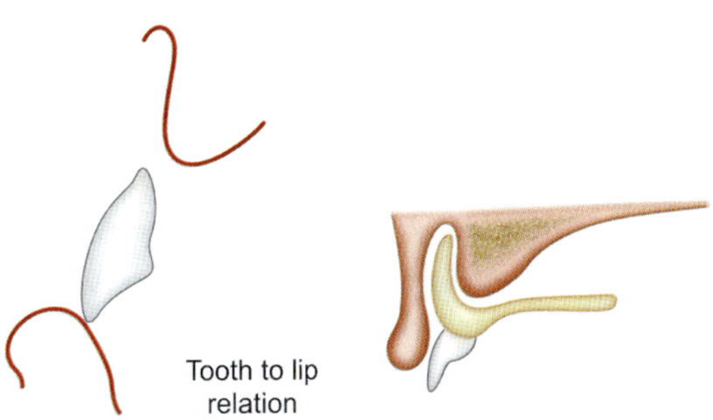

Fig. 9.8: Bisected papilla used to determine forward position of upper central incisor. Tooth and lower lip relation: Length is determined by patient enunciate 'F' and 'V' sounds

The overbite is governed by the type of posterior teeth used and by the amount of overjet established in setting the anterior teeth.

After the maxillary teeth are set according to the esthetic and phonetic guidelines on the maxillary rim, the positions of the incisal edges of the mandibular central incisors can be established with closest speaking space technique. The mandibular anterior teeth are set so that their incisal edges are slightly lingual to the incisal edges of the maxillary incisors (1 to 1.5 mm) when the patient enunciates sibilant sounds. The mandibular incisors are usually be 0.5 to 2 mm above the relaxed lower lip with the labial surface straight up from the peripheral role of the lower cast.

But in case of a retrognathic jaw relation, the mandibular incisors are tipped forward as far as possible for better esthetics, whereas in a prognathic jaw relation they are tipped lingually to prevent or minimize anterior crossbite.

If a patient is provided with a complete denture having same overjet and overbite as in natural dentition it affect the stability of dentures. It is necessary to have shallow incisal inclination to obtain the stability of dentures.

INCLINATIONS

The following rules are related to the setting up of teeth for a basic Angle's class I relationship.

Upper Anterior Teeth (Figs 9.9A and B)

1. *Central incisors*: Its long axis is parallel to the vertical axis when viewed from the front, and sloping slightly labially when viewed from the side. The incisal edge is in contact with the horizontal plane.
2. *Lateral incisors*: The long axis is sloping towards the midline of the mouth when viewed from the front, and is inclined labially to a greater degree than the central when viewed from the side. The incisor edges are about 2 mm above the horizontal plane.

3. *Canines*: Its long axis is parallel to the vertical axis when viewed from both front and side. Its tip is in contact with the horizontal plane.

Lower Anterior Teeth

Labiolingual Inclination (Figs 9.9A and B)

Central incisor: The neck should be depressed slightly.

Lateral incisor: The labial surface should be approximately vertical.
Canine: Slightly prominent at the neck when viewed from the foot.

Mesiodistal Inclination (Fig. 9.9C)

Central incisor: Straight
Lateral incisor: Slightly distal at neck.
Canine: Distal at the neck (when viewed from the side).

Arch Form and Tooth Arrangement

The mesiodistal placement of the upper anterior teeth follows the general form of the anterior ridge to maintain harmony between the artificial teeth and the facial contours. The arrangement of the

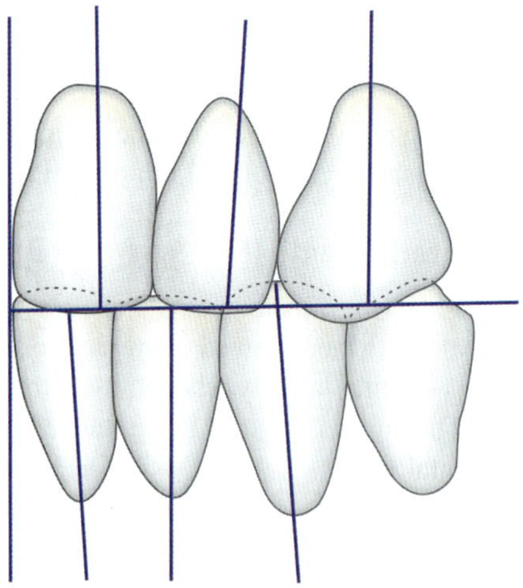

Fig. 9.9A: Sketch showing the normal relationship between the upper and lower anterior teeth in class I jaw relationship when viewed form the front

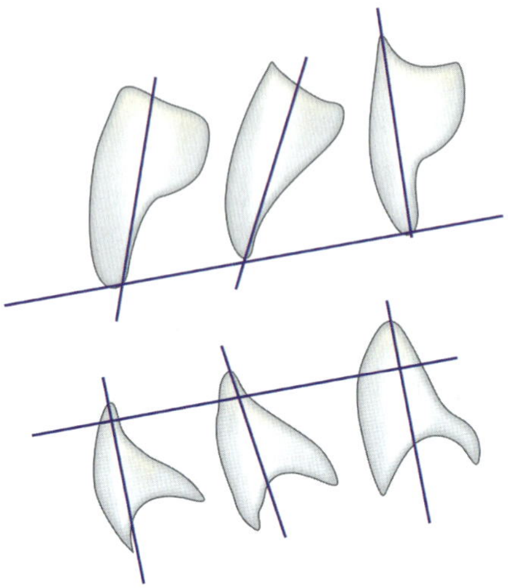

Fig. 9.9B: Normal positions of the upper and lower anterior when viewed from the side

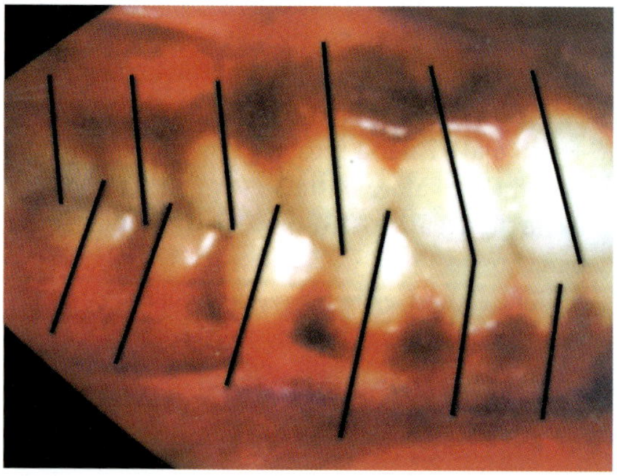

Fig. 9.9C: Mesiodistal inclination of teeth

anterior teeth for a square arch places the central incisors more nearly horizontal with the canines. The arrangement of the anterior teeth for the ovoid arch places the six anterior teeth in a gentle curve. The arrangement of anterior teeth in a tapered arch places the central incisors further forward than the canines.

- In square arch form, the central incisor is nearly perpendicular, whereas the lateral incisor is inclined more distally at the cervical end than the central incisors, and canine is inclined more distally than other anterior teeth to indicate strong personality.

- In ovoid arch form, the central incisor is inclined approximately 2 degrees distally at the cervical end, the lateral incisor is inclined more than the central incisor and the canine is inclined about 5 degrees at the cervical end to provide softness of appearance.
- In tapering arch form, the central incisor is inclined about 3 degrees at the cervical end, the lateral incisor is inclined more than the central incisor and the canine is inclined about 6 degrees at the cervical end to provide delicacy of the personality.

Esthetic Arrangement and Customization of Anterior Teeth

Another general guide effective means of providing realism in artificial teeth is to grind the incisal edges to imitate natural attrition. To reflect the age of the patient, usually longer central incisors than required is chosen to permit incisal grinding. In young patients, this is not advisable, but in any patient of more than 35 years of age this procedure is essential. Horizontal flattening of the incisal edges is not realistic. Some inclination of the incisal attrition in individual tooth is preferred. This can achieve when occlusion is perfected, on articulator after the denture have been processed is to avoid absolute symmetry of right and left sides.

Dissimilarities in inclination, rotation and position of the teeth on each side of the midline provide asymmetric symmetry (Fig. 9.10). The manner in which different esthetic effects can be produced with teeth of same mold by arrangement alone as follows:

"Normal" arrangement: The central incisors of normal size and normal arrangement.

"Soft" arrangement: The central incisors with prominent mesial sides and set back distal sides.

"Bold" arrangement: The central incisors are positioned straight across or slightly ahead of the adjacent teeth.

Modification of a central can be done by:

a. Squaring the incisal edges and corners
b. Rounding the incisal edges.

Customization for Age, Sex and Personality

A flat smiling line is associated with males and increased age. A curved smile line is more appropriate for female and young patients (Fig. 9.11).

Large lateral incisors in relation to central incisors give musculinity while smaller lateral incisors tends to be more feminine.

Lateral incisors lapping the distal of the limbal incisors is generally considered to be a female characteristic. The lapping of lateral by central incisors is more musculinic.

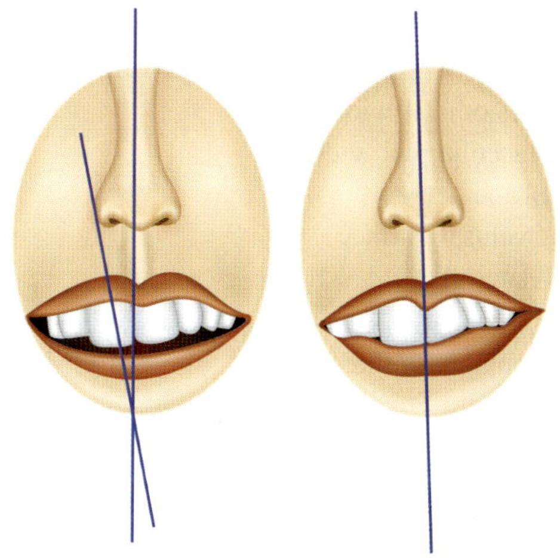

Fig. 9.10: Diagram illustrating asymmetric as related to the midline of the face

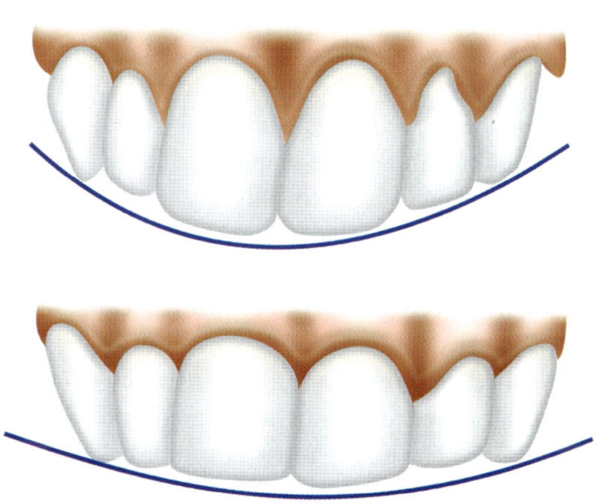

Fig. 9.11: Curved and flat smile line

The incisal edge of incisors and tips of canine grounding to create attrition consistent with ageing. Waxing of papilla producing blunt appearance and exposure of neck of the teeth in older patients creates most naturalness.

SELECTION AND ARRANGEMENT OF POSTERIOR TEETH

SELECTION OF POSTERIOR TEETH

The selection of posterior teeth should not be made until the cast are mounted. It is influenced by factors of articulation of teeth. There are six factors of selection of posterior teeth that include:

1. Occlusogingival length
2. Mesiodistal width
3. Buccolingual width
4. Shade
5. Occlusal surface
6. Material.

1. *Occlusogingival length*: Posterior teeth are available in three lengths, Large (L), Medium (M) and Small (S) moulds. The height of the posterior teeth is determined by the interarch distance. The choosing of the longest tooth that will fits the space without grinding is the rule. Long posterior teeth are usually are esthetically more pleasing than short teeth. Long anterior teeth should not be used with short posterior teeth.
2. *Mesiodistal width*: The mesiodistal width of posterior teeth should be shorter than the distance between the mandibular canine and the ascending area of the mandible. The ascending area is usually situated slightly anterior to the retromolar pad. This should be marked on the landing areas of the cast. Posterior teeth must not be placed on this slope, as it will cause slide of lower denture forward when biting force is applied on posterior teeth. If insufficient space exists, three posterior teeth are used instead of four. The tooth most commonly dropped is the first premolar. Since, this tooth has least occlusal surface. Some dentists prefer to drop the second molar so as not to disturb the buccolingual width in the premolar area. Posterior teeth are available in cards of 28, 30, 32, 34 mm or 29, 31, 33 mm. Smaller posterior teeth transmit less chewing force than larger teeth.
3. *Buccolingual width*: The buccolingual widths of artificial teeth should be less than the widths of the natural teeth they replace. The narrow posterior teeth help in developing the correct form of polished surfaces of the denture and also assist the cheeks and tongue in maintaining the dentures on the residual ridge.
4. *Shade*: The shade of posterior teeth should match that of the anterior teeth. The manufacturers usually have a coding of system that corresponds to the anterior shade and makes selection of posterior teeth easy.
5. *Occlusal surface form*: The selection of posterior tooth occlusal surface forms can be based on the biomechanical needs of each patient. There are various types of posterior denture tooth forms available, varying from 33° cusps anatomical teeth to nonanatomical or cuspless teeth. In between are 5°, 20°and 30° are also known as anatomic teeth. No one form is best for all patients. There are advantages and disadvantages of both anatomic and nonanatomic teeth given below.

In a class I jaw relationship with good size ridge selection of any posterior mould anatomic 30° or semianatomic or zero degree or a combination of mould can be used. In class II or class III relationship zero degree posterior moulds or a combination of zero degree mandibular tooth mould against the maxillary 20° cusp teeth can be used, when a posterior crossbite is encountered, the zero degree mould or a combination of moulds is suggested.

If an anatomical tooth is selected it should have sufficient cusp height so that it can be modified by grinding the transverse ridge of the occlusal surface as needed for freedom in occlusion without destroying the occlusal morphology and without reducing the chewing efficiency of the dentures.

At present there is little scientific evidence to support the use of one tooth occlusal form or arrangement. It is, therefore, seems logical to use the least complicated approach that fulfills the need of the patients. If nonanatomical teeth are used, they should be set in a flat plane, so that not to lose their occlusal details and reduce their chewing efficiency. Both the anatomic and nonanatomic forms have advantages and disadvantages and specific uses that are listed below. To avail the advantage of both anatomic and nonanatomic teeth lingualized occlusion scheme is used, i.e. the maxillary 20° posterior against mandibular zero degree nonanatomic teeth. It is claimed that this occlusal scheme fits all patient. All the advantages (cusp teeth, esthetics, and balanced occlusal concept) are available through the use of the maxillary functional (20°) teeth. The rational or 0 degree mandibular teeth provide the ease of arranging teeth in a classes II or III jaw relation where crossbite situation exist.

6. *Materials*: Porcelain was favored because of hard glazed surface not affected by abrasive food or cleanser and provides efficient mastication throughout the life of the denture. The rapid wear of acrylic teeth causes consequent loss of vertical dimension. Improve hardness of new generation of acrylic resin teeth and fewer composite resin teeth have reduced the use of porcelain teeth. The disadvantage of porcelain is its brittleness and susceptibility to fracture. Additionally they are only bonded mechanically with acrylic base and cannot be set by grinding easily.

Anatomic Teeth (Fig. 9.12)

Advantages

1. They are more natural in appearance and offer better esthetics.
2. They have better chewing efficiency.

Disadvantages

1. They require precise jaw relation records and precise articulator.
2. The vertical force directed against steep incline cusps of an anatomic mould results in more denture movement than that produced in a nonanatomic mould.
3. It is difficult to arrange anatomic teeth in cross-bite ridge relation.
4. Relining and rebasing of dentures is often required with anatomic teeth.
5. Frequent occlusal adjustments are required with anatomic teeth.

Indications

1. To provides good esthetics.
2. In good young healthy patient with good ridges.
3. In denture opposing well preserved natural teeth.
4. In class II, division 2 with large vertical overjet and little or no horizontal overjet.
5. In a case with people chew mainly in vertical mandibular movement, i.e. in choppers.

Nonanatomic Teeth

Indications

1. Shallow resorbed ridge.
2. Knife-edge and flabby ridges.

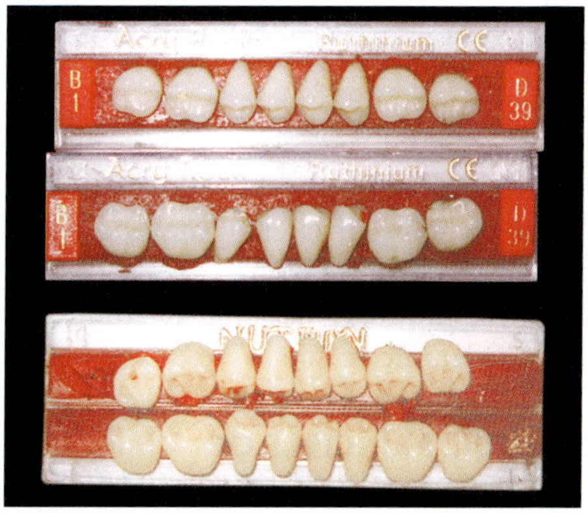

Fig. 9.12: Anatomic and nonanatomic teeth

3. In a case with mainly translatory movements, i.e. in grinders, e.g. class II, division I, and some class III jaw relations.
4. Extreme interridge space.
5. Patient with neuromuscular disturbances, i.e. Parkinsonism's chorea.
6. Denture opposing severely worn natural dentition.
7. In immediate dentures.
8. Great discrepancy in size and relationship of two arches.
9. In habitual eccentric occlusion position.
10. In partial mandibulectomy, and condylectomy cases.
11. In temporomandibular disturbances.
12. In clenching or grinding habits.

Advantages

1. They are easier to arrange and requires less instruments.
2. They permit closure in an area rather than a point, therefore, best suited for patient with difficultly in jaw relation record.
3. They have no inclined plane action to produce horizontal movement.
4. Easy to arrange in class II and class III jaw relations.
5. Relining and rebasing is easily done.
6. Give freedom of mandibular movements to the patient.

Disadvantages

1. Esthetically inferior to anatomic teeth.
2. Their chewing efficiency may be less than that of anatomic teeth.
3. They require more harmful horizontal movement to masticate food.

GENERAL PRINCIPLE OF ARRANGEMENT OF POSTERIOR TEETH

Most of the authors describe setting of upper posterior teeth first. In a normal class I jaw relation it does make any difference whether the upper or lower teeth are set first. But the positioning of the lower posterior teeth first before the upper posterior makes the lower posterior teeth to be easily set in the position of natural teeth because the important landmarks are in the lower ridge. The lower denture is also difficult to stabilized. So, setting the lower teeth first the difficult task of stabilization can be easily be achieved. But setting posterior teeth in tight centric occlusion for try-in is more desirable. The posterior teeth are set without curve and in balanced occlusion until jaw relation is verified. A normal arrangement is best before try-in though crossbite relation may be required for final arrangement. The mandibular posterior teeth are arranged by placing their cusps tips touching a flat plane and the central fossae on a line running from the distal of canines to the center of the retromolar pads.

FACTORS FOR ARRANGEMENT OF POSTERIOR TEETH

The factors which guide the position of the posterior teeth and the number of teeth to be used depend on the type of resorption and the relationship of two arches.

The posterior teeth, like the anterior teeth should be located as nearly as possible to the position formerly occupied by the natural dentition. This position helps to maintain the equilibrium between oral musculature and the lingual and buccal surface of the dentures.

In the absence of pre-extraction records posterior teeth should be arranged in following positions:

1. Anteroposterior position
2. Buccolingual position
3. Superoinferior position.

1. *Anteroposterior position*: The position of the posterior teeth varies with the position of the anterior teeth. The posterior teeth occupy the position between the canines anteriorly and the retromolar pad or inclination of the lower residual ridge posteriorly. Posterior teeth should

not be placed on an incline, as because any force applied to teeth will cause the denture to be displaced anteriorly. Teeth should not be arranged on the retromolar pad as it will not be able to withstand the load during tooth contact. In many cases only three posterior teeth could be arranged in each side.

2. *Superoinferior position*: The tentative occlusal plane was established at the jaw relation records with the help of a fox plane. A line joining the distal surface of the mandibular canine and a point two-thirds up the retromolar pad determines the final position of the occlusal plane. The occlusal plane should be placed at an equal distance between the two ridges. It should not be placed at a level to favor the weaker ridge.
3. *Buccolingual position*: There are several anatomical guidelines which may be used for buccolingual positioning of the posterior teeth:
   - The teeth should be placed in the neutral zone between the forces of the cheek and tongue. These forces dictate the position of the natural teeth. So, artificial teeth should be placed in neutral zone. The width of neutral zone is generally reduced following loss of natural teeth, so narrow posterior than natural will be required.
   - The buccal cusp of the posterior teeth should be placed over the buccal turning point of the crest of the lower ridge to avoid fulcrum action.
   - The lingual cusp should be positioned within the triangle formed by a line drawn from the mesioincisal angle of the lower canine to the lingual corner of the retromolar pad and a line from the same to the buccal corner of the retromolar pad. They should not be placed further lingually. If done these creates a concavity in the lingual flange below the posterior teeth. Tongue movements engage the concavity and causes looseness of the lower denture during function.

LABORATORY PROCEDURES (ARRANGEMENT OF TEETH)

Determination of Jaw Relationship

The relationship of the teeth of lower denture to those of the upper will be decided by the relationship of the jaws. Angle's classification is usually used to designate the three basic jaw relationships as follows:

Class I (Normal) (Figs 9.13A and B)

The maxillary ridge crest is directly above the mandibular ridge. This is the most favorable relation for complete dentures. About 70% of edentulous cases belong to this class.

In this case anterior teeth are set with an overjet and overbite of 1 to 2 mm.

In this case usually the posterior teeth can be set in normal position with 1 mm overjet buccally.

Class II (Retrognathic) (Figs 9.14A and B)

The mandibular ridge is narrower and shorter than the maxillary ridge. The maxillary posterior ridge crest is buccal to the mandibular ridge crest that makes the setting of posterior teeth difficult. About 25% of edentulous cases belong to this class.

In this case anterior teeth are set with an over-jet and overbite of 2 to 4 mm.

In this the posterior teeth are set with more overjet than normal (> 1 mm).

Class III (Prongathic) (Figs 9.15A and B)

The mandibular ridge is larger and wider than maxillary ridge. It projects beyond the maxillary ridge. This patient shows no excursive movement but only open and close hinge jaw movement. This makes balance occlusion unnecessary. About 5% of edentulous cases belong to this class.

In this case anterior teeth are set with overbite 0 mm and overjet 1 mm.

In this case posterior teeth are set with cross-bite, i.e. –ve overjet.

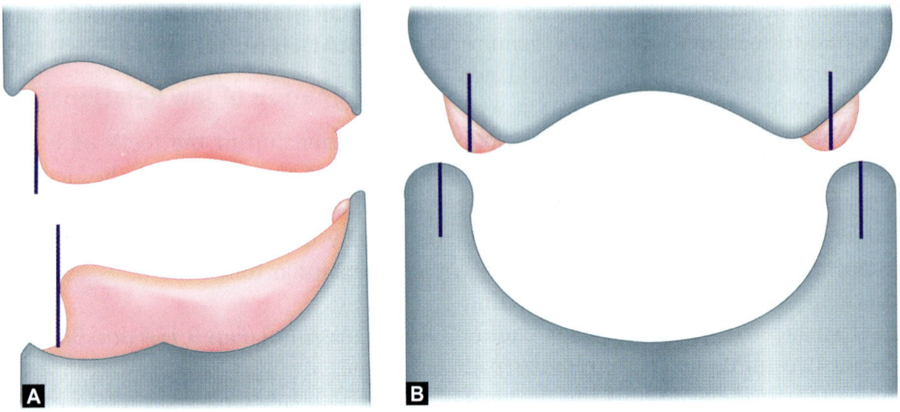

Figs 9.13A and B: Class I jaw relationship: (A) Lateral view (normal); (B) Posterior view (normal)

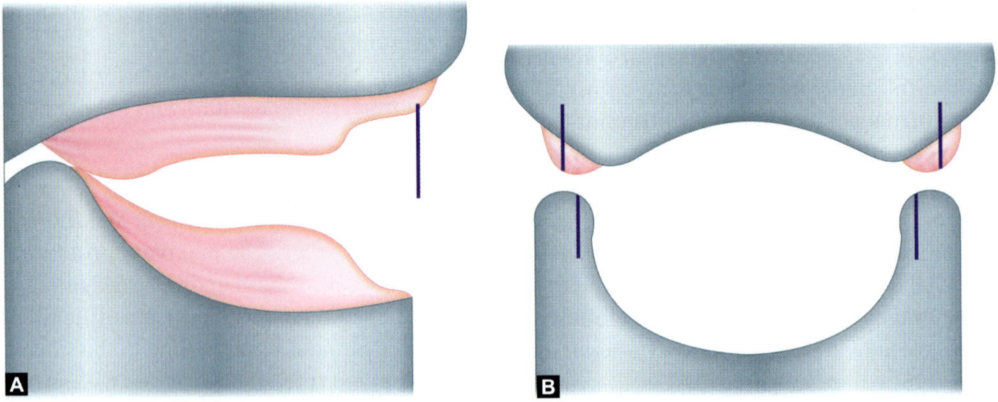

Figs 9.14A and B: Class II jaw relationship—lateral and posterior view (retrognathic)

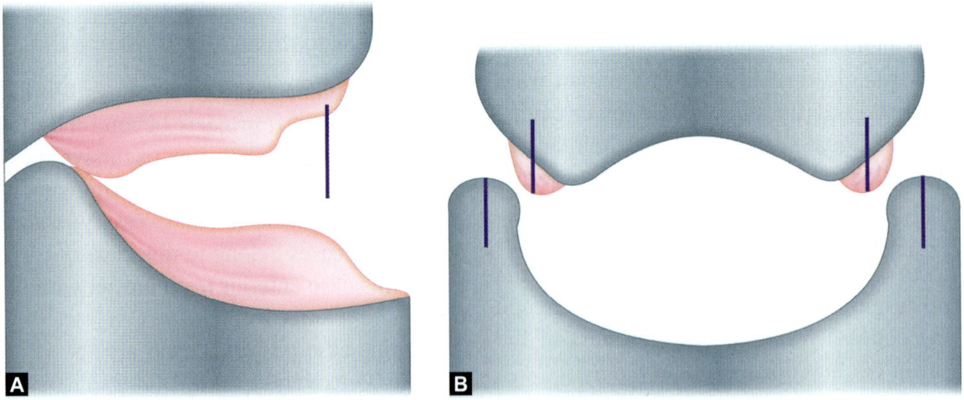

Figs 9.15A and B: Class III jaw relationship—lateral and posterior view (prognathic)

Transformation of Information from Occlusion Rim to Plaster Mounting

The positioning of the artificial teeth is usually done using the occlusal rims as a guide. When teeth are set on occlusal rim the information recorded on the rim is destroyed. Consequently it is desirable to transfer the information to the casts and the mounting plaster on the articulator for further reference.

The technique is as follows:

1. The central line marked on the occlusal rims is continued into the mounting plaster by a sharp blade plaster knife.
2. An arbitrary point is marked on the mounting plaster on the central line. A pair of dividers is opened and the tip of one arm is placed into the point and the tip of other arm rested on the low or normal lip line. This measurement is scribed on top or front of the mounting plaster (Fig. 9.16).
3. The divider are adjusted to record the high lip line in the similar manner (Fig. 9.17).
4. Both the upper and lower rims are removed from the casts.
5. A straight line is drawn on the crest of lower ridge with pencil and the lines are extended down the side of the cast. The lower posterior teeth are set so that the central fossa coincide with the line.
6. The retromolar pads on the mandibular casts are marked with a circle. A horizontal line is drawn through the superoinferior centers of the retromolar pads and extended onto the land areas (Fig. 9.18).
7. The incisive papilla is outlined with pencil. The labial surface of maxillary central incisors are usually set 5 to 7 mm anterior to the center of the papilla. Boley gauge is used to measure it (Fig. 9.19A).
8. A perpendicular line is drawn through the center of incisive papilla which are extended to the both side land areas of the maxillary cast.

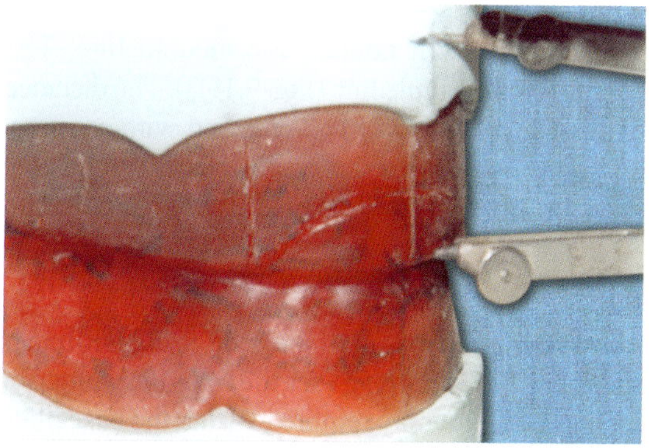

Fig. 9.16: The central line marked on the occlusal rim is continued to mounting plaster by plaster knife. An arbitrary point is marked on the mounting plaster on the central line. The measurement is made from the arbitrary point to lower lip line

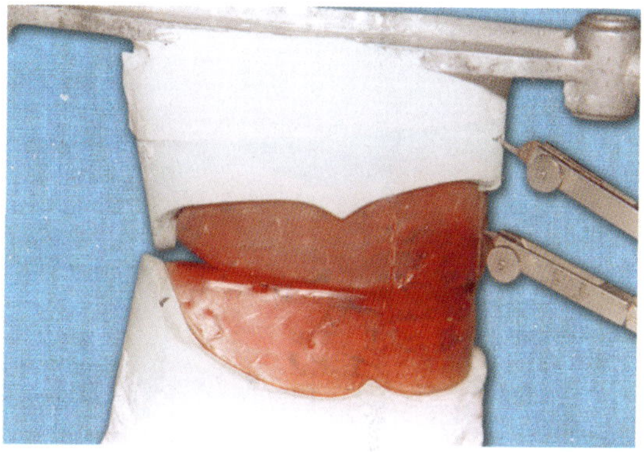

Fig. 9.17: A pair of dividers is opened and the tip of one arm pressed into the mounting plaster along the center line and tip of the other arm on the upper lip line

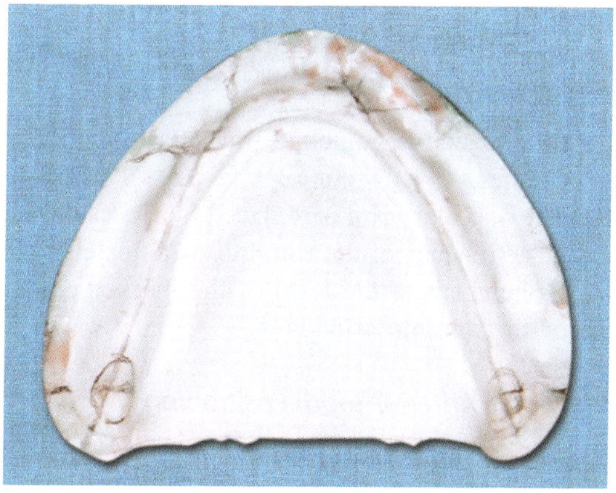

Fig. 9.18: Marked retromolar pads

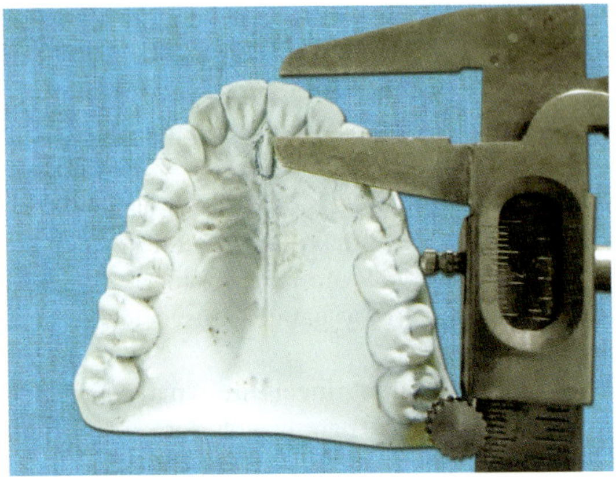

Fig. 9.19A: Gauge is used to measure from center of papilla to labial surface of central incisor

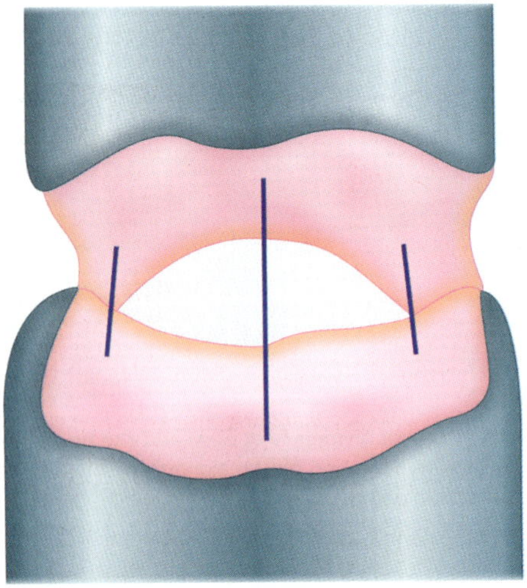

Fig. 9.19B: Information recorded on the occlusal rim and base—median line, canine lines and smile line

It will acts as guideline for setting maxillary canines.

9. The maxillary rim is replaced on the cast. The posterior part of the rim only is adjusted until its height is at the level of the marked center of the retromolar pads.

Individual Anterior Tooth Positioning

The arrangement of artificial teeth for edentulous patients differs according to jaw relationship, i.e.

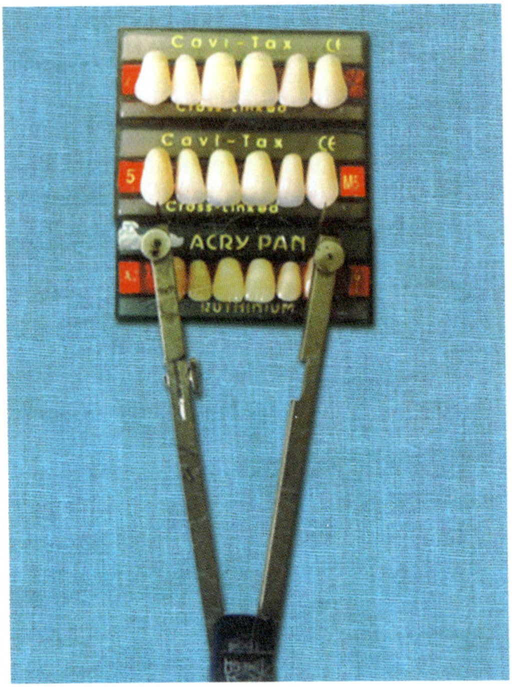

Fig. 9.19C: Upper anterior tooth moulds measured with a gauge between the distance of canine line and tip of canine

class I, class II, and class III. A class I jaw relationship may be regarded as the ideal relationship with the teeth being set in the following manner.

ARRANGEMENT OF TEETH IN CLASS I RELATION

The bite rim will contain the median line. The canine line and smile line (Fig. 9.19B). The distance of the canine line will be measured with a gauge, and considered with the denture teeth moulds for anterior teeth (Fig. 9.19C).

Arrangement of Maxillary Anterior Teeth

The maxillary wax rim of one side of the midline is removed for 25 mm. To set the maxillary anterior teeth properly it may require to grind the base plate to reduce the thickness even if require to create a hole in it than to grind the neck of the teeth. The shape of the occlusion rim should not be destroyed.

Maxillary Central Incisor

The maxillary central incisor is attached to the anterior of record base with a little softened wax using No 7 spatula. The long axis of the tooth should be flush with the mesial and distal surface of the wax rim. The maxillary central incisor is positioned on the bite rim using the length and contour as a guide using a supporting metal template for teeth or wax rim (Fig. 9.20A).

Maxillary Lateral Incisor

The maxillary lateral incisor is set with long axis inclined slightly distally with slight depression at neck. The incisal edge is 0.5 mm above the central, i.e. at the level of the occlusal rim. It may be repositioned with spacing, or lapping for esthetic need (Fig. 9.20B).

Maxillary Canine

The maxillary must be set straight and perpendicular to the occlusal plane with prominence in neck and slight distal tilt in some cases. The mesial half of incisal edge should be in same line of the incisors. The tip of the incisal edge will be placed at the level of the occlusal rim using the same template (Fig. 9.21).

The same procedure will be carried out for the other side (Fig. 9.22A).

Arrangement of Mandibular Anterior Teeth

The wax is removed mandibular occlusal rim for 25 mm. To set the maxillary anterior teeth properly it may require to grind the base plate to reduce the thickness even if require to create a hole in it than to grind the neck of the teeth. The lower anterior teeth are set with 0–1 mm of vertical overlap.

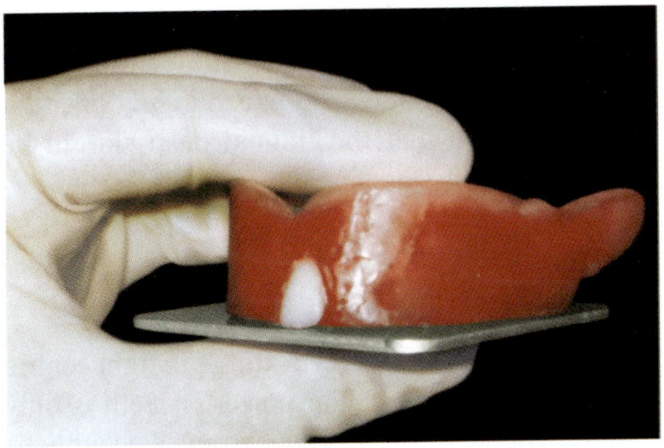

Fig. 9.20A: Arrangement of maxillary central incisor to a template

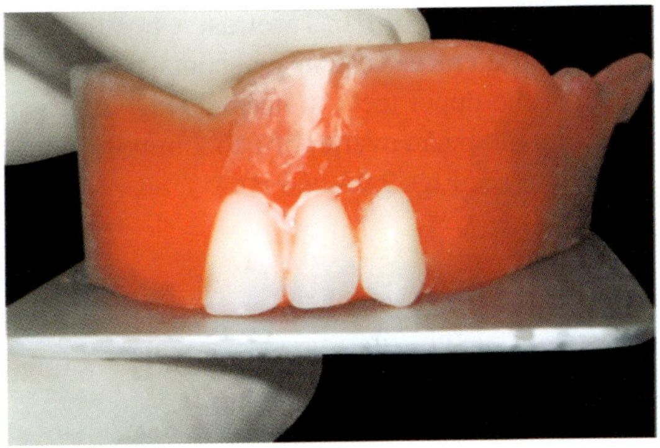

Fig. 9.21: Arrangement of maxillary canine to touch the template

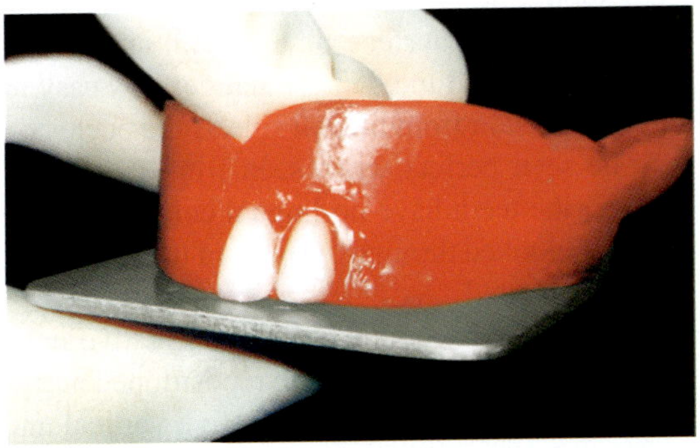

Fig. 9.20B: Arrangement of the maxillary central and lateral to a template

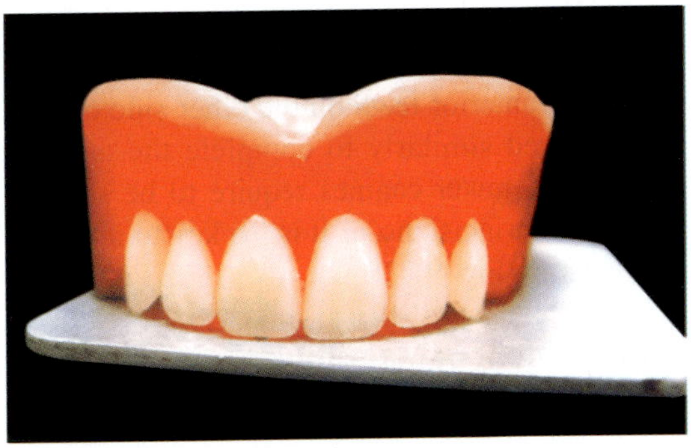

Fig. 9.22A: Arrangement of six maxillary anterior teeth on template

The horizontal overlap should be according to the horizontal jaw relation. There should be no contact of upper and lower anterior teeth in centric occlusion. Although Boucher advocated positioning of artificial teeth in the position occupied by natural teeth such a position will create denture instability due contraction of orbicularis oris muscle. As a general rule, lower anterior teeth should not be set further anterior than the depth of the vestibule. It is advisable to set the canines before the lower incisors, since the formers are the key to the interarch relationship.

Central Incisor

The central incisor should incline slightly towards the midline when viewed from the front and inclined upwards and 5 degrees forwards when seen from the side. The incisal edge is at the level 1 mm above the occlusal rim. In a protrusive position, the central and lateral and canine will contact the incisal edges of the upper teeth in normal ridge relation. There should be an overjet of 1 to 2 mm in centric occlusion (see Figs 9.9A and B).

Lateral Incisor

The lateral incisor is set with the long axis vertical when seen from the side and slightly inclined mesially when seen from the front.

Canine

The canine is set with the long axis vertical with prominence in neck when seen from the side and inclined mesially when seen from the front. The remaining anterior teeth on the other side of arch are arranged similarly to complete the anterior set up. The lower canines require to be set first before lower incisions, as it is the key to interarch relationship (Fig. 9.22B).

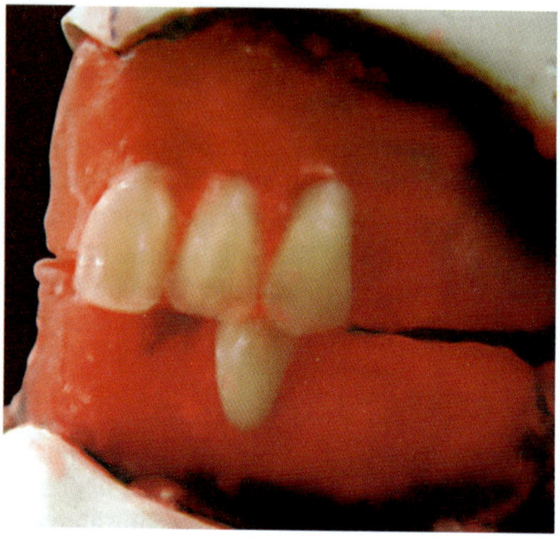

Fig. 9.22B: Canine set first before lower incisors as it is the key of interarch

Arrangement of Mandibular Posterior Teeth

The mandibular posterior teeth are set with the occlusal plane determined by the height of the lower anterior teeth anteriorly and the superoinferior center of the retromolar pads posteriorly. The lower posterior teeth are set so that the central fosse coincide with the line. The buccolingual position should be such that the lingual cusp should be positioned within the single mentioned earlier.

Arrangement of Maxillary Posterior Teeth

The maxillary posterior teeth are set in tight centric occlusion with mandibular posterior teeth is only required for the try-in. This can be checked with the help of articulating paper. The buccolingual position depends on the maxillomandibular relationship. The teeth should be positioned buccal to the residual ridge but buccal surface of the tooth should not be placed beyond the denture flange. It is easy to check occlusion from lingual side as the occlusion may be seen perfect when seen from the buccal side but the teeth have no lingual contacts. These should be looked through the back of the articulator and be corrected.

The arrangements of tooth are tentative now. Probably, teeth will need to be repositioned at try-in slightly. If errors exist in tentative vertical and horizontal jaw relationships significant changes may be required (Fig. 9.23).

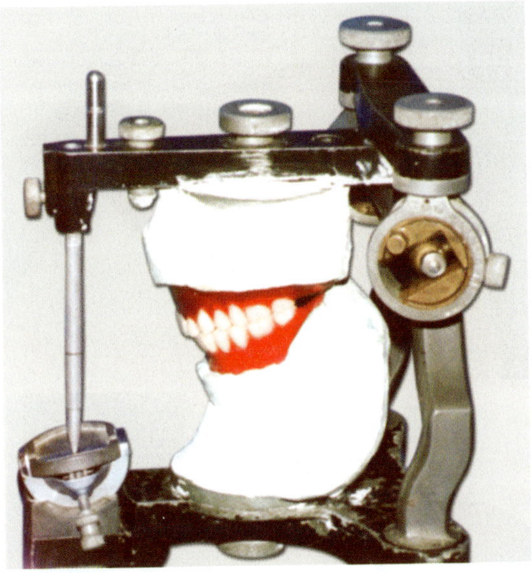

Fig. 9.23: Completed set up in canine position (buccal view)

SELECTION AND ARRANGEMENT OF TEETH IN ATYPICAL RIDGE RELATIONS

Artificial teeth are available in the market in various sizes of normal (Class I) jaw relationship only. For abnormal jaw relationship (Classes II and III) the mandibular anterior teeth should be chosen from different sets, the size of which will depends upon the available space for proper relationship of the upper and lower canines.

In normal Angle's class I jaw relation, the required relationship of upper and lower canines can be controlled by proper selection of the anterior teeth. When the anterior teeth are arranged in their normal position only slight modifications of posterior (size and position) teeth are required to set them in normal teeth and ridge relationship.

In Angle's class II or class III, the upper and lower ridge relationship makes it impossible to set the posterior teeth in normal relationship. The classes II and III jaw relationships can be successfully treated with atypical arrangement of teeth.

ARRANGEMENT OF TEETH IN ANGLE'S CLASS II, DIVISION 1

In class II, division 1, ridge relationship the lower ridge is smaller than the upper ridge. There is always a deep overbite that cannot be reproduced in complete dentures as it causes occlusal imbalance. As the curve of the arch to which the lower incisors are set is of lesser radius than that of the upper incisors, it will be necessary to omit one of the lower incisors or to use somewhat narrower teeth to permit the upper and lower canines and premolars to occlude normally. A more pleasing appearance can be produce by using normal size and number of incisors and canines but the lower first premolar is reduced mesiodistally or omitted if the tooth reduction exceeds one-half of a tooth.

The Angle's class II, division 1 patients may have 2 to 4 mm discrepancy between centric jaw relation position and centric occlusion position. If large discrepancy exists between the two positions (3 to 5 mm), nonanatomic posterior tooth will have to set in centric relation as the patient would like to function anterior to this position. Where the discrepancy is small cusp posterior teeth can be set in balance occlusion.

The "Pleasure curve" scheme of occlusion should be chosen. If anatomical teeth are used, the first lower premolar will be forced by the palatal cusp of the upper premolar to take up a position distinctly outside the lower ridge. This fault can only be corrected by grinding flat surfaces on the buccal cusps of the lower premolars to occlude with similar flat surfaces ground on the palatal cusps of the upper premolars.

ARRANGEMENT OF TEETH IN ANGLE'S CLASS II, DIVISION 2

The relative small overjet and deep overbite of the natural teeth should not be copied in the artificial teeth as this causes severe interference and displacement of dentures. The upper anterior teeth are set at a higher level and the lower anteriors are shortens to reduce the overbite. There are minimum translatory movements of the mandible. So, teeth with high cuspal angulations can be set without balance occlusion.

ARRANGEMENT OF TEETH IN ANGLE'S CLASS III

The anterior teeth should usually be set edge-to-edge in centric occlusion. The incisal edge should be ground so that incision will be proper. In extreme prognathic jaws, the upper anterior teeth may be set inside the lowers. The upper incisors may be inclined outward slightly and lowers slightly inwards. Alternatively, if there is no objection slight spacing in lower incisors may be done.

In class III jaw relationships and in cases of advanced ridge resorption, the lower arch is border than the upper arch. So, the upper posterior teeth cannot be set in the lower central fossae as it would results in setting the upper tooth to much buccal to the upper ridge. The problem may be unilateral or bilateral causing tipping force due to leverage. To avoid this problem teeth are set in crossbite relationship. The upper posterior teeth are crossed over the lower posterior teeth so that instead of lingual the buccal cusp meets the central fossae. To set the teeth in crossbite relationship one cusp of tooth is modified by grinding in which the transition occurs from normal relationship to a crossbite relationship (Figs 9.24A to C). The buccal cusp of upper posterior tooth set in crossbite relation by grounding to give rounded form for mortar pestle type of contact. Alternatively, cuspless posterior teeth can be used more easily.

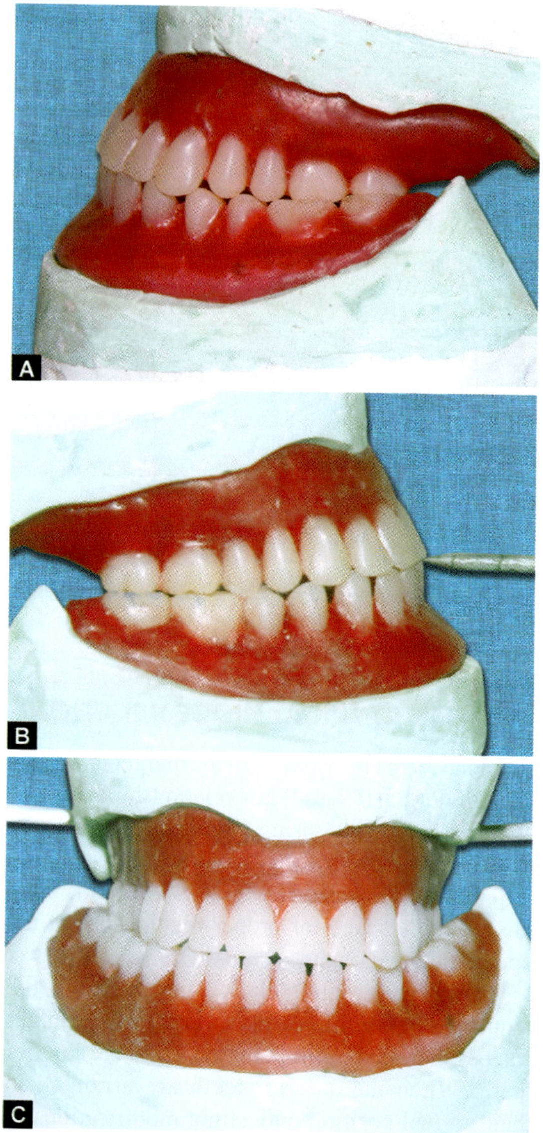

Figs 9.24A to C: (A) Arrangement of teeth in class III jaw relation left sided view showing crossbite arrangement of molars and premolars; (B) Arrangement of teeth in class III jaw relation right sided view showing normal arrangement of posterior teeth; (C) Arrangement of teeth in class III jaw relation (front view)

ARRANGEMENT OF TEETH OF PATIENT WITH OLD DENTURE

The most important factor in setting of teeth in patient having satisfactory old dentures is the tongue space. The new denture should be made with the same amount of tongue space of the old dentures. The tongue space of old denture can be measured with a divider and the teeth in new denture is set according to that measurement.

CONCLUSION

It is extremely difficult to analyze the dental composition when the patient is sitting in dental chair. In addition the dental composition should be criticized from a distance of 6 to 8 feet to obtain the overall effect of the smile. A good rule is to insert the trial denture for a try-in and asked the patient to walk to the door, turn around, and smile. This causes a sudden impact of a pleasing effect and corrections are made from observing the patient at a distance.

BIBLIOGRAPHY

1. Boucher CO. Swenson's complete dentures, 6th end, St Louis, CV Mosby; 1970; pp. 312-7.
2. Boucher CO, Hickery JC, Zarb GA. Prosthodontic treatment for edentulous. Patients, st Louis, CV Mosby Co; 1980.
3. Frush JP, Fesher RD. The age factor in dentogenics. J Prosthet Dent. 1957;7:5-13.
4. Frush JP, Fisher RD. How dentogenics interpret the personality factor, J Prosthet Dent. 1956;6:441-49.
5. Frush JP, Fisher RD. How dentogenics interpret the sex factor. J Prosthet Dent. 1956;6:160-72.
6. Glossary of Prosthodontics Term. J Prosthet Dent. 1994;71:56-107.
7. Herper RN. Incisive papilla—basis of technic. J Dent. Res. 1948;27:661.
8. House MM, Loop, JL. Form and color harmony in the dental art. Monograph: Whittier, California; 1939.
9. Lee JH. Dental Aestheics. The pleasing appearance of artificial dentures. Bristol, John Wright & Sons Ltd; 1962.
10. Pleasure MA. Anatomic versus nonanatomic teeth. J Prosthet Dent. 1953;3:747-54.
11. Pound. Applying harmony in selecting and arranging teeth. Dent Clin North Am. 1962;241.
12. Schiffman P. Relation of the maxillary canines to the incisive papilla. Prosthet Dent. 1964;14:469-72.
13. Sears. Selection and Management of Posterior Teeth. J Prosth Dent. 1957;7:723.
14. Smith BJ. The value of the nose width as an esthetic guide in prosthodontics. J Prosthet Dent. 1975;34:562.
15. Wehner, Hickey, Boucher. Selection of artificial teeth. J Prosth Dent. 1967;18:22.
16. Wilson GH. A Manual of dental prosthetics, 2nd edn, Philadelphia, Lea and Febiger; 1914.

Chapter 10

Occlusion and Articulation in Complete Dentures

INTRODUCTION

The occlusion of teeth affects the denture base movement and affects the objectives of complete denture construction namely:

1. Function
2. Confort
3. Esthetics
4. Preservation of the residual ridge.

NOMENCLATURE AND TERMINOLOGY OF OCCLUSION

Occlusion may be defined as the static relationship between the incising or masticating surfaces of the maxillary and the mandibular teeth, or tooth analogues. A more appropriate term is articulation. There are innumerable occlusion positions out of which our basic positions are clinically used:

1. *Protrusive occlusion*: It is the occlusion exists when the mandible is in the protrusive position.
2. *Right lateral occlusion*: It is the occlusion exists when the mandible moves in right lateral position.
3. *Left lateral occlusion*: It is the occlusion exists when the mandible moves in left lateral position.
4. *Centric occlusion*: It is the occlusion of opposing teeth when the mandible is in centric relation. This may or may not coincide with the maximum intercuspation position.

Articulation

It is contact relationship between the occlusal surfaces of teeth during function. It is the dynamic sliding contact of cusps of upper and lower teeth that takes place during closed gliding movements of the mandible. Articulation is a continuous change from one occlusal position to the other. The term occlusion and articulation are often interchanged.

Centric Relation

The sixth edition of Glossary of Prosthodontic Terms defined centric relation as "a maxillomandibular relationship in which the condyles articulate with the thinnest avascular portion of their respective disks with the complex in the anterosuperior position against the slopes the articular eminence. The position is independent of tooth contact. This position is clinically desirable when the mandible is directed superiorly and anteriorly. It is restricted to a purely rotary movement about the transverse horizontal axis".

Christensen's Phenomenon

It is a space that occurs between opposing occlusal surfaces during mandibular protrusion (Fig. 10.1).

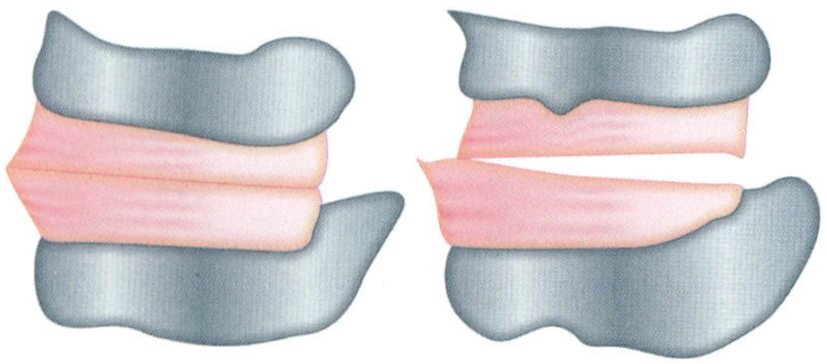

Fig. 10.1: Christensen's phenomenon

Curve of Spee

Anatomic curvature of the occlusal alignment of the teeth beginning at the tip of the lower canine and following the buccal cusp tips of the natural premolar and molars, continuing the anterior border of the ramus, ending with anterior most portion of the mandibular condyle (Fig. 10.2).

Curve of Wilson

The mediolateral curve in the mandibular arch, as viewed in the frontal plane, is concave inferiorly and contacts the lingual and buccal cusps of the maxillary molars. The curve formed by the facial and lingual cusp tips on both sides of the dental arch (Fig. 10.3C).

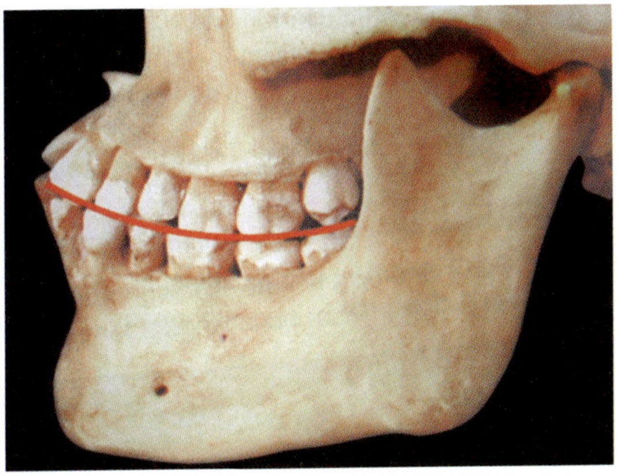

Fig. 10.2: Curve of Spee: A line from the tip of lower canine following the buccal cusps of the posterior teeth (natural)

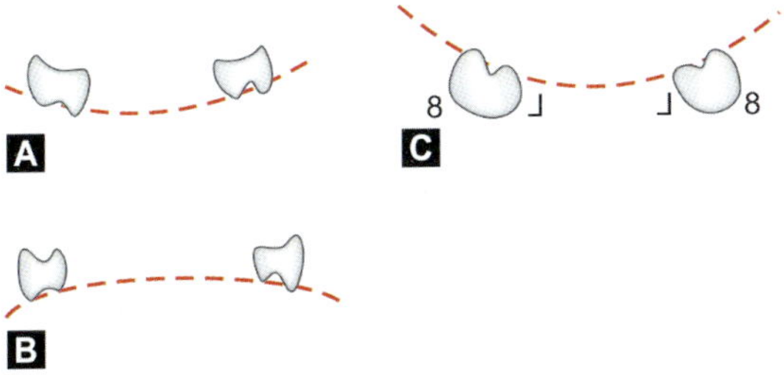

Figs 10.3A to C: (A) Monson curve; (B) Anti-Monson curve; (C) Curve of Wilson

Curve of Monson

The curve of occlusion in which each cusp and incisal edge touches or conforms to a segment of the surface of the sphere 8 inches in diameter with its center in the region of the glabella (Fig. 10.3A).

Curve of Pleasure

Sync: Anti-Monson curve, frequency curve, probability curve, reverse curve.

A helicoidal curve of occlusion that, when viewed in frontal plane, conforms to a curve that is convex superiorly, except for the last molars which reverse that pattern (Fig. 10.3B).

Requirements of Complete Denture Occlusion

The research fails to identify a specific occlusal concept or a posterior tooth form or arrangement but the following five factors affect the requirements of complete denture occlusion.

Maximum Intercuspation at the Centric Relation Position

Centric occlusion coincides with centric relation.

Absence of Deflective Occlusal Contacts Between Opposing Teeth in Eccentric Movements

The presence of deflective occlusal contacts occurring during functional and parafunctional movements will cause movement of denture bases may lead to trauma, discomfort and loss of function.

The Presence of Tooth Forms with Enough Cuspal Height for Selective Grinding

The tooth form with some cuspal height is indispensable for occlusal reshaping to develop freedom in movements by avoiding deflecting occlusal contacts.

Natural and Pleasing Appearance in Tooth Form and Arrangements

The anatomic form of posterior teeth is essential for a pleasing and natural appearance in patient's mouth.

Concepts of Complete Denture Occlusion or Articulation (Table 10.1)

The principal concepts of occlusion are:
1. Bilateral balanced
2. Monoplane or nonbalanced
3. Lingualized articulation.

Various tooth moulds are selected by the clinician and arranged in a particular occlusion scheme to achieve one of these concepts. The balanced occlusion concept utilizes either cusp or cuspless form of posterior teeth arranged in balance in the centric and eccentric jaw positions, at least a tripod type of contact of teeth is utilized. Monoplane concept utilizes either cusp less form or cusped posterior teeth arranged on a plane. Lingualized occlusion concept is a compromise between the balanced and monoplane occlusion. It utilizes both types of teeth, upper anatomical and lower nonanatomical moulds marketed by several manufacturers viz. Myerson lingualized integration (MLI) by Austenal Inc., Chicago.

BALANCED ARTICULATION

The "Glossary of Prosthodontic Terms" defined balanced occlusion as "the bilateral, simultaneous, anterior, and posterior occlusal contact of teeth in centric and eccentric positions". The more appropriate definition of balanced occlusion would be "the occlusal contacts of maxillary mandibular teeth initially in maximum intercuspation and their continuous contacts during movement from this initial position along specific working, balancing, and protrusive guidance pathways developed on the occlusal surfaces of the teeth". A balanced articulation allows developing a balance occlusion in the mouth resulting less denture base movement and reduction in inflammation and bone loss. This is done by modifying the teeth by grinding so that all are in functional harmony with the incisal and condylar guidance.

In this concept, teeth are to glide evenly over each other on the working side. No single tooth should interfere and cause the others to lift out of articulation. Contacts on the balancing side must exist and must not interfere with smooth gliding

Table 10.1 Comparison of the three major occlusal schemes

Parameter	Balanced	Monoplane	Lingualized
1. Esthetics upper	Favorable due to cusped teeth	Unfavorable due to cuspless teeth	Favorable due to upper visible cusped teeth
2. chewing	Efficient due to cusped teeth	Relatively poor due to cuspless teeth	Efficient "mortar and pestle" action of opposing teeth
3. Stability in lateral excursions	Good due to both working and balancing contacts	poor	Good
4. Technique of teeth set-up	Requires skill	Simple	Easy, more so with "Myerson's teeth"
5. Freedom in centric	Have to be achieved by grinding on the articulator	Incorporated in the scheme	Incorporated in the scheme
6. Post-insertion adjustment	Required usually undetected deflective contacts are present	Minimum	Minimum
7. Lateral stresses	Higher, particularly if deflective contacts are present	Minimum	Minimum

movements of the working side. Posterior tooth contacts must exist simultaneously with anterior tooth contact for protrusive and lateral movements.

Necessity for Balanced Articulation

The necessity of balanced occlusion has been debated for many years. Prosthodontists unanimously agree that equal contact or balance in centric occlusion is essential but differs in opinion regarding the essentiality of bilateral eccentric balance. Prosthodontists primarily concern with the retention of dentures during mastication and proposed eccentric balance as an aid in retention. To them balance is necessary because of the bodily movement of lower teeth away from the upper teeth in protrusion. If anterior teeth are held together, a space is created between upper and lower posterior teeth named Christensen's phenomena. So, lateral and protrusive balance was achieved by incorporating anteroposterior and mediolateral compensating curves.

Soon, it becomes apparent that during mastication the smallest grain of food on the working side eliminated the balance on the nonworking or balancing side. So, Sheppard remarked "Enter bolus, Exit balance". But eccentric balance was not abandoned, but the rationale for its use has changed. Balance is necessary for the health of the mucosa during the countless excursive contact that occurs between meals during swallowing, mastication, and parafunctional movements of the mandible. So, Hanau's law of balance occlusion and theories remain valid today.

Laws of Articulation of Balanced Occlusion

The laws of articulation are purely physical laws which must be observed in the formation of the masticatory surfaces of natural and artificial dentures, whenever it is the aim to establish or produce that function which we accept as balanced articulation. Balanced articulation comprises a continuous change from one balanced occlusion into another for all occluded mandibular excursions.

Stansbery (1932) advocate this balanced occlusion concept. Kurth (1954) refers to balanced occlusion creating balance when the mandible is in centric relation to the maxillae. This is known as balance in centric. No eccentric balance is present.

In 1920 and 1930, Rudolph L. Hanau an engineer developed articulators and theories of occlusion. He presented nine "factors governing articulation" in a paper before the American Dental Association that was published in ADA journal in 1926. Of these nine factors the most important in practice are the following five factors which is known as "Hanau's Quints" (Fig. 10.4).

1. The inclination of the condylar guidance.
2. The prominence of the compensating curve.
3. The inclination of the plane of orientation.
4. The inclination of the incisal guidance.
5. The height of the cups.

Thelmam propose the following equation represents the relation between them.

$$\frac{HCG \times IG}{CC \times CA \times OPP} = K$$

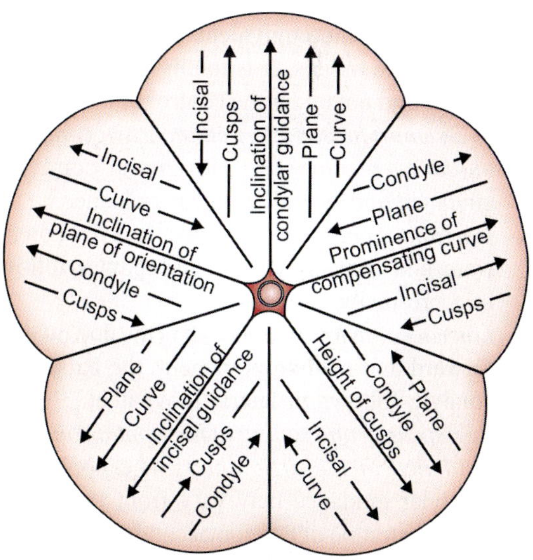

Fig. 10.4: Hanau's Quints: Arrow pointing towards the center indicates decrease. Arrow pointing away from the center indicates increase

HCG = Horizontal condylar guidance
IG = Incisal guidance
CA = Cusp angle
CC = Compensating curve
OPP = Orientation of occlusal plane
K = Balanced occlusion (constant)

Balance is achieved when the above five factors are in harmony. A change in any one requires change in any one of the remaining four factors. The dentist can only change four out of five factors. The condylar guidance cannot be changed by him. Of the other four factors he can alter two to smaller degrees—incisal guidance and inclination of occusal plane. The other two factors—the compensating curve and cusp angles can be modified by the dentist to obtain harmony among the five factors.

Condylar Guidance

It is an anatomical concept transferred to the mechanical device on a articulator intended to produce guidance in articulator movement similar to the paths of condyles in the temporomandibular joints. It is not the geometrical replica of anatomical inclination, but the equivalent for it and due to "realiff" of the tissues. It is totally obtained from the patient and not under the control of the dentist.

1. *In a semi-adjustable articulator, two condylar guidance are present*: Horizontal condylar guidance and lateral condylar guidance.
2. *Horizontal condylar guidance*: It is the downward and forward slope, the condyles follow in a protrusive movement.
3. *Lateral condylar guidance*: It is the downward, forward and medial movement, the balancing condyle follows in lateral movement.
4. *Registration and setting of horizontal condylar guidance in the articulator*: The horizontal condylar guidance may vary from 0–60º.

The registration of horizontal condylar guidance is obtained from the patient by means of protrusive record and transferred to a semi-adjustable articulator such as Hanau, Whip-Mix or Dentatus articulator. It is made with recording material placed between the teeth at try-in stage after the vertical and horizontal relationships are confirmed. A minimum six millimeter of protrusion will produce a record for setting the articulator. The horizontal condylar setting of 0–20° is low, 20–30° medium and above 30° is high. For lower or medium 0°, 20° or 30° or combination and for high setting 20° or 30° or combination of moluds are chosen.

Registration and setting of lateral condylar guidance (Bennett angle):

There are three ways of registration of Bennett angle as follows:

a. *Recording lateral movements*: This is recorded by placing recording material in between the posterior teeth and the patient is asked to close in lateral relationships with the upper and lower cuspids come edge-to-edge position. Two intraocclusal records of two sides are obtained and arcon type articulator can be set with this records as done in setting the horizontal condylar guidance.
b. *Using Hanau's formula*: The formula is **L = H/8 + 12, L** is lateral condylar guidance and **H** is horizontal condylar guidance.
   This formula is embossed under Hanau's articulator (Fig. 10.5).
c. By average setting the angle as 15–17 degrees for complete denture.

The condylar guidance is not under the control of the dentist. The other two factors tooth inclination, and compensating curve are controlled

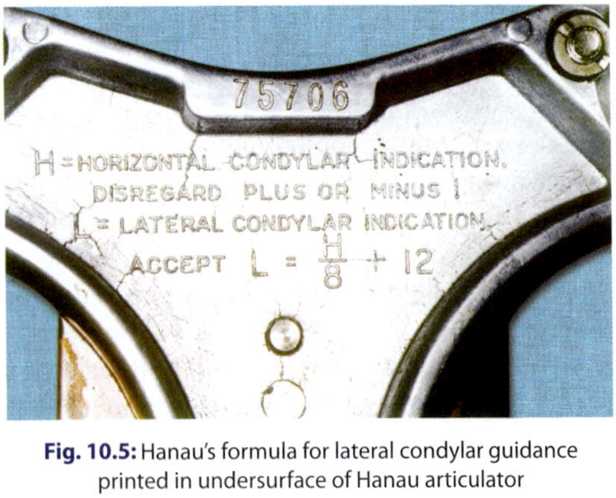

Fig. 10.5: Hanau's formula for lateral condylar guidance printed in undersurface of Hanau articulator

and modified by him to obtain harmony among the five factors. Articulator movements are fixed with these records may not be replicate the actual movements but acceptable simulations.

Pantographic records with fully adjustable articulator having custom made condylar guide paths to reproduce the curvature of the condylar guidance accurately to obtain balanced occlusion was tried. But it was found that the movement of the denture on soft tissues exceeds the fine adjustments.

Inclination of Incisal Guidance

It is defined as, the influence of the contacting surfaces of the mandibular and maxillary anterior teeth on mandibular movements (GPT). It is the angle of the lingual surface of the incisors with the accepted horizontal plane. The incisal guidance can be set by the dentist considering the amount of horizontal and vertical overlap of anterior teeth for proper esthetic and functional result. It set by adjusting the incisal guide table when the anterior teeth are in an end-to-end relation and tip of the incisal pin touches the incisal guide table. If the resulting angle exceeds 10°, the anterior teeth should be modified until a smaller angle is achieved. The incisal guide table should be as nearly parallel to the occlusal plane as possible this creating a small incisal guide angle and low cusp angulation.

Incisal guidance and condylar guidance, the two factors are known as end controlling factors determine the movements of the articulator. That will affect the cusp height needed to achieve a balanced occlusion. If the end controlling factors of condylar guidance and incisal guidance are steep (particularly the incisal guidance because of its proximity to the posterior tooth), then anatomic tooth will be require to achieve balance. If the incisal guidance is less than 10 degrees, the nonanatomic teeth can be arranged to achieve balance.

Prominence of Compensating Curve

A compensating curve is the anteroposterior and lateral curvature in the alignment of the occluding surfaces and incisal edges of artificial teeth which is used to develop balance occlusion. This curve compensates for opening that occurs in the posterior region when a protrusive movement is made. This is known as "Christensen's phenomenon. It also compensates for the opening that occurs when a lateral movement is made. The anteroposterior curve is used to creating protrusive balance and the lateral curve is used to provide lateral balance. The value of the compensating curve allows the dentist to alter the cusp angulations by changing the inclination and therefore without changing the form of the artificial teeth.

Cusp Angle/Cusp Height

Trapozzano has pointed out that the cusp angle and not the cusp height is the factor involved as the mandible moves in three-dimension. The cusp angle is the angle made by the slopes of a cusp with the mean occlusal plane, measured mesiodistally or buccolingually. It is designated in degrees. It is the inter-relationship between the incisal guidance, the condylar guidance, the comparing curves, and plane of occlusion. A particular tooth may be of 30 degrees inclination but by tilting the tooth in relation to the mean occlusal plane one may create inclination greater or less than 30 degrees.

Inclination of Plane of Orientation

It is the average plane established by the incisal and occlusal surfaces of the teeth. Generally speaking it is not a plane but represents the planer mean of the curvature of these surfaces. The anterior part of the occlusal plane is determined by the position of the anterior teeth which is determined by the esthetic and phonetic requirements. The posterior part is determined by the height of the retromolar pad. So, it is not under the control of the dentist.

The above mentioned five factors when analyzed show that each consists of an increased or decreased factor. These ten main laws of articulation were presented as follows:

1. An increase of the inclination of the condylar guidance increases the prominence of compensating curve.

2. An increase of the inclination of the condylar guidance increases the inclination of the plane of orientation.
3. An increase of the inclination of the condylar guidance decreases the inclination of the inclisal guidance.
4. An increase of the inclination of the condylar guidance increases the heights of the cusps, progressively towards the posterior.
5. An increase of the prominence of the compensating curve decreases the inclination of the plane of orientation.
6. An increase of the prominence of the compensating curve increases the inclination of the incisal guidance.
7. An increase of the prominence of the compensating curve decreases the heights of the cusps, progressively towards the posterior.
8. An increase of the inclination of the plane of orientation increases the inclination of the incisal guidance.
9. An increase of the inclination of the plane of orientation increases the cusp height equally or so.
10. An increase of the inclination of the progressing incisal guidance, increases the cusp heights towards the anterior.

The meaning of the large arrow in the middle is given in each sector of the Quint. The four small arrows two on each side of the large middle arrows of each sector, relate the influence or change caused. All arrows pointing away from the center indicate an increase, while those pointing towards the center indicate a decrease of the property or character of the indicated factor. The dot near the head of an arrow indicates—progressively towards the anterior. The dot near the tail of an arrow indicates—progressively towards the posterior. Dots near both ends of an arrow indicate—equally or nearly so anteroposteriorly. All dots indicate the changes of cusp height only.

Advantages of Balanced Articulation

The advantages of balanced articulation can be summed up as follows:

1. Improved stability of the dentures, especially in nonfunctional contacts between teeth.
2. Better force distribution over the ridges.
3. Better esthetics due to use of anatomic tooth forms.
4. Improved chewing efficiency.

Disadvantages of Balanced Articulation

1. A balanced articulation compromise esthetic, as it does not allow for sufficient overbite of maxillary anterior teeth. The mandibular anterior teeth are often not visible enough unless the vertical dimension is raised to the correct height. Usually aged persons should display more of the mandibular teeth but more of the maxillary teeth are made visible.
2. Sheppard stated that "Enter bolus, Exit balance". He explained that whenever food is present between occlusal surfaces on one side, the other side is separated. So, effort to produce balancing side contact is rendered useless.
3. Balancing of occlusion is done in a specific movement range on the articulator. But in the mouth, the mandible may make greater range of movements, so balance become useless.
4. If balanced articulation is not refined, deflective contacts during functional and nonfunctional movements may lead to inflammation of the mucosa.
5. The character of the supporting tissue makes it impossible to harmonize teeth arrangement with jaw movements and to maintain this harmony.
6. A costly semi-adjustable articulator with face-bow is needed.
7. More chair side and laboratory time increases the cost of treatment.

ARRANGEMENT OF ANATOMIC (CUSP) TEETH TO BALANCED ARTICULATION

Bilateral balance is obtained by incorporating anteroposterior and mediolateral compensating curves by altering the cusp angles of teeth by slightly tilting mesiodistally or buccolingually.

The final refinement is done by selective grinding. The balance is done in two stages—protrusive and lateral balance.

Protrusive Balance

The two end controlling factors—condylar and incisal guidance control the movement of the articulator. The condylar guidance is obtained from the patient by means of protrusive record and not under the control of the dentist. The incisal guidance is set by the dentist considering the esthetics. The rest three factors are altered by dentist to obtain harmony among the five factors providing protrusive balance. Protrusive balance should not be achieved at the expense of having unstable tooth positions, or unesthetic appearance. Only in cases where the anterior teeth can be set with an incisal angle of 20 degrees or less (with little overbite) protrusive balance can be obtained with advantage.

Lateral Balance

The lateral balance is easily obtained between the lower buccal and upper lingual cusps with a slight lateral tilt because correctly set posterior teeth have very little buccal overbite.

Balance in lateral occlusion is also governed by five factors. Two end controlling factors for obtaining lateral balance similar to protrusive balance. Condylar guidance influenced the balancing side cusps. Incisal guidance influenced the cusps on working side. It is set on the articulator by raising the butterfly wings on the incisal table at 10 degrees. The compensating curve in buccolingual direction known as curve of Wilson.

ARRANGEMENT OF NONANATOMIC (CUSPLESS) TEETH TO BALANCED ARTICULATION

Nonanatomic teeth are usually are arranged with a flat occlusal plane without balance. But balance may be achieved by:

1. Arranging with compensating curves which enable the teeth to maintain contact during the mandibular excursion.
2. Tilting the second molars creating an inclined plane.
3. Placing balancing rams distal to lower second molars.

Regardless of the method selected, balancing is not undertaken till try-in appointment.

Arranging Teeth with Compensating Curve

Noncusp teeth can be used to balanced occlusion if the teeth are set with an anteroposterior buccolingual compensating curve. The buccal cusps are set higher than the lingual cusps and the distal cusps are set higher than the mesial cusps. A 20° template can be used to aid informing the curves.

Tilting the Second Molars

All teeth are arranged in a plane except the second molars. The second molars are set with their destal cusps higher than mesial cusps and the buccal cusps. The amount of the tilt is dictated by the condylar guidance and incisal guidance.

Balancing Rams

All the posterior teeth are arranged in a straight line, i.e. in monoplane occlusion. A pair of wax ram is created distal to the mandibular second molars during the excursive movements to achieve a three point contact (anterior point in incisor region) (Fig. 10.6).

Monoplane Articulation

It is defined in Glossary of Prosthodontic terms as "the arrangement of teeth by which they are positioned in a single plane". The more precise definition is "the occlusal contacts of the maxillary and mandibular teeth initially in maximum intercuspation, and the disocclusion of the posterior teeth as a result of their arrangement in a single

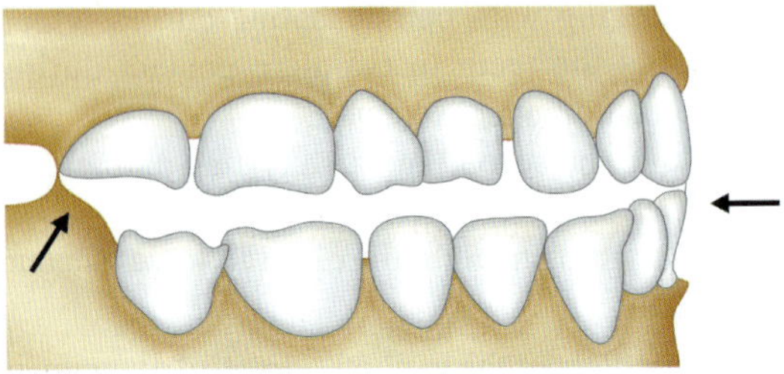

Fig. 10.6: Balancing rams

plane, and the contacts of the anterior tooth during movements of the mandible.

De van was the main propagator of this concept, which gained much importance due to enthusiasm of the non-believers of balanced articulation concept. This concept relies on two key words—"neutral" and "central" which imply: (1) neutralization of all inclines and (2) centralization of forces on the basal seat.

Neutralization of the inclines is achieved by use of flat ('0' degree) teeth and abandoning all attempts to secure balance by setting teeth in a flat plane.

Centralization of forces is achieved by reducing the size and number of artificial teeth.

This concept in practice is used on four parameters:

1. *Position*: Teeth are positioned in as per as centrally with respect to medial and lateral forces, i.e. in the neutral zone as described by fish.
2. *Proportion*: The teeth size is required to be reduced up to 40% to achieve centralization of forces. The tooth size is reduced buccolingually. The number of teeth is also reduced by omitting the lower second molars or by keeping them out of occlusion, in order to dircet masticatory forces to the premolars and first molars. This also avoid the placing teeth on the inclined portion of the ridge.
3. *Pitch*: The inclination or tilt of teeth and the occlusal plane is pitch. It has to be eliminated. So, cuspless teeth are set in one plane to make the occlusal plane parallel to both the upper and lower ridge planes. Condylar guidance has no role in this type of occlusal scheme and can be set to 0 degree. So, a hinge articulator may also be used.
4. *Form*: The cuspless 0 degree teeth or rational posterior teeth (low cusp) are used to avoid cusps or projections that may cause interference with eccentric movements. In this concept of posterior occlusion the plane of occlusion is a flat plane parallel to the ridges without any anteroposterior or mediolateral curve.

This concept gained popularity due to the its supporter who claimed that there were some demerits in balanced articulation as listed above.

Advantages of Monoplane Articulation

1. Minimum horizontal forces are generated and there is preservation of ridges.
2. No interference in lateral excursive movements.
3. Easy to create "freedom in centric".
4. Easy to set up teeth for class I, II, III jaw relationship.
5. No protrusive or laterotrusive cheek records and use of a hinge articulator makes the procedure easier.
6. As stability of the denture is adequate patient can learn to use the denture easily.

Disadvantages of Monoplane Articulation

1. The lack of chewing efficiency of zero degree teeth.
2. Unesthetic appearance of cuspless teeth.

These disadvantages can be avoided using low cusp rational teeth.

Lingualized Articulation

It is defined as "the form of denture occlusion articulates the maxillary lingual cusps with the mandibular occlusal surfaces in centric working and nonworking mandibular positions".

In lingualized articulation the maxillary lingual cusp only contacts the mandibular occlusal surface as a centric holding cusp. It is this cusp which also functions in the eccentric movements. The posterior teeth selected for lingualized articulation differ depending on whether the balanced or non-balanced (monoplane) arrangement is used. In a balanced arrangement maxillary tooth with sharp and pointed lingual cusps are used against shallow cusped occlusal table. In nonbalanced arrangement monoplane mandibular teeth are used.

In 1927, amidst the arguments between balanced and monoplane occlusion, Gysi first came up with the concept of lingualized articulation. Later Payne (1941) suggested that the maxillary buccal cusps of posterior teeth should be reduced so that only lingual cusps would be in contact. Pound (1970) proposed nonbalanced lingualized occlusion.

Arrangement of Teeth to Lingualized Articulation

Both anatomical and nonanatomical teeth are used in this. Usually maxillary anatomic posterior teeth (30 or 33 degrees) are selected to oppose mandibular nonanatomical teeth (zero degree) for a lingualized occlusion. An anatomic tooth with shallow cusp (ten to twenty degrees) can also be used for the mandibular posterior teeth. The steps of arrangement are as follows:

1. The mandibular posterior teeth are arranged either according to monoplane concept or balanced articulation concept.
2. A slight groove or trough is cut down the center of the mandibular occlusal surface or in the position where the lingual cusp of the maxillary teeth touches the mandibular occlusal surface.
3. Each maxillary teeth is so positioned that the lingual cusps are set into the cut groove. The buccal cusps are raised higher so that they do not touch the mandibular teeth during any excusions. They will not be locked into a centric position and will produce a mortar and pestle action (Fig. 10.7).

Advantages of Lingualized Articulation

1. The main advantage of lingualized articulation is its flexibility.
2. Artificial teeth with cusp forms that lock against their antagonist during articulation are unacceptable for a patient with compromised muscle control. The lingualized articulation is a better choice because it permits development of maximum intercuspation at centric jaw relation position yet provides some freedom of movement forward from this recorded position.
3. Edentulous patients rarely present classic class I jaw relationship. When using anatomic teeth some freedom of movement must be provided by occlusal reshaping procedures during. It is possible in lingualized articulation.
4. Patients with resorbed ridge or flabby ridge usually restored with monoplane occlusion and zero incisal guide angle presented with unesthetic appearance. The lingualized articulation in such cases can be used to improve esthetics.
5. The lingual cusp of posterior teeth penetrates the bolus in a holding and grinding fashion

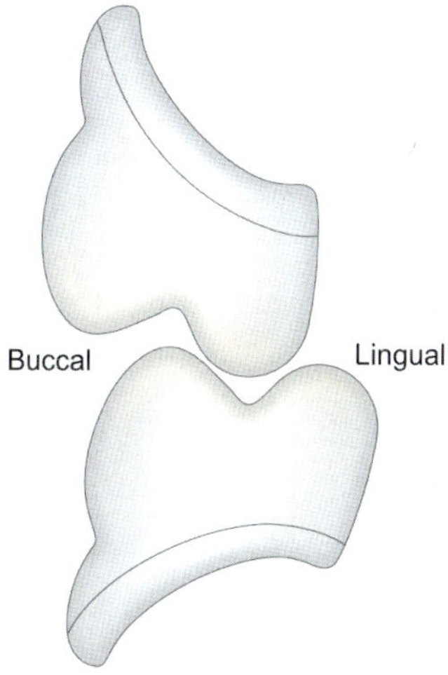

Fig. 10.7: Lingualized articulation

similar to the action of a mortar and pestle (Mehringer).

6. Trapozzano (1960) found that 70% of patients have no preference for balance or nonbalance articulation and only 20% preferred balanced articulation over nonbalanced articulation.
7. Clough et al (1983) compared the chewing efficiency of monoplane articulation with lingualized articulation. The majority of the patient (67%) prefers lingualized articulation for better masticatory efficiency. Patients quoted that lingualized articulation "to chew better, look better and there was no cheek biting".

CONCLUSION

No longitudinal clinical study as yet provides with a simple solution to the complete denture occlusion.

Prosthodontists unanimously agree that equal contact or balance in centric occlusion is essential but differs in opinion regarding the essentiality of bilateral eccentric balance. Posthodontists do agree that for long-term success of complete denture prosthesis continuous monitoring is essential whatever the occlusal form and concept is selected.

BIBLIOGRAPHY

1. Beck HO. Occlusion as related in complete removal prosthodontics. J Prosthet Dent. 1972;27:245-56.
2. Clough HE, Knodle JM, Leeper SH. A comparison of lingualized occlusion and monoplane occlusion in complete dentures. J Prosthet Dent. 1983;50:176-79.
3. Devan MM. Synopsis, Stability in full denture construction fern Dent J. 1955;22:8.
4. Gysi A. Masticating efficiency in natural and artificial teeth III. The bites in natural and porcelain teeth. Dental Dig. 1915;21;139-45.
5. Gysi A. Practical application of research results in denture construction. J Amer Dent Assoc. 1926; 16:199-223.
6. Jones PM. The monoplane occlusion for complete dentures. J Prosthet Dent. 1972;85:94-100.
7. Kurth LE. Balanced occlusion, J Prosthet Dent. 1954;4:150.
8. Lang BR and Razoog ME. A practical approach to resorting occlusion for edentulous patients, part I guiding principles of tooth selection. J Prosthet Dent. 1983;50;455-58.
9. Lang BR, Kelsey CC, Ann Brbort (MI). The University of Michigan School of Dentistry; 1973.
10. Lang BR, Razoog ME. A practical approach to resoring occlusion for edentulous patients, Part II arrangement of the functional and rational mold combination. J prosthet Dent. 1983;50:599-606.
11. Levin B. A review of artificial posterior tooth forms including a preliminary report on a new posterior tooth. J Prosthet Dent. 1977;38:3-5.
12. Ortaman HR. Complete denture occlusion—Essentials of complete denture prosthodontics: Winkler; 2nd end. 1988. p. 217.
13. Pound E. Utilizing speech to simplify a personalized denture service, J Prosthet Dent. 1970;24;586-600.
14. Stansberry CJ. Balanced occlusion in relation to last vertical dimension. JADA. 1932;24:288.
15. Zarb AG, Bolender CL. Prosthodontic treatment of edentulous partients, 11th edn, Mosby; 2004.

Chapter 11

Try-in of Complete Dentures

DEFINITION

A preliminary insertion of a complete denture wax-up in the patient's mouth to evaluate fit, esthetics and maxillomandibular relationships.

It is essential to try the waxed-up dentures in the patient's mouth before acrylization because it is laborious and difficult to do any alteration after processing the denture. The clinical try-in provides the last opportunity to make alterations, as a time of approval and acceptance to both the dentist and the patient.

OBJECTIVES

1. To identify and correct any portion of the denture that interferes with the retention and stability of dentures.
2. To identify and correct any part of denture that is esthetically unpleasant.
3. To verify the jaw relation records.
4. A clear communication between the patient and the dentist which begins at the first appointment is continued during this critical phase of treatment. The dentist knows what the patient wishes, and the patient expectations, because it is necessary to have a clear understanding of desires and possibility for successful treatment.

INSTRUMENTS AND MATERIALS (FIG. 11.1)

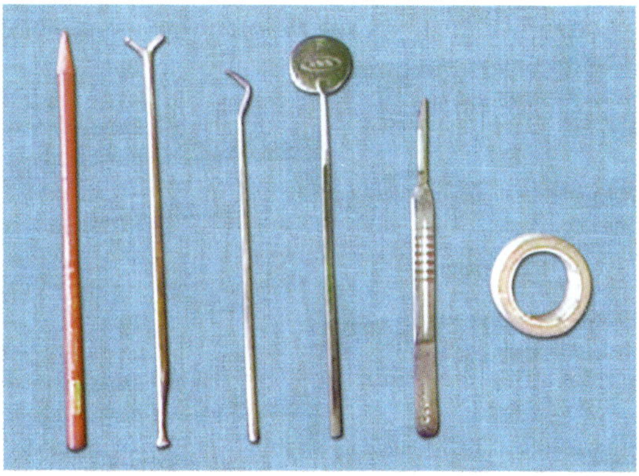

Fig. 11.1: Instruments and materials for the posterior palatal seal

1. Waxed-up dentures on articulator
2. Denture bowl
3. Bunsen burner
4. Waxing instruments
5. Millimeter ruler
6. Sticky tape
7. Sticky wax
8. Patient card
9. Base plate wax
10. Alcohol torch
11. T-ball burnisher
12. BP knife
13. Indelible pencil
14. Mouth mirror

TRIAL DENTURE PROCEDURES

The try-in of denture is the most significant step in denture fabrication because it is the last stage for the dentist to evaluate all previous steps prior to the processing. The steps are:

Examination of Trial Denture on the Articulator

There are several points about waxed dentures that will be considered. It is essential that the patient should be able to visualized the dentures in their final form (Fig. 11.2).

a. To ensure the necessary fit of the denture bases to the casts.
b. To remove the mandibular denture from the cast to assess the relation of the maxillary posterior teeth to the mandibular ridge. The palatal cusps of the maxillary premolars and molars should lay over the crest of the mandibular ridge.
c. Both the dentures removed and the verification of the occlusal plane level.

Examination of Trial Dentures in the Mouth

This is carried out in four stages:

Insertion of Dentures

The mandibular denture may be inserted in patients mouth first because if the maxillary denture is inserted first, the two buccinator muscles which restore the functional width of sulcus are stretched causing discomfort to the patient and dislodgement of maxillary denture at the time of insertion of the mandibular denture. It also help to verify the mandibular denture stability and patients training for tongue to control the mandibular denture.

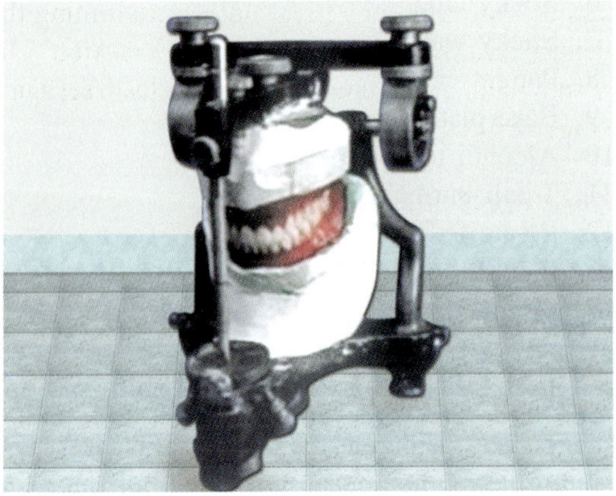

Fig. 11.2: Complete denture waxed-up on articulator

- *Checking the stability of the dentures*: If stable in master cast and unstable in mouth, the fault in impression must be considered and a new final impression is indicated.
- *Checking the retention of the dentures*: The poor retention is determined by sitting the dentures on the ridges when the dentures move in occlusal direction after the sitting pressure is removed. The causes of poor retention are:
  a. *Over-extension*: The border tissue is displaced excessively and the tension in the tissues causes displacement of the denture. The over-extended detected should be removed by trimming the periphery of the base.
  b. *Under-extension of the periphery*: The lack of elastic strain is not developed in the border tissues. The border molding of the base with green stick compound and remaking of the final impression with zinc oxide eugenol is indicated.

Checking the Vertical Dimension

1. The patient is asked to relax with lips closed. While watching the point of chin the patient is asked to close the teeth together; the chin should move slightly upward but in definite amount. If this movement is absent in spite of repeated attempt, it indicates that the vertical dimension is too great.
2. On measurement of vertical dimension of rest and vertical dimension of occlusion by nose chin method if the error found is small, it can be adjusted within the range of plus or minus 3 mm by raising or lowering the articulator pin and resetting the teeth to the correct vertical dimension. This may be done in all cases where the arrangement of cusped teeth associated with face bow record was secured.
3. If the error of vertical dimension is greater than 3 mm. It is necessary to remove the teeth from

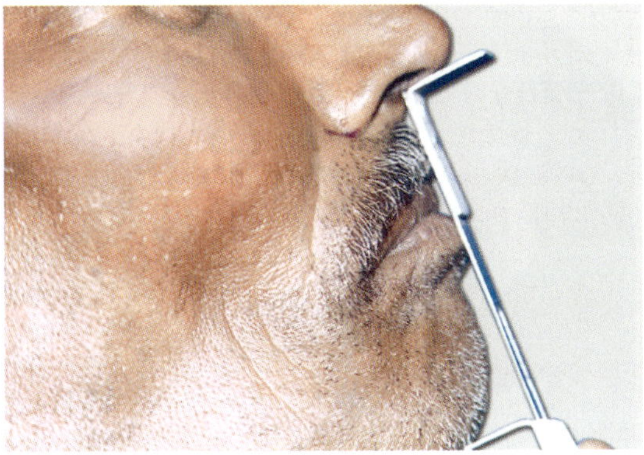

Fig. 11.3: Checking the vertical dimension

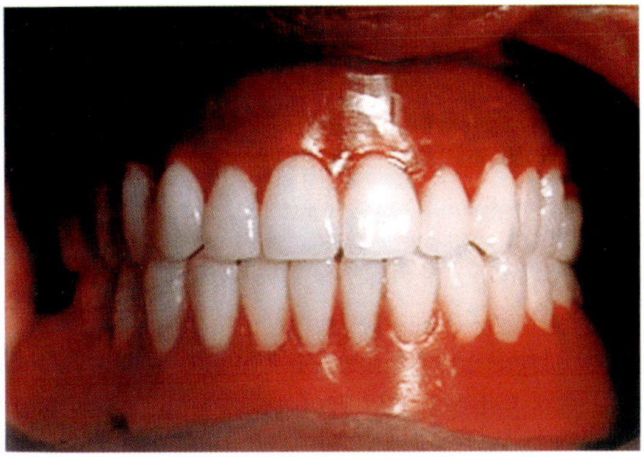

Fig. 11.4: Patient closes in centric relation to check accuracy

the lower denture, and a wax occlusal rim is constructed on the lower base to a required height. It is necessary to take a new vertical dimension and the new centric record and to remount the lower cast on the articulator (Fig. 11.3).

Checking the Centric Relation Record

Centric relation should be the first thing in verifying jaw relation records. If this is done, the patient will not be able to become accustomed to any discrepancies in the occlusion. The patient should not be allowed to make tooth contact until the operator is ready to check the centric. Before proceeding with this stage of try-in, it is necessary to confirm that retention of the trial dentures is adequate. Where this is not so, then the use of gum tragacanth is recommended. There are two commonly used methods for verification of centric relation as:

1. Tactile determination.
2. Extraoral articulator method.

1. *Tactile determination*: The dentures are placed in the patient's mouth, and he is asked to close slowly on the back teeth just until the first even contact of the upper and lower occlusal surfaces occur. The presence of deflective contact should be determined by touch. There must be an even occlusion with maximum interdigitation of the cusps, at the correct vertical dimension. If the centric relation record was correct the opposing cusps interigitate in the mouth in the exactly in the same manner as on articulator and there will be no movement of the denture bases. It is necessary for the dentist to test the centric relation several times to prove himself wrong. If he cannot prove himself wrong, it can be assumed that the articulator mounting is correct (Fig. 11.4).

2. *Extraoral articulator method*: The trial dentures are returned to the articulator and the lower posterior teeth removed and replaced by a wax occlusal rim. Using a little soft wax over the surface of the lower occlusal rim, a new centric relation is established in mouth. The lower anterior teeth are retained *in situ* as their presence is an aid in determining the centric relation in correct vertical dimension. The mandibular cast is remounted and the teeth set again (Fig. 11.5).

Checking Occlusal Planes

There are four planes may be considered, incisal plane, left and right occlusal planes, and plane of the mandibular teeth.

a. *Incisal plane*: It should be parallel to inter-pupillary line.
b. *Right and left occlusal planes:* These should be parallel to the ala-tragus line. A fox plane guide may be used (Fig. 11.6).

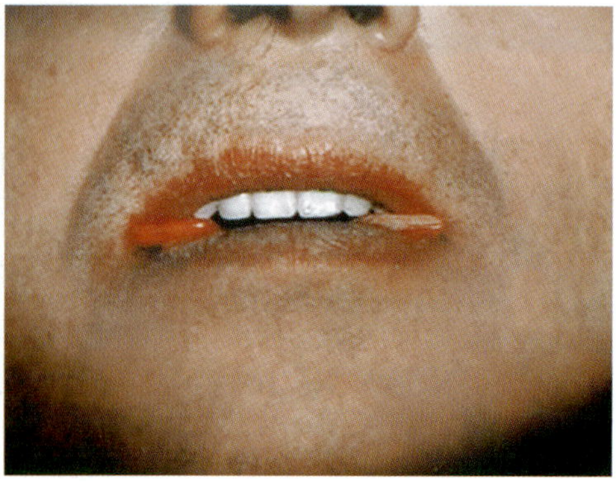

Fig. 11.5: The patient closes in centric relation on softened wax rolls placed on lower posterior teeth

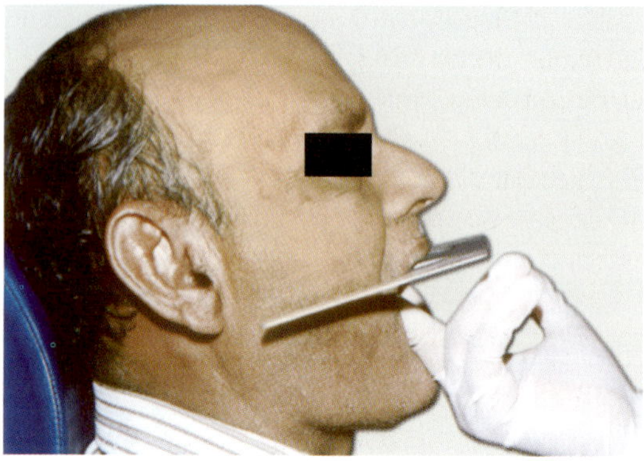

Fig. 11.6: Using Fox's plane to check the orientation of the occlusal plane both with ala-tragus line and interpupillary line

c. *Plane of the mandibular teeth:* The resting tongue should overlie the lingual surface of the lower teeth.

Checking the Simultaneous Tooth Contacts

It is checked by placing thin celluloid strips between the posterior teeth one on each side and requesting the patient to close on these and try to pull the strips simultaneously. Any difference in force indicates uneven occlusal contact. It is necessary then to take a new jaw relation record. A well-retained acrylic base is helpful when examining the occlusion as there is no tendency for the lower denture to lift on the side opposite to that on which there is a premature occlusal contact, and giving an apparent even occlusion.

Checking the Tooth Arrangement for Phonetics

The phonetics may be used to determine the proper placement of artificial teeth as difficulties with speech are uncommon if they are placed in proper positions. Those are concerned are the labial sounds, 'p' and 'b', labiodental sounds 'f' and 'v'; and the linguodental sounds, 'th', linguopalatal 't', 'd', 's', 'ch' and 'j'.

Labial Sounds

The sounds 'p' and 'b' are made totally by the lip and therefore known as labial sounds. If the lips are not supported properly by the artificial teeth, these sounds may be defective. Therefore, antero-posterior tooth position must be evaluated from the point of view of phonetics as well as esthetics.

Labiodental Sounds

The labiodental sounds 'f'and 'v' are produced by contact between the maxillary anterior teeth and the wet/dry line of the lower lip. If the incisal edges contact and lingual side of the lower lip, either the maxillary teeth are set too far lingually or the lower anteriors too far labially. The reverse is true if the incisal edges contact too far forward on the lower lip.

Linguodental Sounds

The linguodental sounds such as 'th' are produced by extending the tip of the tongue between the upper and lower anterior teeth. The normal extension of the tongue beyond the incisal edges during this sound is 2–4 mm. If less than 2–4 mm of tongue is visible, the anterior teeth may be placed too far anterior, if more than 4 mm of tongue is visible, the anterior teeth may be placed too far lingually.

Linguopalatal Sounds

The sounds 't' and 'd' are formed by contacts of the tip of the tongue with the anterior part of the palate. If the teeth are placed too far palatally, the 't' will sound like a 'd' and if they are set too far labially. The 'd' will sound like a 't'.

The difficulty in pronouncing 'S', 'CH', and 'J' sounds occur due to an excess overjet which can be corrected by moving the upper or/and lower anterior teeth forward or back. During production of these sounds the upper and lower anterior teeth should approach each other in end-to-end relation just short to make contact.

Checking the Tooth Arrangement for Esthetics

With both dentures in mouth:

1. The position of the anterior teeth to lip is checked. The upper anterior teeth should provide suitable lip support. In absence of support the nasolabial and mentolabial sulci are deepened, the philtrum is flattened, the amount of visible vermilion border is decreased, and the commissures droop. In case of over support there are shallow sulci, and obliteration of curvature of philtrum.
2. The lower anterior teeth should be placed to provide adequate lip superior for the lower lip. The lower lip should rest against the incisal one-third of the labial surface.
3. The orientation of the occlusal plane should be parallel to the interpupillary line anteriorly and ala-transit line posteriorly.
4. The shape of the arch and shape of face in harmony.
5. The shade, mould of teeth should be checked for satisfactory appearance.
6. The individual rotations and inclinations of teeth for harmony with face form.
7. The smile line should be consistent with age, sex and personality.
8. Midline of the denture should be same as the midpoint of the forehead, sore and chin.
9. Central line: A piece of dental floss is stretched over the midpoint of the forehead, nose and chin. The central line should be directly behind the floss.
10. The resting tongue should over lie the lingual aspects of the lower teeth. It is done to place the lower teeth in the neutral zone. It can be better achieve by a denture space impression. The lower denture base is adapted with a rim of silicone putty or modified tissue conditioners and patient is asked to read aloud a selected passage of prose 'A quick brown fox jumps upon the lazy dog'. This will mold the surface of rim compatible with the requirement.

Patient Approval

The patient's main concern at the trial stage is the appearance of the dentures. The patient should be satisfied with the appearance because, however, technically satisfactory the dentures are, they will not be acceptable to the patient unless the appearance is up to their choice. The patient should be left with trial denture in front of a large mirror at a normal speaking distance. The patient should be encouraged to make suggestions. Many fine dentures failed due to patient dissatisfaction with very minor esthetic reasons. It is better to allow some close relative or friend in the final approval only. When the dentist, the patient and friends are satisfied with the appearance, a written consent is signed and placed in the patient's chart.

POSTDAM/POST-PALATAL SEAL

Definition: The posterior palatal seal is defined as "the soft tissues along the junction of the hard and soft palates on which pressure within the physiological limits of the tissues can be applied by a denture to aid in the retention of the denture" (GPT).

The retention of a complete upper denture is largely dependent upon the effective posterior palatal seal against the ingress of air. In the sulcus the peripheral seal is developed by the elastic displacement of the soft tissues by the rounded border of the base but it must be continued across the posterior palatal border. The degree of displacement depends on the consistency of the tissues in that area. In the midline the mucosa and periosteum are glands and fibrous tissue interposed between them. The polymerization shrinkage of acrylic resin base causes a space in this area. The postdam (PPS) is used to compensate for the shrinkage and occurring during processing.

The posterior palatal seal is created between the two vibrating lines—the anterior vibrating line and posterior vibrating line.

Anterior vibrating line: It is the line at the junction of the hard and soft palates determined by having the patient attempt to blow through nose while holding it closed. The maxillary denture must extend to or beyond this "blow" line.

Posterior vibrating line: It is the line of flexure of soft palate when the patient say "ah".

In a class I soft palate, the denture may be terminating in a wide area. Whereas in class III soft palate, the "ah" and "blow" lines almost coincide (Fig. 11.7).

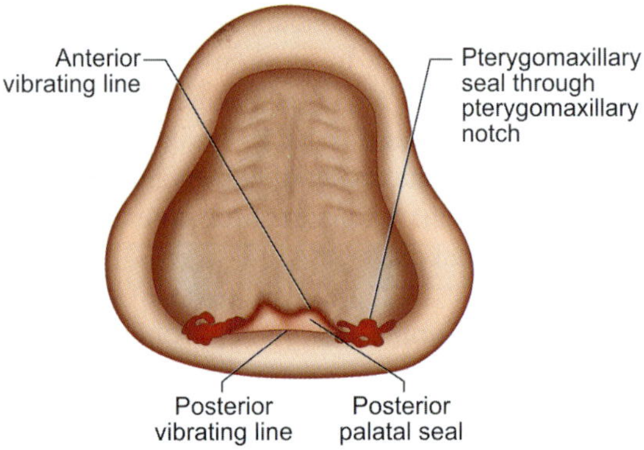

Fig. 11.7: Posterior palatal seal

Clinical Procedure

Posterior Palatal Seal

1. The posterior part of the palate of the patient is dried with a 2" × 2" gauge piece. The patient is asked to say "ah" repeatedly and the moving line is marked with an indelible pencil. The patient is then asked to blow through the nose when holding it closed (Fig. 11.8). This line is also marked with indelible pencil. The relationship of both the lines are accessed (Fig. 11.9). When satisfied with the position of two lines an adhesive plaster tape is adapted in the posterior palatal area of the maxillary denture (Fig. 11.10A). The denture is then placed in the patient's mouth and asked the patient to blow through nose while holding it closed (Fig. 11.10B). The soft palate will flex downward transferring the blue lines to the adhesive plaster on the base (Fig. 11.11).
2. The denture base is trimmed up to the posterior blue line. The record base is placed on the moistened cast to transfer the line on the maxillary cast. This line is extended laterally 3 mm beyond the crest of the hamular notch (Figs 11.12 and 11.13).

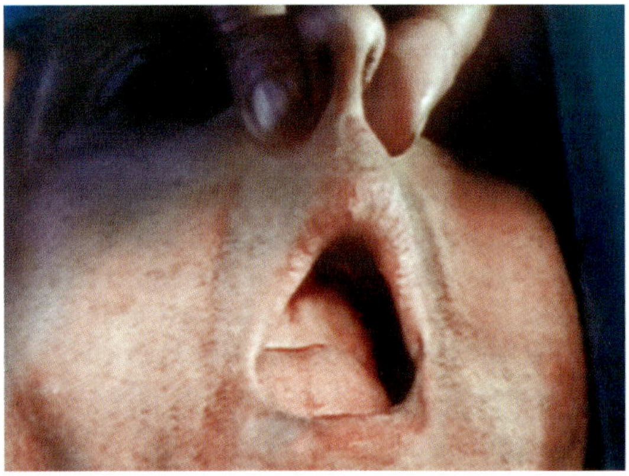

Fig. 11.8: Valsalva maneuver which requires that both nostrils be held firmly while the patient blows gently through the nose, one way of locating anterior vibrating line

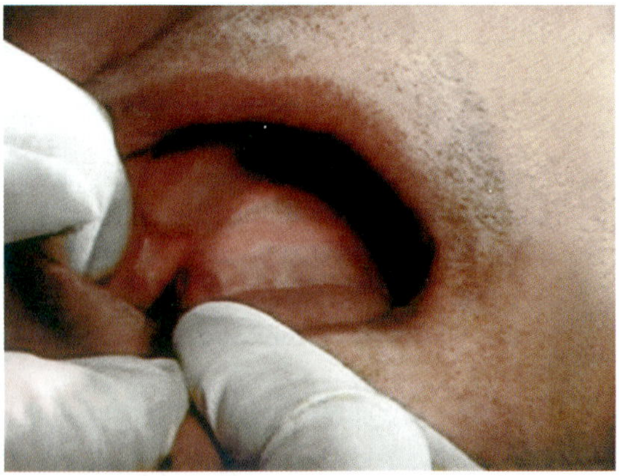

Fig. 11.9: The anterior and posterior vibrating lines are marked on the palate

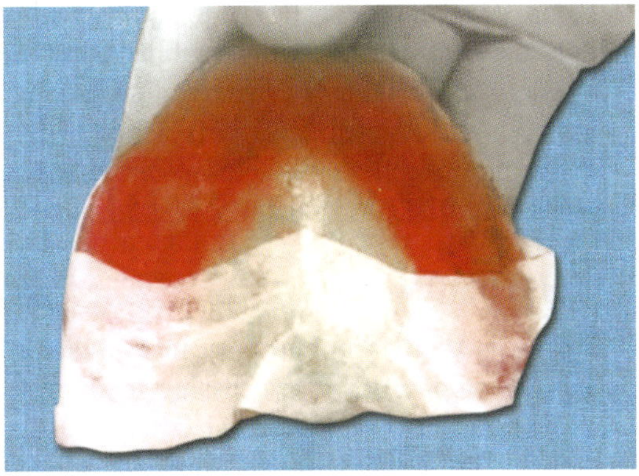

Fig. 11.10A: A stripe of adhesive tape was adapted to the posterior part of maxillary denture base

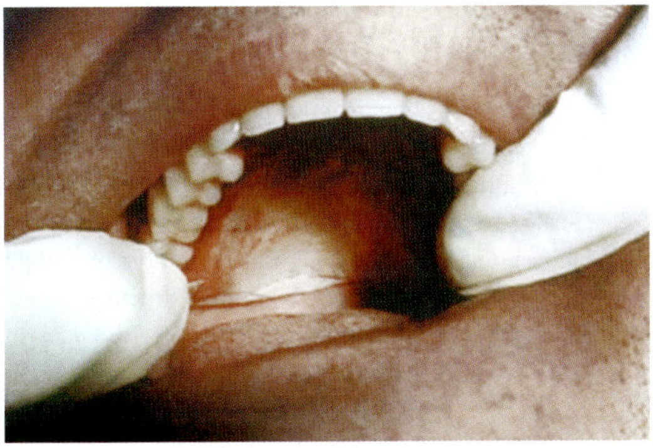

Fig. 11.10B: The maxillary denture base with the tape is placed in the patients mouth properly seated

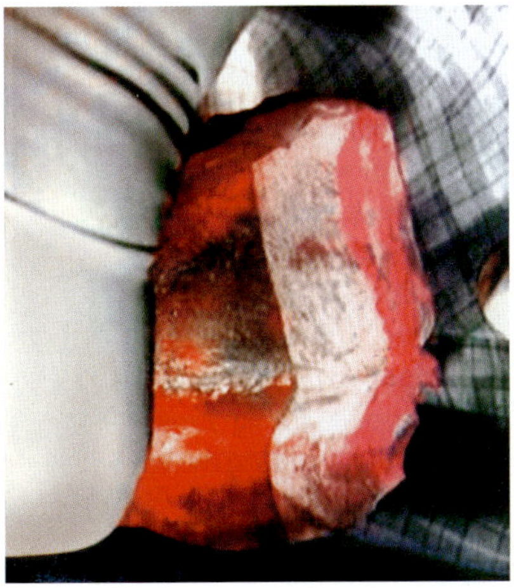

Fig. 11.11: The vibrating lines marked area transferred on the base

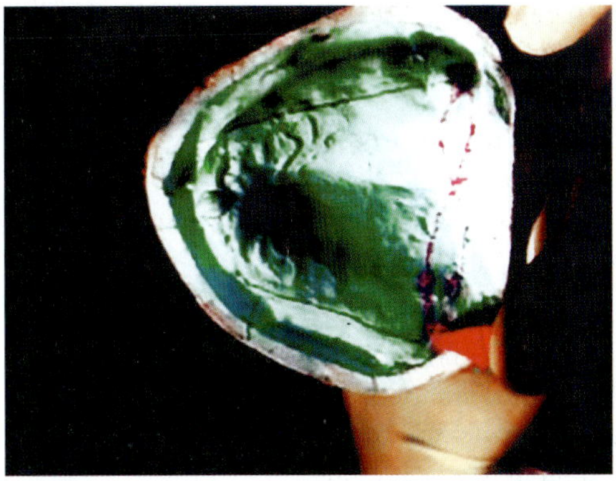

Fig. 11.12: The vibrating lines are transferred to the cast

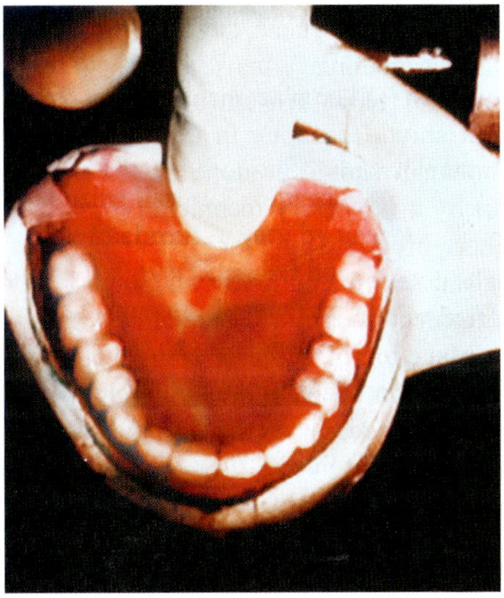

Fig. 11.13: The maxillary denture base with the marked tape was placed on the cast and pressed with finger

3. The whole area marked between the anterior and posterior vibrating lines is scraped with Kingley's, knife as follows:

   1–1.5 mm depth on both side of the midline and 0.5–1 mm over the midpalatine raphe area. The maximum depth at the posterior end and feathering progressively anteriorly. The depth depends on the tissue displacebility.

   Tissue displacebility should be determined by palpating with a ball burnisher, because of individual variation in tissue displacebility

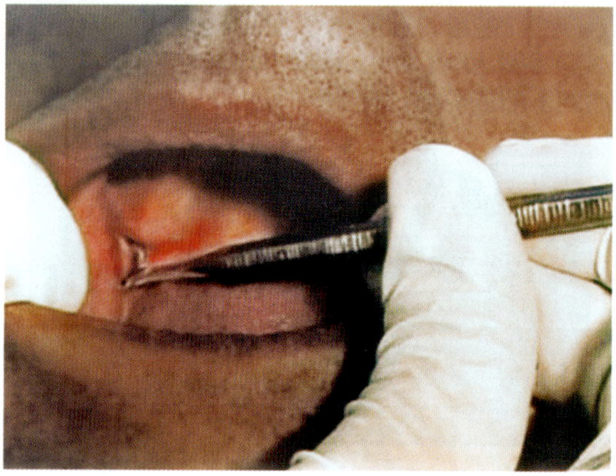

Fig. 11.14: A T-burnisher is used to palpate for the displaceability of tissue

(Fig.11.14). The placement of the post-palatal dam should be done in the presence of the patient. It should be done by the dentist and not by a laboratory technician.

4. The appropriate time for placement of the post palatal seal is controversial. Some believe in placement of the post palatal seal should not be placed until try-in is completed and final varification of maxillomandibular records are made. The reason is that the displacement of the trail base by the tissue causing the base to move downwards when first stated in the mouth. The base should be placed in the mouth for at least for 5 minutes each time before ascertain the occlusal contact. Thereafter only the post-palatal seal is established. Some operator established post palatal seal in the impression stage only. It will depend upon the operators choice in which stage of denture fabrication the post palatal seal is to placed.

CONCLUSION

The try-in is the last opportunity to evaluate all the clinical steps prior to processing. It is better to assume that errors exists in all areas and that need correction after the denture is processed in acrylic resin when chances of correction of errors are limited.

BIBLIOGRAPHY

1. Avant WE. A comparison of the retention of complete denture bases having different types of posterior palatal seals. J Prosth Dent. 1973:29:484-93.
2. Hardly LR, Kapur KK. Posterior border seal—its rationate and importance. J Prosthet Dent. 1985;8:386-97.
3. Hold HR. Variable denture-limiting structures of the edentulous mouth. Parti maxillary border areas. J Prosth Dent. 1959;9:978-87.
4. Landa JS. Troubleshooting in complete denture prosthesis. J Prosth Dent. 1964;9:978-87.
5. Millsap CH. The posterior palatal seal area for complete dentures. Dent Clin N Am. 1964;8:663-73.
6. Silverman SJ. Dimensions and displacement patterns of the posterior palatal seal. J Prosth Dent. 1971;25;470-88.
7. Winland RD, Young JM. Maxillary complete denture. Posterior seal; variations. J Prosth Dent. 1973;29:256-61.

Chapter 12

Laboratory Procedures—Final Arrangement of Teeth, Waxing, Processing and Finishing of Dentures

INTRODUCTION

At the end of try-in step rearrangement of teeth is done for developing lateral and protrusive balance. So, the teeth should be finally arranged on articulator to achieve balanced occlusion.

There is no proof that bilateral balance occlusion is necessary, though most prosthodontists believe that it will slow down the process of ridge resorption. It is more important that the teeth be placed in their correct relation to the ridges and the surrounding soft tissue than they placed in any form of ideal occlusal concept. The advantage of the use of an adjustable articulator is not as much for balance occlusion but for the avoidance of premature balancing contacts. It is easy for class I jaw relation. But it is difficult to achieve in class II jaw relation which requires lots of modification of cusp tooth by occlusal grinding. In class III jaw relation the patient can only make open and close movement. So, no eccentric balance is necessary.

FINAL ARRANGEMENT OF TEETH

Final arrangement of the teeth should be done in balanced occlusion after try-in and setting of condylar guidance is done. When the dentures are moved out of centric occlusion into lateral or protrusive occlusion, there is contact both on the working side and on the nonworking or balancing side, the occlusion is said to be balanced.

In protrusive occlusion, the anterior teeth are edge-to-edge, and balancing contacts will be present between the posterior teeth. In lateral occlusion, the teeth on the working side will be in buccal cusp to buccal cusp interdigitation and on the nonworking side contact will be between the upper palatal cusps and lower buccal cusps of the posterior teeth.

This intercuspation should be even and accurate which has a stabilizing effect on dentures during initial contact. Inclined plane or premature contacts will produce possible instability of dentures.

Bilateral balance means that there is simultaneous contact of protrusive and lateral phases of occlusion. Bilateral balance occlusion is obtained by tilting the teeth mesiodistally and/or buccolingually. The final refinement of bilateral balance is done at the delivery appointment by selective grinding and milling. The reasons for obtaining balanced occlusion and balanced articulations are to produce efficient mastication to help in stabilization of dentures and to prevent their movement during chewing.

To achieve these ideals the lower teeth should glide smoothly across the surface of the upper teeth during all movements of the articulator. There should be no interference when the articulator moves laterally 2 mm in premolar areas in an average.

There are many techniques for arranging posterior teeth in balanced occlusion in a semi-adjustable articulator. The technique described below is used because it maintain the preliminary arrangement of the mandibular teeth to the tongue level determined at the trial stage.

Balance in Protrusion

Protrusive balance is generally absent in natural dentition due to high degree of incisal angle

(60–70 degrees). In setting the denture teeth like natural anterior teeth protrusive balance will be difficult unless incisal angle is 20 degrees or less. So, protrusive balance in denture should not be used at the expense of unstable tooth positioning or unsatisfactory esthetics.

Arrangement of tooth: The six anterior maxillary and six anterior mandibular teeth one set up in the arrangement dictated by the patients esthetic (lip support) and phonetic requirements. This is done by arranging teeth using the occlusal rim as guide.

It depends on the class, on the esthetic position of the incisors and depth of the curve of Spee.

Balance in protrusion is only possible when incisal guidance is set 20° or less. It is obtained in the following steps:

1. The articulator is fixed to the protrusive relationship so that the incisor teeth are positioned edge-to-edge. It shows no posterior tooth contact (Fig. 12.1). In protrusive balance there should be contact of all the maxillary and mandibular anterior and posterior teeth simultaneously.
2. The balancing contact between the upper and lower second motors are made by tilting down the mesial side of upper second molars slightly and tilting up the distal side of lower second molars (Fig. 12.2). The articulator is returned to the centric relationship and the teeth are adjusted until they make centric contact.
3. Then the articulator is again fixed to the protrusive relationship and balancing is done by tilting down the mesial side of upper first molars and tilting up the distal side of lower first molars until contact is made (Fig.12.3). The articulator is returned to the centric relationship and the teeth are adjusted until they make centric contact.
4. The premolars are similarly adjusted. They require very little adjustment. All the posterior teeth have now been adjusted to obtain contact in protrusion (Fig.12.4).

Balance in Lateral Occlusion

Working side: The side on which the patient is masticating (the side of no lateral condylar

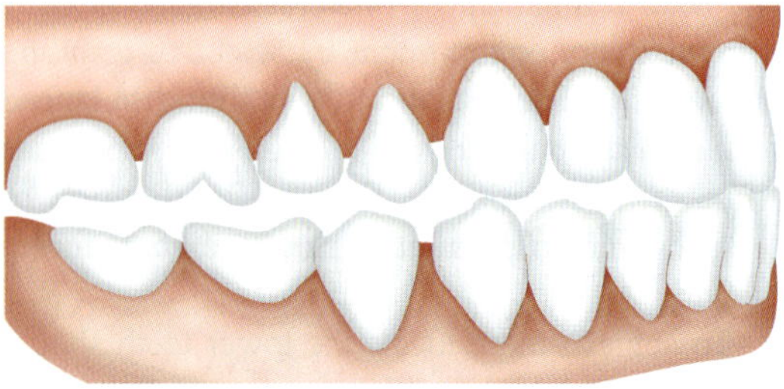

Fig.12.1: Protrusive relationship showing no posterior contact

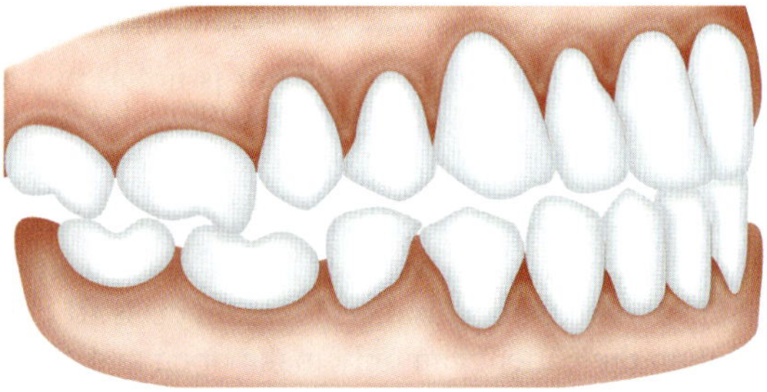

Fig. 12.3: Protrusive balance is provided by contacting the posterior teeth by tilting posterior 1st and 2nd molars

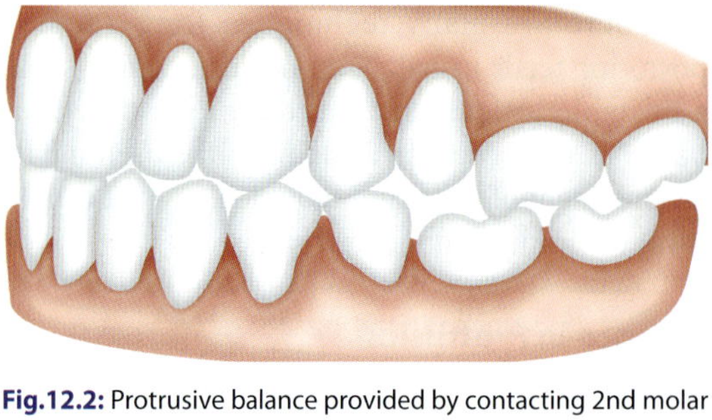

Fig.12.2: Protrusive balance provided by contacting 2nd molar

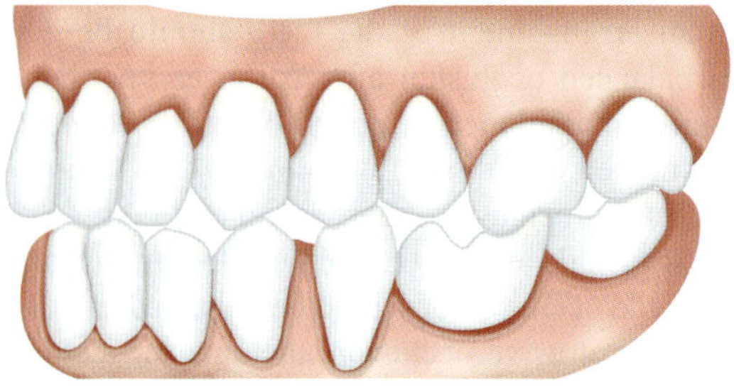

Fig.12.4: All the posterior teeth adjusted for contact in protrusion

translation) is known as the 'working side'. There is contact between similar cusps: Upper buccal and lower buccal.

1. The articulator is fixed in one lateral occlusion by unscrewing one condylar stop screw and bringing buccal cusps of working side edge-to-edge (Fig. 12.5). These buccal cusps should interdigitate and if not adjustments are made by slight grinding the cusps inclines preferably the upper buccal cusps as they are not used in centric occlusion (Fig. 12.6).
2. The articulator is returned to centric occlusion and checked for centric contact.
   Note: The incisal pin may slightly raised from the table due to the cusp inclines. This should not be eliminated by grinding because it will cause excessive grinding of the buccal cusps.
3. The same procedure is repeated for the opposite lateral occlusion.

Balancing side: The side on which the patient is not masticating (the side condyle moves down and medially is its articular fossa) is known as 'non-working or balancing side.

1. There is separation of teeth on the balancing side because of the condylar drop occurred (Fig. 12.7A). This separation should be eliminated by tilting the palatal side of the upper second molars down and the buccal side of the lower second molar up until contact is made (Fig. 12.7B).
2. The articulator is then returned to centric position and necessary adjustment is done if required for centric contacts.
3. The same procedure is repeated for the first molars and for premolars.
4. The whole procedure is repeated for the opposite lateral occlusion.

WAX CONTOURING (WAXING) OF COMPLETE DENTURES

It is defined as "the contouring of a pattern in wax, generally applied to the shaping in wax of the

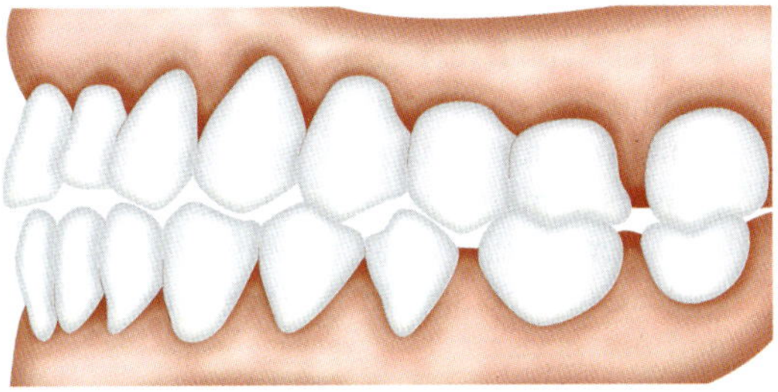

Fig. 12.5: In lateral excursion, inadequate interdigitation of working side buccal cusps

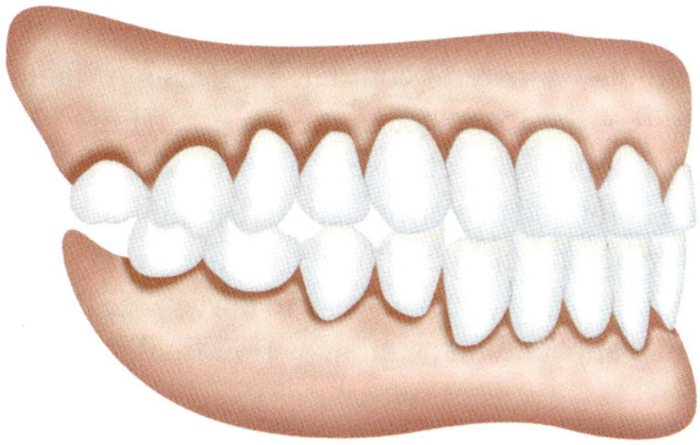

Fig 12.7A: In lateral excursion no balancing contact present

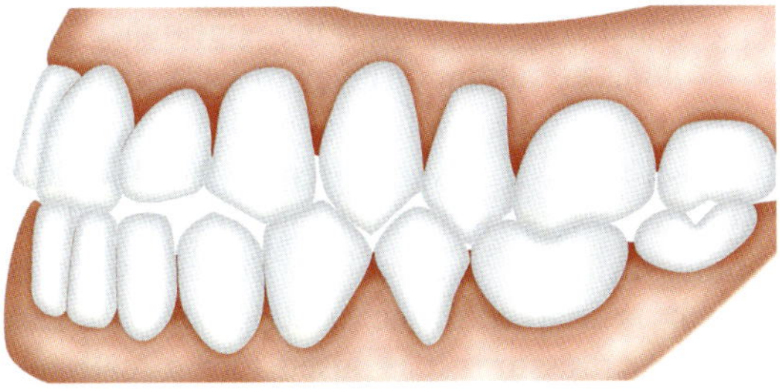

Fig. 12.6: In lateral occlusion, buccal cusps of working side interdigitated properly

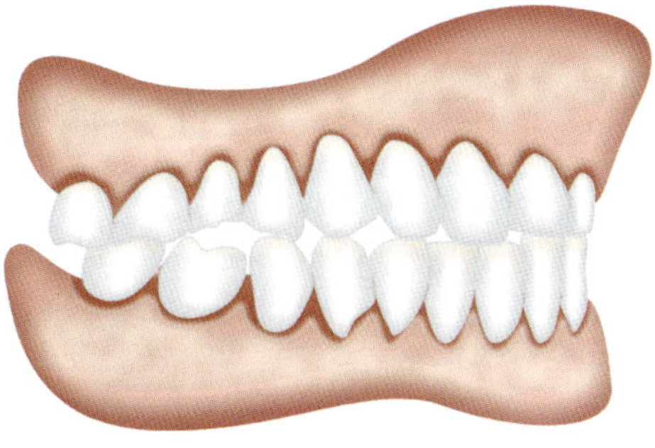

Fig.12.7B: In lateral excursion balancing contacts provided by the tooth movement

contours of a trial denture". After all the teeth are arranged waxing is done prior to try-in. The form of the polished surfaces of a denture is important for comfort, stability, retentive, phonetic, and hygienic and the esthetic quality. The form of waxing surrounding teeth should resemble the form of tissue around the natural teeth.

The wax is contoured and smoothed to make it compatible with the movable oral tissues. For this the following general principles should be followed.

There are two methods of waxing-up the polished surface of a denture:

a. Free hand or conventional method. This is the common method.
b. Physiologic method or flanged method. This method utilizes functional movements of sucking and swallowing to form the polished denture surface in wax, zinc oxide paste, alginate or other impression materials.

CONVENTIONAL METHOD

The external surfaces of complete dentures are most commonly developed by conventional method to produce a natural contour. The casts of natural teeth can be excellent guide for this (Fig. 12.8). It is important to choose a hard wax of pleasing pink color and perform waxing resembling natural tissue before the appointment for the try-in. It will distort less in mouth and easy to curve. The denture should appear to the patient as if in final form. The waxing is simply the contouring the trial denture in wax. The contours should be compatible with the tongue, cheeks, and lips as they function. The bulk of final wax-up must be sufficient to provide for restoration of normal tissue contours. The wax-up should not be bulky also as it lead to the porosity and poor esthetic.

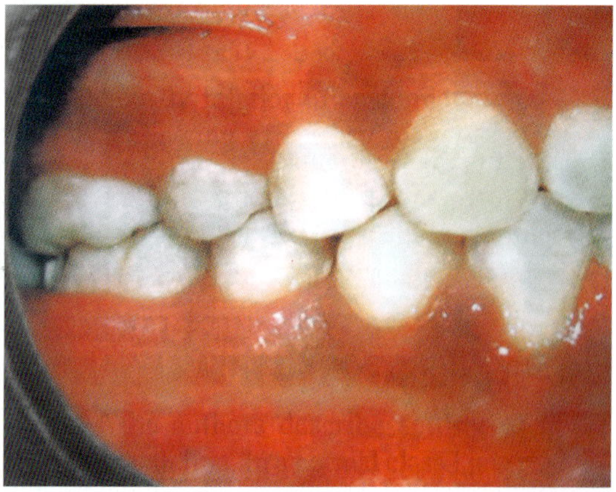

Fig. 12.8: Natural teeth can be excellent guide for waxing

Laboratory Procedure

When the teeth have been arranged in their correct positions and occlusion, the wax surrounding them is rough and irregular. This is smoothed and shaped like natural tissues surrounding the natural teeth. The borders of the upper denture must be thick and rounded, with a thin down post-palatal border to prevent tongue interferences. The buccal and labial surfaces must be concave to allow the buccinators and orbicularis oris to function.

Maxillary Denture

1. *Buccal and labial surface*: The denture base is closely extended to the periphery of a cast which has been poured from a border moulded final impression.

   The labial surface is generally thickened around the neck of the central incisors and canines to form the neck omitting the lateral incisors. This forms a slight depression over the laterals, known as the lateral fossa. The buccal surface should be facing downwards and outwards.

   The wax contouring is less important for the U-shaped large, well-preserved residual ridge whereas, extensive wax contouring should be performed in the case of severely resorbed residual ridge to restore the appearance. This is done by adding a layer of base plate wax over the buccal and labial areas of the record base. This wax covers the entire facial surfaces and extends from the necks of the teeth to the vestibular borders. The strip of softened wax is adapted to the existing contours with finger pressure. It is fused to the teeth and the record base with a hot No. 7 wax spatula. Excess wax is curved from around the neck of each tooth with an Ash No. 5 carver or Lecron carver or No. 7 wax spatula, starting from the second molar. This carving is done by holding the carver at an angle of 30–40 degrees to the surface of the anterior teeth and 45 degrees to the surface of the posterior teeth and should expose each tooth crown down to their junction with the ridge lap.

The wax is scrap away from the buccal and labial surfaces to produce shallow grooves in the inter-radicular space using a No. 11 BP blade. The final rounded form should be produced by flaming the dental papilla with alcohol torch.

These grooves between the roots of the maxillary anterior teeth particularly in lateral incisors should be accentuated and root prominence over the canines should be formed. These grooves must not extend up to the gingival margins which should be slightly raised in the interdental space in the form of a papilla. The shape of the gingival crevice can be imitated by passing a probe around the gingival margin, the point of the probe pointing to the root apex and at an angle of about 20 degrees to the tooth axis. The modifications of rounded gingival margins and interdental papilla can be made by passing floss silk through the contact points.

The healthy tissue should have stippling spreads in a band of one centimeter wide around the arch between the marginal gingivae and free alveolar mucosa. No stippling should be present at the following areas:

a. Canine eminence.
b. Palatal and lingual surfaces.
c. Interproximal grooves.

The stippling is done by using a toothbrush with all bristle removed except only 2–3 tufts at the end shortened to about half. The stippling is done by jabbing the surface of wax with the brush in the required area. The area is lightly polished with water and cotton wool. Stippling may also be produced during finishing and polishing of dentures by slowly rotating an eccentric round bur mounted on a straight handpiece (Fig. 12.9).

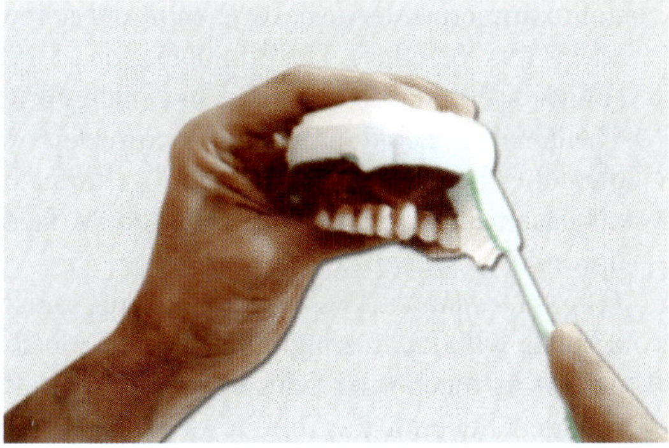

Fig. 12.9: Stippling done by using a toothbrush

2. *Palatal surface*: The palatal surface area of the maxillary denture should have thickness of about 1.5 to 2 mm (including the record base) and should follow the contours of the palate. The anterior S-shape of the dented mouth becomes concave due to loss of teeth and tissues in the edentulous mouth. The contour of the palatal area should be curved in a S-shape. If not done phonetic disturbances with the sibilant sound 'S' or explosion sound 'T' will occur. The posterior palatal part of the denture base should have least amount of bulk in order to allow space for tongue. The palatogram of the sounds, 'S' and 'T' should be used to duplicate the palatal form of the natural dentition. Palatal rugae can be produced on the denture as slightly wider rounded rolls than natural rogues. These should not be formed unless they are present on previous denture and patient needs them contouring. The lingual festooning of the six maxillary incisors should be given a natural lingual contours with cingula. This type of contouring is important for certain speech sounds.

Mandibular Denture

1. *Labial and buccal surfaces*: The buccal surface should be flat and faces outwards and upwards. The labial and the buccal flanges are kept as

thin as practicable (usually 2 mm and some places less than this). The pronunciation of the sound 'so' tends to raise the lower denture. The labial wax contour should be corrected by phonetic method in try-in stage to eliminate displacement. The labial surface should face upwards.

2. *Lingual surface*: The lingual surface must descend without creating bulk below the teeth except at the border which should be well rounded beneath the tongue. The posterior lingual areas must be thin down to prevent interference with the tongue. They should face upwards and inwards. The tongue will rest on the medial extension of the lingual surface of the molar region.

The final step is to seal the trial denture to the cast with molten wax. All the excess wax must be removed from the teeth and land area of casts prior to investing. The following steps should be reviewed:

1. The wax is melted around the teeth to attach them firmly. The rough areas are smoothened with a hot wax knife.
2. The wax is added rounded the necks of teeth to form a gingival roll with the wax knife or No. 7 wax carver holding like a pen. The edge of globule of wax placed in the requisite area and the role is drawn by trailing the globule of wax around the neck of each teeth. The roots are also formed in the similar way.
3. The gingival wax is trimmed with a inlay carver held at an obtuse angle to the cervical margin of the tooth to create a ledge of uniform thickness of 1 mm. All wax should be removed from the exposed area of teeth.
4. The ledge is curved back to a uniform thickness of 1 mm. The cingulum of anterior teeth are exposed and the wax given a natural contour. The flame is brushed over the surface of wax which takes on a sheen. Any air holes appear on the surface of wax are filled and the surface is smoothened by reflaming.
5. *Contouring*: The buccal and labial flanges are contoured to a thickness 2 mm labially and 3 mm buccally in a normal case. In a tight lipped case only 1 mm of labial thickness may be allowable and where excessive thickness is required it should not exceed 4 to 5 mm. A check of occlusion of teeth is required as contraction causes slight movement of some teeth. The lost contact is restored in occlusion.
6. *Smoothening the wax*: At the time of setting and curving all effort should be to maintain the smoothness of wax. The final smoothening is accomplished by brushing a fine flame quickly over the wax to melt its surface momentarily. The excessive heat should be avoided to cause run of wax and destruction of contouring. When acrylic teeth are used the flame must be kept away from it.
7. *Stippling*: This is done with a toothbrush with reduced to about 5 mm length. The bristles are jabbed into the surfaces of wax to produce stippling. The stippling can also be done during the denture finishing with the help of a exocentric bur moving on the laboratory handpiece.
8. *Polishing the wax*: The smoothed wax denture is placed in cold water to harden, and then rubbed with wet cotton wool to obtain high polish.
9. The casts are cleaned of wax by pouring on boiling water after removing the waxed dentures from it. They are returned to the articulator.
10. The final checking the occlusion and discrepancies correction should be done before presenting the dentures for investing.

Physiologic or Flange Method

The main objective of conventional waxing-up of denture is to produce the surfaces as an ideal without regards to the detailed surrounding of oral structures. But in a physiologic or flange technique, the impressions of oral structures that come in contact with the surfaces of the denture base made in soft flange wax or alginate in try-in stage.

These contours are then incorporated in the polished denture surfaces. Advantages of physiologic technique are as follows:

1. Physiological alignment of arch form of anterior and posterior teeth on the occlusal rim is possible.
2. Accurate reproduction of the oral structures produces accurate adaptation of the tissues to the denture bases.
3. Improves masticatory efficiency, retention, esthetic and phonetics.

The principals are scientific and incorporation of them in the conventional method of waxing-up produces comfortable and successful denture experience.

PROCESSING COMPLETE DENTURES

It is the conversion of wax pattern of a denture into resin or other material. There are various methods of processing acrylic resin denture bases for complete dentures, such as compression molding, injection molding, and pouring fluid resin into a vented mold. The continuous injection molding method shows less processing error than the standard trial-pack compression molding method. However, the equipment is very costly to use in most dental clinics. Turk et al (1992) found no significant difference in dimensional accuracy in dentures processed with conventional heat cure compression molding, microwave, and light cure procedures for polymerization of resin. Microwave processing requires a microwave oven, special resin and nonmetal flasks which deteriorate more rapidly than metal flasks.

The fluid resin procedure is quite technique sensitive. The voids are difficult to eliminate. The most important drawback is the high amount of residual monomer that remains in the dentures after polymerization. Therefore, compression molding with external heat application for polymerization is the method of choice for denture fabrication.

Processing of complete dentures consists of following steps:

1. Preliminary preparation for investing.
2. Flasking and removing the wax.
3. Packing.
4. Polymerization.
5. Deflasking and remounting.
6. Finishing and polishing.

Preliminary Preparation for Investing

The trial dentures, after waxing are prepared for flasking. The flask should be coated with separating media. The casts should be socked in slurry water for 5–10 minutes. A three piece (ejector type) flask containing three parts is convenient for the removal of the denture after processing without damage. The pieces are known the drag (bottom), cope (middle) and cap (Fig. 12.10). Flask should be in good condition.

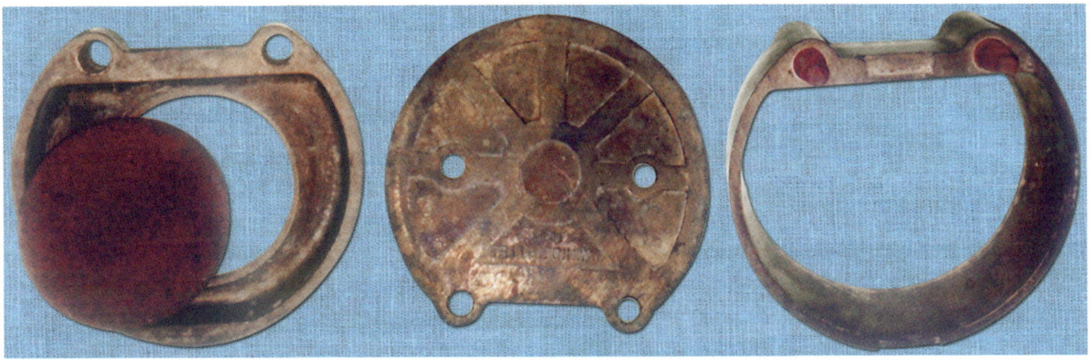

Fig. 12.10: The three piece flask (ejector type)

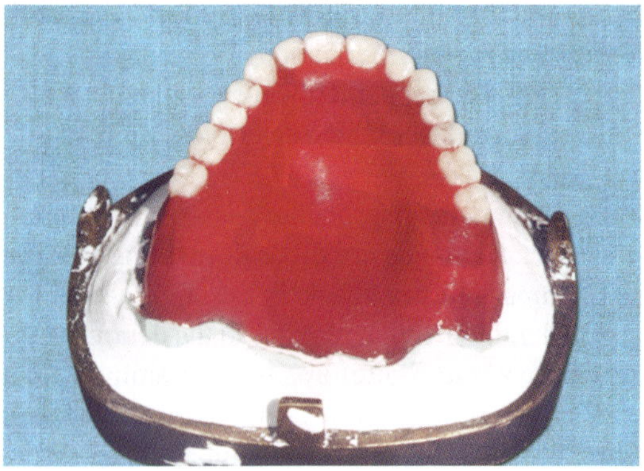

Fig. 12.11: The first pour up to the levels of land area in lower half of flask

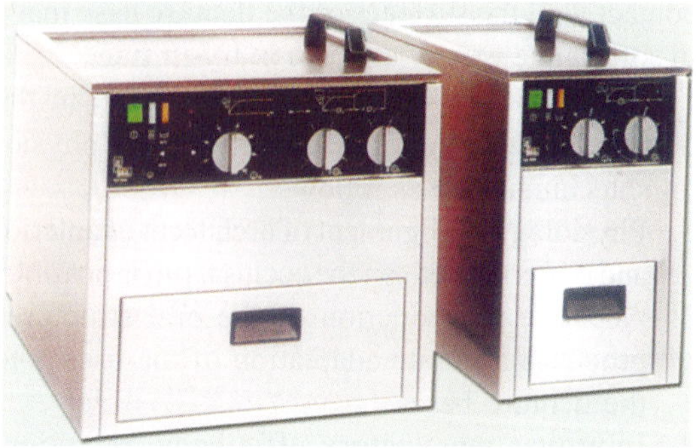

Fig. 12.12: An electrical time and temperature acrylizer and a dewaxing bath

Flasking

It is the act of investing a pattern in a flask. The procedure of investing the cast and the wax denture in a flask to mould the denture base material into the denture.

Three pour techniques gives best result. The first pour is up to the level of the land area in the lower half of flask (Fig. 12.11). The second pour is up to the occlusal surfaces and incisal edges of the teeth. Third one should fill up mould. Dental stone is used to invest the dentures in the bottom (shallow) half of the flask until the rim of the cast is near the top of the rim of the flask. A posterior tilt to the lower denture reduces the chance of damage of the cast due to undercut. The wet stone is smoothed from brass edge towards the land of the cast so that no undercuts exist. When the stone is set the separating medium is painted on the plaster and the land areas of the cast.

The top half of the flask is set in position making certain that it is completely seated on the lower half. The flask is now filled by vibration with 50:50 dental stone and plaster mix. The investment is painted with a brush into the interproximal spaces. It is then poured up to the level of the incisal edges and occlusal surfaces of the teeth, so that none remains on these surfaces. Before exothermic heat is developed in the investment, the flasks are submerged in cold water. This will dissipate the heat of the stone and prevent wax expansion and teeth movement. The rest of the space is filled with dental stone and the cap of the flask is set in position. When excess comes out through holes on it. The stone is cleaned away from the side of the flasks and from one hole at the top of the flasks, but allow to remain over the other hole. Excess stone is forced back into hole to prevent voids in stone formed due to initial shrinkage before set hard and expand.

Removing Wax

When the investing stone has set (1 hr), the flask is placed in boiling water exactly for 5 minutes to soften the wax so that the two halves can be separated. An electrically time and temperature controlled wax bath is available for complete removal of wax (Fig. 12.12).

Types and uses of denture base materials are shown in Table 12.1.

Table 12.1 Types and uses of denture base materials

Class I	Metallic	Cobalt-chromium alloy
	Nonmetallic	Acrylic resins, vinyl resins
Class II	Temporary	Shellac base plate, base plate wax hard, autocare acrylic resin
	Permanent	Heat-cure acrylic resin, cobalt chromium alloy, injection molded acrylic resin, injection molded polycarbonate
		a. Conventional
		b. High impact

The flask should not be overheated as the wax is liquefied and run into investment pours. It is almost impossible to remove this wax completely after it has penetrated the investment.

The residual wax is removed with a stream of boiling water. The mold is washed again with a stream of boiling water containing a powder detergent (liquid detergent leave residue on acrylic teeth effect polymerization). Then the investments are cleaned thoroughly by flashing with the boiling water. This is repeated in the other half of the flask.

The both halves of the flask are prop up on a board so that they stand on end to allow the water to drain out. When the flasks are still quite warm, two coats of separating medium is applied with a medium-sized camel hair brush (with pointed ends) to all the plaster surface using the point of the brush to paint in between the teeth and allowed to dry. The separating medium should be avoided over the teeth as much as possible. A larger size brush can be used to paint the large sections such as the land areas.

The flasked molds are allowed to stand overnight to allow the investment to reach its full strength.

Packing

Denture-base material shadeguide is available for characterization hand (Fig. 12.13). The monomer and polymer is mixed according to the manufacturer's direction in a glass or porcelain jar with lid. The ratio of polymer to monomer is 3:1 by volume or 2:1 by weight. Sufficient amount of acrylic resin for one denture only (10 ml liquid and 30 cm powder) should be mixed to pack whatever the convention is used.

The lid of the jar should not be removed until full doughy stage has been reached to prevent contamination. When the mixture has reached doughy consistency and does not adhere to the walls of the mixing jar, it is placed between two cellophane sheets and formed a 6 mm thick role that is flattened and cut into pieces and packed over the teeth in the flask with finger pressure. The mould is packed with the dough in several stages of closure to ensure the complete filling.

The flask is closed in a hand (Figs 12.14A and B) press with a sheet of cellophane separating sheet between two halves until almost completely closed. Then the flask halves are separated and the excess flash resin is cut away precisely at the denture border and additional resin is added at any places where no flash is visible. The trial packing is repeated until no flash is formed (three times). The two halves of the flask is then closed completely to make metal-to-metal contact without separating

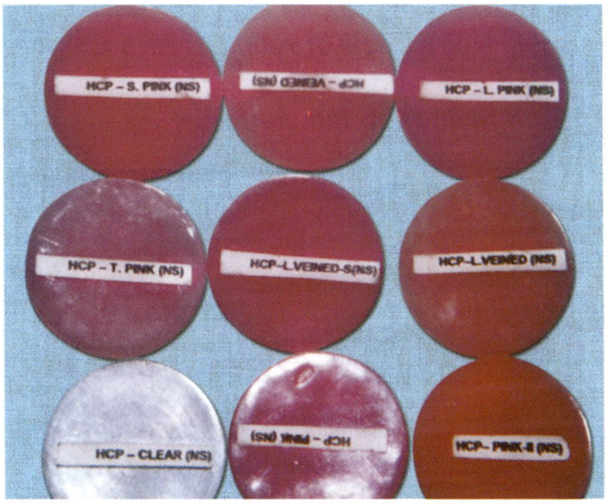

Fig. 12.13: Shade guides for denture base materials

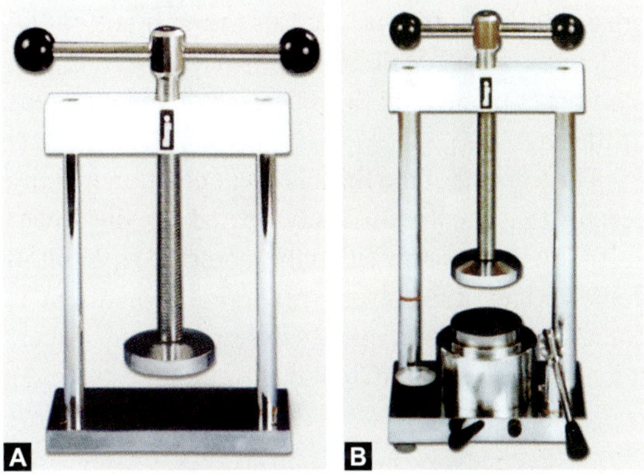

Figs 12.14A and B: (A) Denture press; (B) Hydraulic denture press

sheet but applying separating media. The slightest discrepancy in closure of the two halves of the flask will cause occlusal discrepancy.

The flask is closed with a spring clamp closed tightly but not fully. This will allow the resin to expand and contract still under pressure during polymerization. If the clamps are firm, the expansion will be compensated for by an expansion of the mold space.

If this expansion goes beyond the limit of expansion of investment it will cause teeth movement. To prevent this compensating press is of value (Fig. 12.15).

Polymerization

Definition: It is the process of converting of heat cure acrylic resin dough into a hard mass by raising the temperature of the mould. Following 30 to 60 minutes of bench curing, the dentures may be polymerized by either one of two accepted methods.

Long polymerization cycle: The acrylic resin is processed for 9 hours in a water bath at 73.5 degree centigrade followed by 30 minutes boiling.

Short curing cycle: The flask is immersed in water at 73.5 degree centigrade temperature for 1.5 hours, then boiling for 30 minutes. A quick cure acrylic resin requires only 20 minutes boiling (Fig. 12.16).

The long polymerization cycle is the method of choice. Both the cycle should end with a boiling period to remove residual monomer. An electrical time and temperature controlled acrylizer is available commercially to ensure correct curing is cut.

Deflasking

The flask should be removed from the curing bath and allowed to bench cooled for 30 minutes before placing it into cold water for 15 minutes to avoid warpage, because there will be a difference between the shrinkage of the denture base and the gypsum.

The whole content of the flask is removed in one piece. The investing stone is cut piece by piece. The flask should not be strike with metal hammer to prevent damage of the denture flasks. The use of wooden mallet prevent the damage.

A cut is made with a sharp knife, down the front of the investment opposite the labial surfaces of the

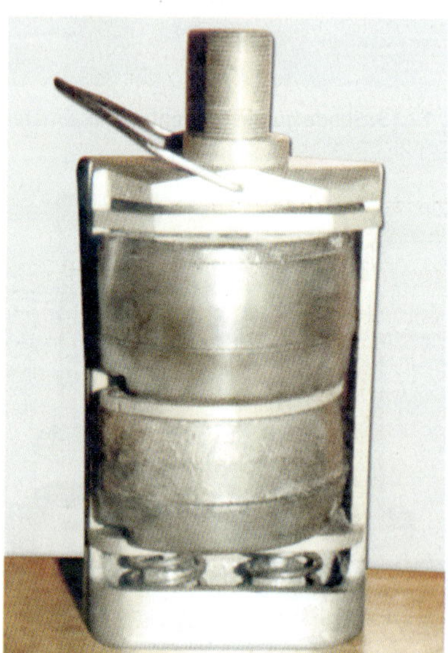

Fig. 12.15: Hand compress with two flasks, use of hand compress minimizes packing pressure

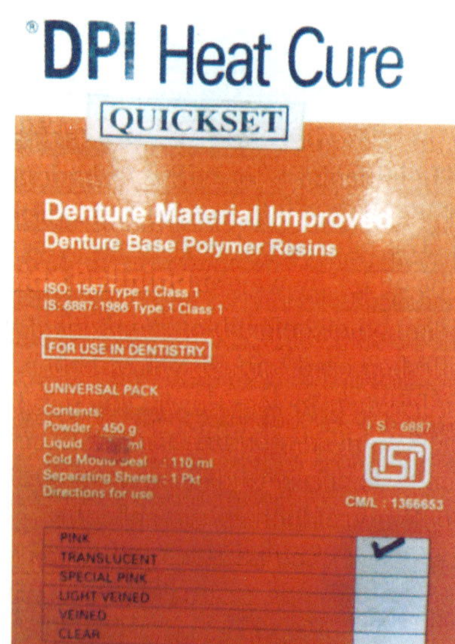

Fig. 12.16: The quick cure acrylic resin. It requires only 20 minutes boiling

two central incisors and sections of investments are removed by prying both the right and left sections of investments. The care should be taken to avoid the cutting of the teeth or labial surface of the denture.

The investments of the lingual and palatal surface of the dentures are removed with the help of the knife.

The dentures should not be removed from the casts. The casts and the dentures should be made free of investment particles by using a hard bristle brush and air blast (Fig. 12.17).

Remounting

The casts and dentures are fitted back onto the articulator mountings by means of index notches that were cut before mounting (Figs 12.18A and B). They are sealed and the processing errors are observed. The correction of processing errors are usually done at this time. Usually, the incisal pin will show a sight opening. Articulating paper is placed between the teeth, and articulator opened and closed in the centric position. The marks of articulating paper indicate which areas should be ground. This is continued until the original vertical dimension has been restored. The same procedure is repeated with the articulator moved into eccentric positions. During the all lateral and protrusive excursions and in centric relation there should be contacts of incisal pin on the guide.

Finishing and Polishing

The dentures are now removed from the casts. As most of the dentures have undercuts and the plastic is weaker than cast, injudicious prying will results

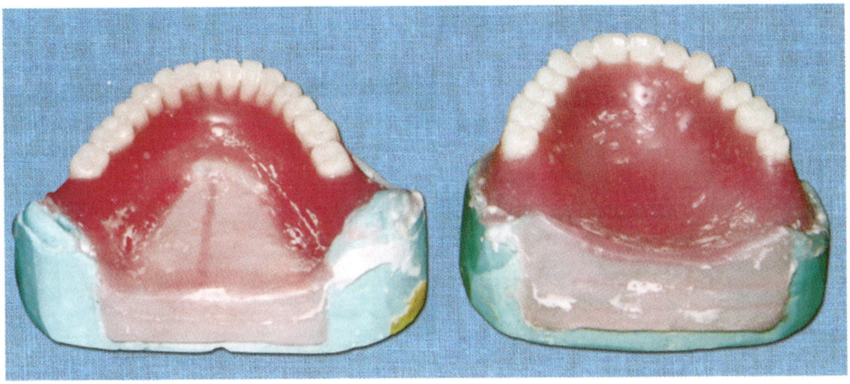

Fig. 12.17: The denture should not be removed from the casts which should be intact

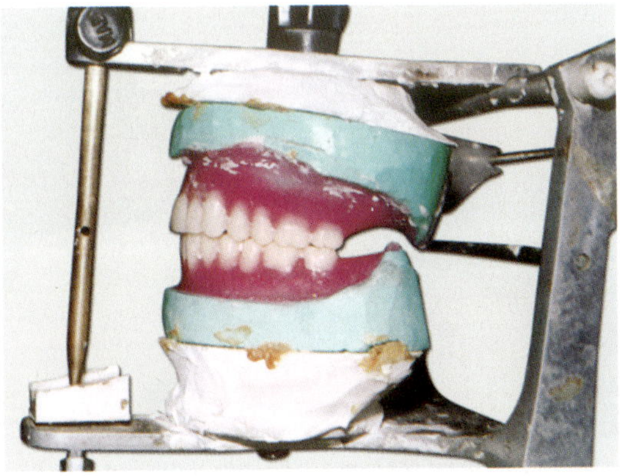

Fig. 12.18A: Dentures and casts remounted on articulator

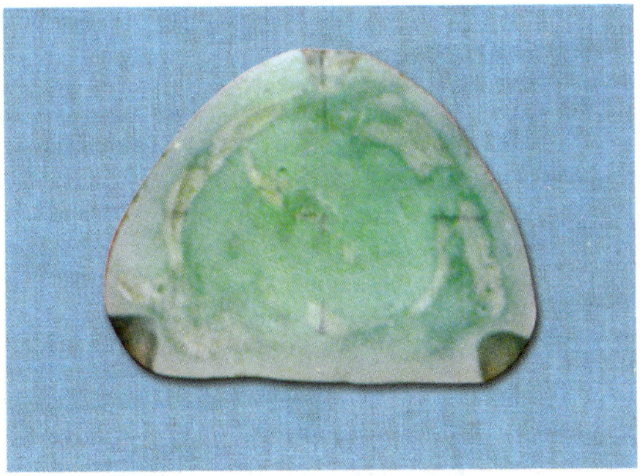

Fig. 12.18B: Three V-shaped notches are cut in three widely separated area at the base of the cast for correct remounting

in breakage of denture. The undercut areas should be cut with small disc or saw or removed with a "shell blaster". The base is cut with a circular saw in many pieces and small parts are removed until the denture is completely free of all stone. A knife may be used as a wedge between cuts for removal of pieces. The pieces should be removed first from posterior part of the cast and preceding forward (Fig. 12.19).

After removing the denture from plaster, the flash is trimmed of with arbor bands or wheel stone on dental lathe (Fig. 12.20). The borders should be round and not left square or sharp. The feather edges of the denture base around the gingival line are removed with burs and the surface is shaped to produce a smooth, clean surface without any plaster or scratches (Fig. 12.21).

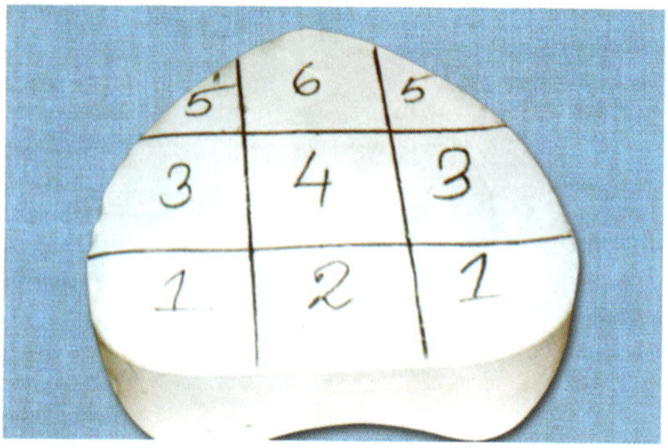

Fig. 12.19: Many cuts with saw to remove small parts of the cast without exerting pressure in denture base

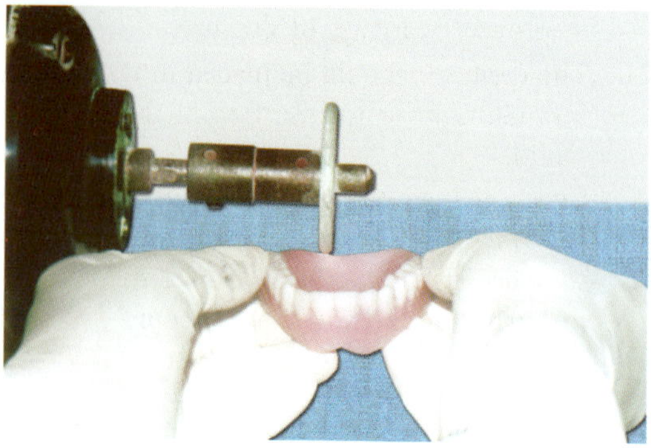

Fig. 12.20: Wheel stone on dental bathe

The borders are now polished using wet rag or black brush wheel (Figs 12.22A and B) with pumice. For palatal areas not accessible to wheel a felt cone is helpful. The polishing should be done

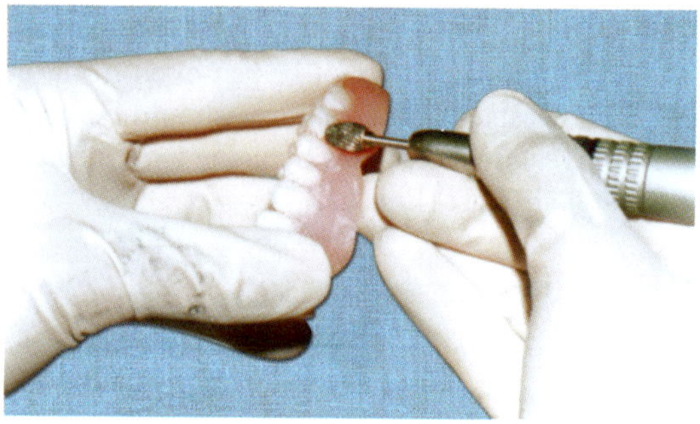

Fig. 12.21: Carbide trimmer on St handpiece

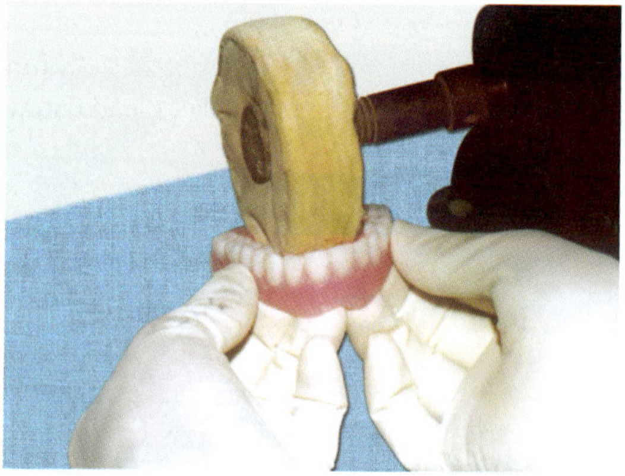

Fig. 12.22A: Polishing with wet rag wheel with pumice

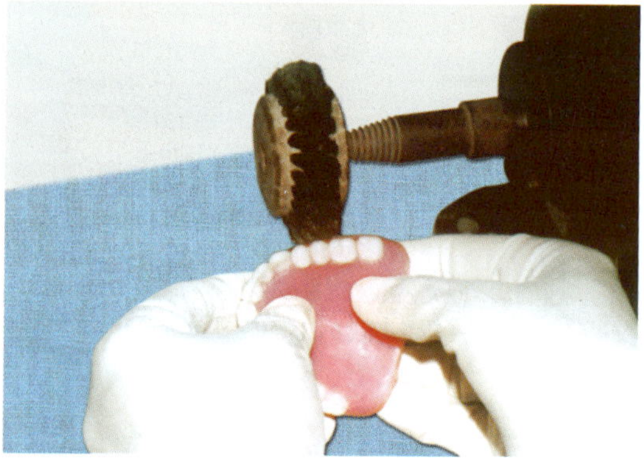

Fig. 12.22B: Polishing with black bristle brush with pumice

without overheating or burning. The interproximal spaces can be polished with acrylic polishers (Fig. 12.23) in a handpiece. The final polishing is done with a resin polishing compound applied on dry wheel. Highly polished denture helps the patient to clean it to maintain tissue health.

The tissue fitting surface of the denture is finally examined by eye and by finger for any sharp projections which should be removed and smoothed.

The dentures should be washed with warm water, soap and a denture brush and stored under water until delivered to the patient. The following tips should be followed for successful processing of acrylic dentures.

1. The relationships obtained from the patient must be mechanically and physiologically sound, i.e. the impression recorded of rested mucosa with proper border extension, proper vertical dimension and centric relation; correctly mounted on articulator, and correct tooth dentures.
2. The waxing contour of trial denture should be a replica of final denture. The borders should be sealed with wax. The palatal coverage should be uniformly 2.5–3 mm thick (2 thickness of wax). All wax should be removed from the teeth surface.
3. Flasking should be done with dental stone. Silicone mould release should be used instead of vaseline.
4. The dewaxing must be timed so that wax is not to sock into the stone from prolong heating. The wax is removed as one piece by lifting. Some house hold detergent should be used to wash inside the flask followed by cleaning with warm water.
5. The tin foil substitute one coat should be painted when the flask is still warm to the tissue fitting surface of the casts The opposite surface should be painted with two or three coats of tin foil substitute. This extra coating of separator will cause the acrylic to shrink towards and hug the cast for optimum tissue contact. So 6 percent of shrinkage will be towards the polished surface and not toward the fitting surface.
6. During packing the powder-to-liquid ratio should be accurately measured, no more than two flasks should be packed at a time.
7. The processing should be done using recommended time temperature curing cycle recommended by the manufacturers.
8. The inside of the flask must be cooled at room temperature before pressure is released on the clamp.
9. Polishing and finishing should be minimized to prevent warpage of denture.
10. The dentures should be placed in water for a few hours prior to insertion in the patient's mouth.
11. Every new set of denture should be checked for tissue adaptation in the mouth with pressure-indicating paste and remounted on the articulator from a new centric record before the patient wear them home.

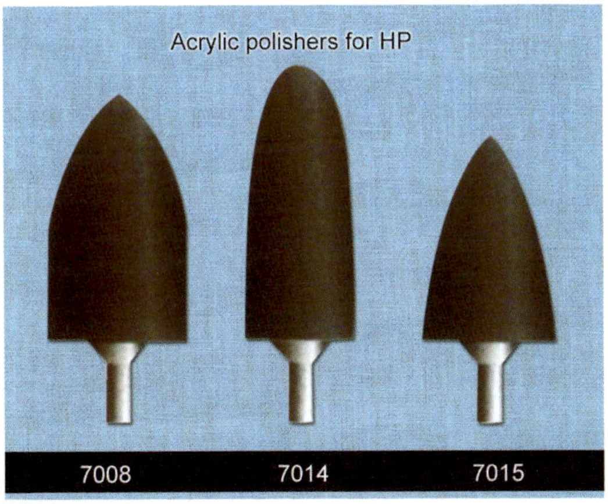

Fig. 12.23: Acrylic polishers

CONCLUSION

It is very difficult if not impossible to achieve perfect centric, protrusive and lateral balance for all cusps of all teeth.

The desirability of balancing contacts is essential. Solid contact in centric relation must receive highest priority, working and balancing contacts are next in competence. Protrusive balance is of least importance in denture construction. All contacts should be checked with the help of thin articulating paper.

BIBLIOGRAPHY

1. Fish EW. Principles of Full Denture Prosthesis, 6th edn, Charles C Thomas Publisher, Springfield; 1964. pp. 32-66.
2. Lott F, Levin B. Flange technique: an anatomic and physiologic approach to increase retention, function, comfort and appearance in dentures, J Prosthet Dent. 1966;16:394.
3. Morrow RM, Rudd KD, Rhoads JE. Dental laboratory Procedures: complete Dentures, Vol I, 2nd edn, St Louis V Mosby; 1986. pp. 339-63.

Chapter 13

Correction of Occlusal Discrepancies

INTRODUCTION

The efficiency and comfort in wearing complete dentures rests on the occlusal harmony. A proper impression procedure, correct jaw relation records, facebow transfer and the use of a semiadjustable articulator to build a balanced articulation will usually produce comfortable dentures. But in actual practice occlusal errors are often crypt in resulting a uncomfortable and painful denture that cause damage to the supporting tissues. The errors in occlusion should be checked and be corrected before the dentures are delivered to the patient. This becomes an essential step in complete denture construction.

CAUSES OF OCCLUSAL DISCREPANCIES

1. Incorrect registration of jaw relations.
2. Errors occurring during mounting of casts on articulator.
3. Errors in the setting of the denture teeth.
4. Tooth movement occurred during flasking packing and polymerization.
5. Incomplete flask closure.

Methods

Two methods are generally used in correcting occlusal discrepancies. In both the methods occlusal surfaces of teeth are altered by selective grinding.

Method I: Laboratory remounting and correction of occlusion due to processing errors by selective grinding before recovering the dentures from their casts.

Method II: Clinical remounting dentures with check-bite records (a new jaw relation records) and adjustment of the occlusion is necessary at the time of delivery of complete dentures to eliminate errors, which may not be found at the try-in of the trial denture.

The laboratory remounting procedure will not correct for clinical errors in recording maxillo-mandibular relation records.

So, correction of occlusal discrepancies are done preferably by patient check record remounting and selective grinding at the time of delivery.

Laboratory Remounting Method

This is done by using split cast mounting plates or by notching casts to create keys in the mounting plaster. The split cast has got several advantages:

a. Processing errors introduced by movement of teeth are easily detected.
b. Deflecting contacts can be removed easily by grinding.
c. Original vertical dimension can be restored.
d. The centric occlusal relation position of cusps to the opposing teeth can be re-established.

Procedures

1. Any chips of investment or acrylic flash that prevent accurate sitting of the casts should be

removed first from the base of the casts. The upper and lower dentures on their original casts are remounted on the articulator. They are attached to the original plaster mountings with stricky wax added to the sides.
2. The remounting shows the changes that occurred in the teeth during processing and makes it helps to restore the original vertical dimension of occlusion that exist in wax-up dentures. It may be found that the incisal pin fails to contact the incisal table to about 0.5 to 1 mm (Fig. 13.2).
3. It is corrected by placing a fine articulating paper in between the teeth, and the articulator is closed in centric position several times. The marks are ground by the process of selective grinding until the original vertical dimension is restored as evident by the contact of the incisal guide pin to the incisal guide table. When the occlusion is perfected on the articulator, the amount of work in the mouth is reduced substantially.

Clinical Remounting Method

The clinical remounting method is to remount the dentures on an articulator by means of interocclusal records made in the patient's mouth. This is most accurate method. It has the following advantages:
1. It allows the dentist to observe the procedures better.
2. It eliminates patient participation.
3. It provides a stable mounting casts and bases those are not shifted on resilient tissues.
4. The saliva will not remove the markings of articulating paper.
5. The correction made in absence of the patient is advantageous.
6. It may be done in recall appointments from 24 hours adjustment to one year appointment. Of course delay of occlusal adjustment until the denture settle in patients mouth may cause excessive tissue injury, instability and unsatisfactory retention.

Procedures: This method maintains the articulator settings for various records used in setting and the facebow index of the maxillary waxed cast before processing.

After processing the dentures are recovered from investment and carefully finished and polished. All the undercuts are blocked with modeling clay. The fitting surface is lubricated with petroleum jelly and mounting casts are poured.

The maxillary cast is attached with plaster to the articulator with facebow index produced on the remounting jig. With both the dentures a wax check-bite centric relation record is obtained from the patient are joined securely with sticky wax. The upper arm of the articulator is opened up and maxillary denture is seated on the upper mounted cast on the articulator. The plaster is placed on the lower mounting disk and the articulator is inverted and closed as plaster sets.

Selective Grinding

Definition

'The intentional alteration of the occlusal surfaces of teeth to change their form.'

Grinding of the occlusal surfaces of the artificial teeth at selected points is carried out to ensure that the centric occlusion of the teeth coincides with the centric relation and also to have balanced eccentric contact in all position. The elimination of the deflective contacts of the teeth with provision of balanced occlusion is one of the most important stages in the fabrication of dentures carried out as a clinical remounting after the dentures have been tried in the patient. It is an corrective process that should be carried out after a thorough knowledge of balanced occlusion is required. This procedure is to correct minor errors in clinical and/or laboratory procedures. It is not effective in elimination of gross error where a wrong centric relation has been obtained. The attempt to correct the large errors by occlusal grinding will cause loss of occlusal form which is not desirable. Large errors needs removal and replacement of teeth with cold cure acrylic resin. Final correction of occlusal errors are made by selective grinding. So that simultaneous contact around the arch in centric and eccentric contacts is made.

Selective grinding helps in preservation of tooth form and occlusion.

The process is carried out in two stages:
a. Correction of centric occlusion at a correct centric relation.
b. Development of eccentric balancing contacts.

Correction of Occlusal Errors in Anatomical Teeth on Articulator

Instruments (Fig. 13.1)

1. Red and blue thin articulating paper.
2. Green stones or diamonds.
3. Laboratory handpiece.
4. Rubber points.
5. Gauze moistened with alcohol.

Rules for Selective Grinding

1. A centric cusp tip should never be grind unless prematurely in all excursions of the mandible. The oppositioning fossa should always be grind.
2. The BULL rule should be used for working occlusion by grinding the buccal cusp inclines of the upper and lingual cusp inclines of the lower.
3. In balancing occlusion cusp inclines should be grind and not the cusp tips.
4. In protrusive interferences in anterior teeth grinding of lower labial and upper lingual teeth in recommended. In posterior teeth the upper buccal cusp slopes and lower lingual cusp slopes should be grind.

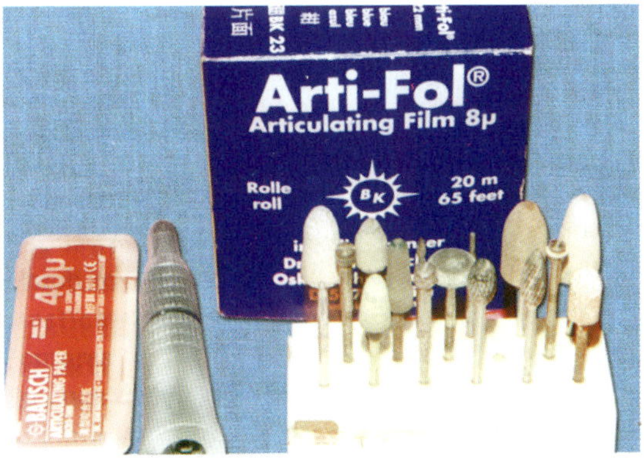

Fig. 13.1: Instruments for occlusal correction

Selective Grinding for Centric Occlusion

1. Articulating paper of minimum thickness is placed between the posterior teeth bilaterally and the teeth are tapped together. The articulator should be locked with centric lock so as to make centric closure only.
2. The markings are observed for premature contacts that are to be relieved depends both in centric and eccentric relationships as follows:
   a. If tip of cusp is high in centric contact only, the opposing fossa should be deepened.
   b. If tip of cusp is high both in centric and lateral excursions, it is reduced.
3. The marking and reduction is repeated until even, bilateral, cusp/fossa markings occur. The marking of premature contacts should be identified as dark spot with a light center.
4. The anterior contact if any should be removed as required. There should be no contact of anterior tooth in centric relation.
5. The incisal guide pin is set against the incisal table and locked in this position.

Selective Grinding for Working and Balancing Occlusion Contacts

Selective grinding for working and balancing occlusions must be done at the same time.

To improve the stability and retention of the dentures it is necessary to ensure that there is balance in lateral movements and that there is no cuspal interference both in working and balancing occlusion.

The lateral wings of the incisal guidance are raised until only slight contact exists in lateral excursions with the incisal post.

The premature contacts are removed by grinding and the lateral wings are lowered slightly.

1. The articulating paper is placed bilaterally between the teeth. The articulator is moved in right and left lateral excursions placing articulating paper between the teeth bilaterally (Fig. 13.2).
2. Blue color articulating paper is placed between the teeth and tapped sharply together in centric relation. The marks should not be removed during selective grinding for eccentric balance.
3. The premature areas are identified and removed by grinding according to the following rules:
   a. *On working side*: It is essential that the proper alignment of the opposing cusps and their opposing embrasures are reestablished. It is done by reducing the lingual inclines of the upper buccal cusps and the buccal inclines of the lower lingual cusps (BULL RULE) (Fig. 13.3).
   b. *On the balancing side*: The buccal inclines of the upper palatal cusps are reduced and the lingual inclines of the lower buccal cusps are saved (Fig. 13.4).
4. The process of marking and grinding is repeated until there is even bilateral contact for both right and left lateral movements.
5. The anterior contact occurs, the lingual surface of the maxillary anterior teeth and labioincisal surface of mandibular anterior are reduced. The lateral wings should be lowered as far as possible without much grinding of teeth. The incisal guide pin must stay on the incisal guide table during lateral movements.

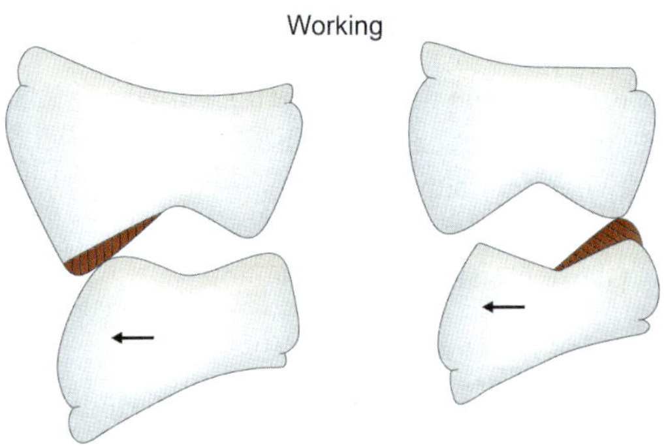

Fig. 13.3: Selective grinding for working side occlusion

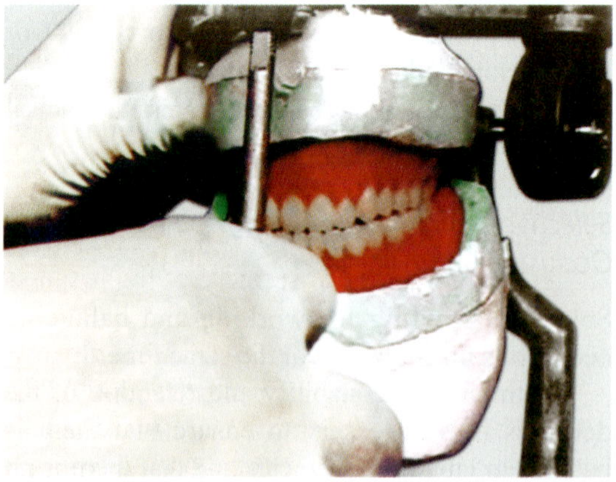
Fig. 13.2: Checking and occlusal correction errors in lateral balance (working side)

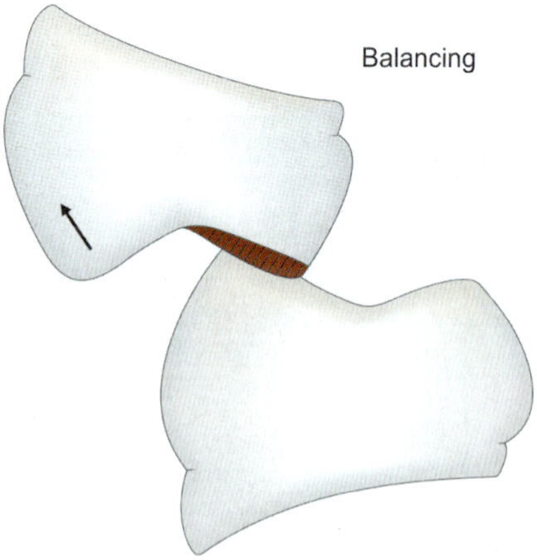

Fig. 13.4: Selective grinding for balancing side occlusion

Selective Grinding for Protrusive Balance

Protrusive balance is least important in denture occlusion. It is desirable but not so important to sacrifice esthetics.

1. The red articulating paper is placed between the teeth bilaterally and the articulator is moved anteriorly in edge-to-edge position (Fig. 13.5).
2. The blue articulating paper is placed between the teeth in centric relation contacts.
3. The premature contacts are identified and removed by grinding according rules:
   a. If teeth contact anteriorly only and not posteriorly, the lingual surface of the upper incisal edges of anterior teeth and the labial surface of the incisal edges of lower anterior teeth are reduced.
   b. If the teeth contact posteriorly but not anteriorly, the distal inclines of upper buccal cusps and mesial inclines of the lower buccal cusps are reduced.

Evaluation of Occlusal Adjustment

After the occlusal adjustment is over it should be checked observing the following points:

1. Maximum tooth contacts bilaterally in centric and eccentric positions.
2. No contact of anterior tooth in centric closure.

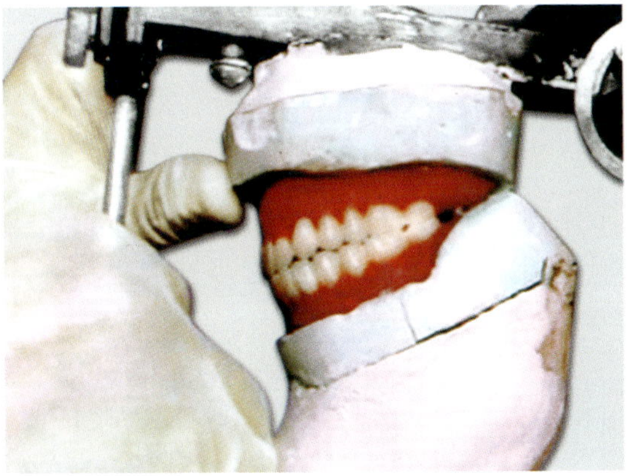

Fig. 13.5: Checking and correction of occlusal errors in protrusive balance

3. Incisal pin remains in contact with incisal table during its movements.
4. Light contact between posterior teeth during protrusive movement.
5. Tooth contact when incisal pin moves 2 mm on incisal table.
6. The occlusion is fully balanced during the movements of the articulator.

Correction of Occlusal Errors in Nonanatomical Teeth

After the centric relation mounting of the lower cast has been proved to be correct, the occlusal grinding should be done in the laboratory. This is done as follows:

1. The flat occlusal table of the mandibular denture is grounded by gently rubbing the occlusal surfaces and incisal edges over flat sandpaper block. This is done as the mandibular teeth are arranged to a flat plane and the maxillary anterior teeth may be set slightly below the occlusal plane for esthetic reasons.
2. The dentures are placed on the articulator and a 10 cm square articulating paper is placed between the teeth, and tapped together gently several times.
3. The premature contacts of the denture bases between the tuberosities and retromolar pads are removed by grinding.
4. The premature contacts of the maxillary teeth are removed with a large diameter wheel instead of a small diameter bur as it will removes the contacts between two flat occlusal surfaces of teeth.
5. All the anterior contacts are removed by grinding the lingual surfaces of the maxillary teeth.
6. The gross lateral interferences are removed without sacrificing the esthetics although no horizontal condylar inclination are usually determined (condylar guidance set parallel to the occlusal plane and incisal guidance at or near zero) when using cuspless teeth and monoplane occlusion.

The removal of wrong surfaces may cause reduction of vertical dimension and loss of balance surfaces. All the marks are washed away and removed with gauze moistened with alcohol.

Providing Smooth Articulation

All the ground tooth surfaces should be smoothened with a brush wheel applying wet pumice. This will remove any uneven contact along the paths between the centric and eccentric position. In case of porcelain teeth silicon carbide paste No. 150 is applied on the lower posterior teeth and lateral and protrusive movements are performed to produce smoothness.

Milling: It is a process of removing the irregularities of grinding with a slight abrasive paste.

Polishing: The surfaces of teeth is then polished using rubber wheels, with pumice.

CONCLUSION

The fabrication of complete dentures with anatomic teeth and balanced occlusion are technically difficult to construct than dentures with nonanatomic teeth and monoplane occlusion. Moreover, due to precise cusp fossa relations dentures with cusp teeth and balanced occlusion patient requires frequent recall visit to the practitioner. So, they should be informed before the treatment is started.

BIBLIOGRAPHY

1. Beck HO. Occlusion as related to complete removable prosthodontics. J Prosthet Dent. 1972;27:246.
2. Glossary of prosthodontic terms (6th edn). J Prosthet Dent. 1994;71:41-112.
3. Lang BR, Kelsey CC (Eds). International Prosthodontic Workshop on Complete Denture Occlusion. Ann Arbor; MI; University of Michigan, School of Dentistry; 1973.

Chapter 14

Delivery and Adjustments of Complete Dentures

The insertion of complete dentures needs only a little time if all previous steps in the fabrication of the new dentures have been done with attention. Of course, the dentist must verify that the dentures are acceptable and the patient is educated properly in care and use. Ideally the patient should be instructed to remove the previous denture out of mouth for 12 to 24 hours immediately before the insertion of new denture. Many patients will not accept these and in that case the existing dentures should be relined with a tissue treatment material or tissue conditioner to minimize tissue distortion problems. It is advisable to have an attitude that errors exist in every principle steps of denture fabrication that results in errors in every parts of the denture. During the delivery of the new dentures the old dentures should be retained by the dentist until the patient has adjusted to the new ones. If it is not followed, patient may continued to use the old dentures or may attempt to use one old and one new denture together. The patient should learn how to speak, eat and smile with their new dentures. The experienced old denture wearers even need to know that new dentures will feel different from the old ones.

OBJECTIVES

The routine of complete denture service includes the following objectives:

1. To locate and relief of pressure areas in the denture bases.
2. To identify and correction of overextended or sharp and square shaped borders.
3. To test the retention of dentures.
4. To check the accuracy of the jaw relations and adjustment of occlusion when required.
5. To give instructions to the patient on the proper use and care of dentures and its supporting structures.
6. To advice on the limitations of artificial denture.

INSTRUMENTS AND MATERIALS (FIG. 14.1)

1. Completed dentures
2. Denture bowl containing cold water
3. Mouthwash glass
4. Pear-shaped carbide cutter
5. Laboratory handpiece
6. Articulating paper
7. Modeling wax or silicone material
8. Vernier caliper or ruler
9. Patient history form
10. Glass slab

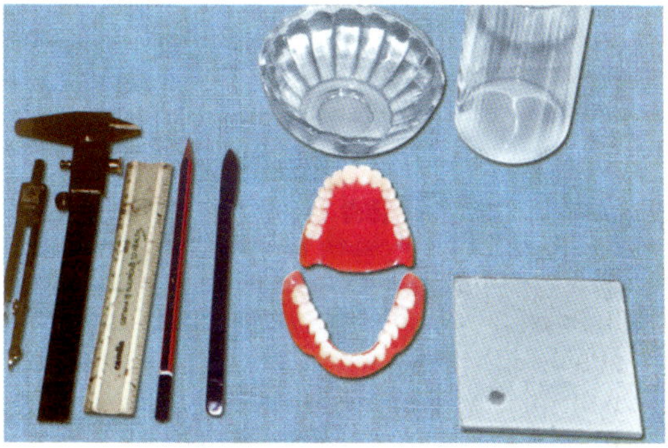

Fig. 14.1: Instruments and materials

11. Mouth mirror and napkin
12. Wax knife
13. Medium grit sand paper
14. Indelible pencil

Steps of Insertion of Complete Dentures

Insertion of complete dentures consists of the following steps:

1. Delivery of the dentures: The insertion appointment
2. Postinsertion adjustments.

PREPARATION FOR INSERTION

The processed dentures are recovered from flasks but not separated from their casts immediately but are first remounted on the articulator using the index that have been preserved for this purpose.

1. *Restoring the vertical dimension*: Usually the processed denture shows an increase in vertical dimension of slight to moderate degrees. This is due to dimensional changes of the denture base material as well as previously undetected clinical and laboratory errors. These occlusal discrepancies are eliminated when the dentures are prepared for insertion. The split cast techniques is utilized to return a denture to its original mounting to restore the original vertical dimension of occlusion. This eliminate the occlusal error to some extent but fails to remove the dimensional changes in the denture base which occurs when the denture is removed from the cast for polishing and finishing. That is why apart from the laboratory procedures, occlusal adjustment is usually required during delivery of the dentures to the patient.
2. *Construction of the mounting casts*: Undercuts are blocked out with wet asbestos, or coarse pumice or plasticine and cast are poured using quick-setting plaster. The maxillary denture on the cast is seated in the remounting index and attached to the upper member of the articulator with plaster. The dentures are then removed from the mounting casts cleaned off.
3. *Preservation of facebow record*: The facebow record is preserved after final wax-up so that there is no need for making a new orientation relation record at the time of insertion. This is done by attaching a remounting jig to the lower member of the articulator. A quick setting impression plaster is placed on the jig and a mounting index of the occlusal surfaces of the maxillary teeth obtained. The jig is removed from the articulator after the plaster set and maintained for future use. The dentures may now be removed from the casts for finishing. and polishing.

An occlusal index should be made after the final wax-up so that the maxillary denture can be related to the opening and closing axis of the articulator. The maxillary denture is repositioned into the remounting cast. The occlusal surfaces of the teeth placed on the occlusal index. The maxillary denture on cast should be remounted on the articulator in the same position.

INSERTION PROCEDURE

Inspection of Dentures

After completion and when awaiting fitting, the dentures should be stored in cold water.

The dentist has the ultimate responsibility for the quality of the dentures. The dentures should be examined under strong light for defects such as checked or damaged teeth, cracks in the base, sign of repair, and porosity or other signs of poor processing. The dentures should be examined before insertion as follows:

1. *Fitting surfaces*: The fitting surface of the dentures is first examined under a magnifying glass, to verify nodules or spiny fins resulting from air bubbles or irregularities of the cast. Failure to inspect a denture carefully results in overlooking a small irregularity produce serious problems for the patient and needlessly requires time for denture adjustment. The surface roughness arises in various ways and steps should be always taken to obtain a smooth surface. The complete dentures may

have sharp nodules of acrylic resin on the fitting surfaces. These defects arise from cut and scratches on the cast; arise from damage by knife when setting up the teeth. A rough surface over the entire fitting surface of a denture arises from bubbles present just below the superficial surface of cast which break under the pressures of flasking and packing acrylic resin dough. These numerous small elevations on the denture surface may hardly be visible to the naked eye but can be felt with a finger drawn across the surface. The large nodules can be removed by a sharp knife, while the numerous tiny projections are best treated by lightly holding the denture surface against a pear-shaped carbide cutter running in slow speed. The sharp edges also if present require to be removed by grinding. Such edges are found on the border of a relief area, deep rugae, at the midline of a steep palatal vault, and in mucosal flaps of anterior sulcus of upper denture. In the lower denture a sharp edge is found in the anterior lingual undercut area. All sharp edges should be rounded of by grinding. Sharp edges on the fitting surface of a denture cause small mucosal ulceration during functional movement. Such ulcers become infected to form chronic inflammation causes denture sore mouth.

The stops of impression trays sometimes produce high pressure areas. These areas must be removed before insertion.

2. *Denture periphery*: Denture borders are carefully examined outside the mouth. The denture border should reproduce the borders of the final impression as recorded in the master-cast. The operator secures an impression of the sulcus in the functional form with border moulding technique with much difficulty. It is, therefore, essential to preserve the denture periphery which should not be reduced by the technician to produce a pleasing symmetrical shaped periphery. The borders are reduced to their original functional height and width by removing excess flash material. The entire periphery especially the frenal notches should be rounded and properly extended. It should be only lightly polished otherwise there is a danger of destroying the peripheral seal. The posterior edges of the maxillary denture should be thinned to a knife edge. The edges of all relief areas should be rounded and not left square or sharp.

   Labial and buccal frenal attachments areas should be enlarged to provide freedom of their functional movements. When doing these, the labial frenum will be relieved in a vertical direction in sagittal plane and the buccal frenums are relieved in an oblique anteroposterior direction.
3. *Polished surface*: The polished surface should be evaluated by inspection of the denture contour and polish. The polished palatal, lingual, and buccal surfaces are inspected for irregularities. The polished surfaces should be developed in convex fashion. This form is utilized most effectively the retentive action of facial musculatures. The labial and buccal areas of lower denture facing in relation to the anterior and premolar region are usually thinned down. The polished surface should always be absolutely smooth and very highly polished. Any slight rough areas attracts attention of tongue may cause a mild glossitis. The rough surface may produce a unhygienic denture due to accumulation of plaques and calculus on denture surface. These rough areas should be removed with stones and burs and adequate finishing and polishing done.

   The finish of the gingival margin area is very important. This is a potential stagnant area and a high degree of surface finish must always be present here. There are two forms of finishing the gingival margin in the upper anterior region are possible. The first is the contoured finish for esthetic reason in case with good oral hygiene with a free flow of thin or medium saliva. The rolled effect of natural gingival margin is reproduced here. The second type is smooth-cut gingival shape, which is more self-cleansing and require less skill than contoured form. It is indicated where the oral hygiene is poor or there is a thick mucoid saliva causing accumulation of plaque in the gingival crevices.

Test for Retention of Dentures

The dentures are tested for retention as follows:

1. *Maxillary denture*: The denture should be seated in the mouth with firm upward and backward pressure and the patient allowed keeping them for a few minutes before any checking is done.

   The buccal surface is gripped between thumb and fore finger in the premolar region and a downward pull is applied and resistance is assessed.

   The denture is reseated if required. The forefinger is placed on the palate behind the upper anterior teeth and a forward leverage is applied to dislodge the posterior border of the denture. The resistance to this force is assessed.
2. *Mandibular denture*: The retention of the mandibular denture is checked by applying an upward and backward pull with a probe inserted in between the lower incisors. If the retention is poor the base must be corrected.

Checking the Centric Relation (Fig. 14.2)

The patient is asked to close the jaws in centric relation and the manner the opposing teeth comes in occlusion is noted. Irrespective of presence or absence of an error it is always necessary to record the centric relation by cheek-bite because displacement of the soft tissue and movement of the denture base may mask the error from being seen. It is for the same reason it is not possible to detect the occlusal errors by using articulating paper in the mouth.

So, the error of centric relation should be recorded making 'check-bite' or check record and adjustment is carried out on an articulator.

CHECK RECORD

1. Silicon, impression material is mixed and placed on the posterior teeth of the lower denture on each side (Fig. 14.3).
2. With upper denture in mouth, the lower denture is placed in mouth and the patient is instructed to close in centric relation without penetrating the silicon material.
3. The lower denture together with the bile record is worked and dried.
4. The bile record is reinserted in the mouth to verify the jaw relationship.
5. When a repeated record has been obtained this is used to remount the mandibular denture on the articulator by remounting the lower cast (Fig. 14.4).
6. The detection of error and its correction is done in laboratory (See Chapter 13, Correction of Occlusal Discrepancies).
7. After the occlusion is adjusted the dentures are reinserted in the patient mouth.

Instructions to Patient

Instructing the patient in the use and care of complete dentures is an essential but often neglected phase of treatment.

The primary objectives, at the time of complete denture insertion are:

1. The limitations of dentures should be stressed, that the maximum occlusal load which may be

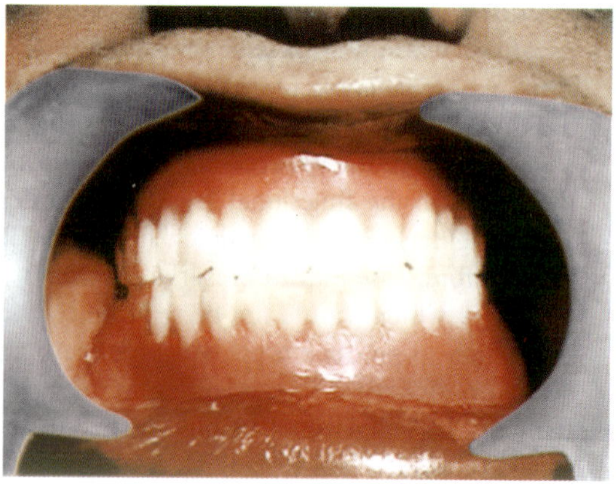

Fig. 14.2: Denture in centric relation

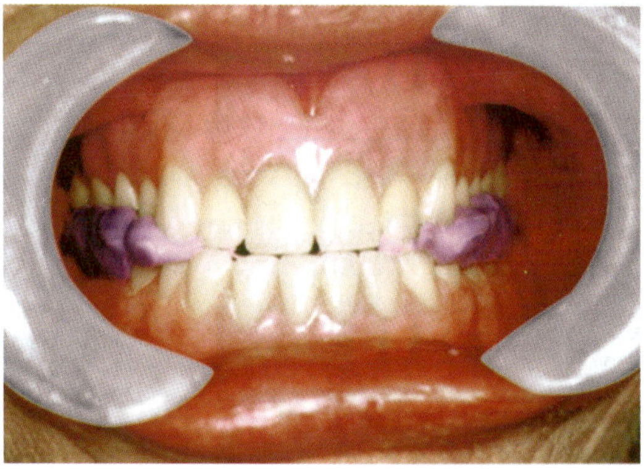

Fig. 14.3: Check-bite record with silicon material

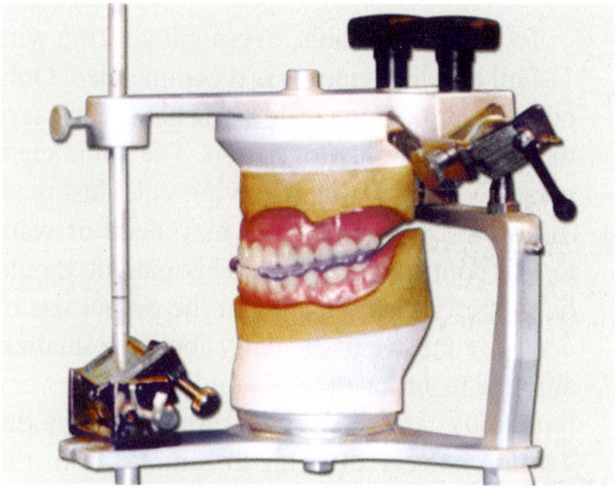

Fig. 14.4: Mandibular denture remounted on articulator cast

developed in one-tenth of that possible with natural teeth.

2. In early stage it is wise to limit to food which require less mastication. They should cut up their food in small pieces and chew them in both side.
3. The dentures must be regularly checked and refitted or replaced time to time as the existing ridges continue to resorb a little.

Instruction should be provided to the patient verbally and also in form of informatory booklet on what to expect with the new dentures and how to care for them. It should be explained that the patient might experience an increase in saliva flow due to body's reaction to foreign body in the mouth. This increase is only temporary and become normal within a week or two. The younger the patient more readily the adaptation in this abnormal situation. Patient from 20 to 30 years of age may learn dentures in 10 days, whereas those from 30 to 40 years of age may learn in three weeks, and those from 40 to 50 years of age may require 2 to 3 months.

Education of the patient should begin with the initial interview and should continue throughout the complete denture service. The patient should be explained about his responsibility in complete denture service so that he should not considers the dentist to be solely responsible for the success or failure of the dentures. The use of visual aids to understand his oral problem is helpful for both, the patient as well as the dentist. The dentist has the professional obligation to instruct the patient in the following items:

- *Talking*: The problem of phonetics is not too difficult because of adaptability of patients to dentures. The position of the teeth in relation to the denture base and the retention can vary from patient-to-patient yet not cause serious speech problem. Patients are told to speak calmly and avoid excessive movement in speech. Speech may be altered for a time particularly the production of 'S' sounds. The tongue gradually adapts to changes and the patient mast speech with new dentures within a few weeks. The practice is required to speak normally with new dentures. The patient should read aloud from a book or the newspaper to practice with the new dentures

  The speech problems usually arise from faulty setting of teeth and that should be corrected by phonetic tests in trial stage.
- *Eating*: The patient should start eating with soft and crisp foods and taking small bites. They should cut their food into small pieces and chew on both sides of their mouth carefully and slowly before swallowing. The first meals will take longer than usual and slow learning to eat is required. The dentures will tend to move

at first, but will become firm after a few days. Patients should maintain good nutrition and balanced diet for healthy body and gums which support the dentures.

- *Night wear*: Patients are counseled not to wear the dentures at night. They are also advised not to clench their teeth which produce excessive pressure on the underlying mucosa. The dentures should be stored in a glass of cold water during night and never letting them complete dry. Patient without habit of bruxism may wear their dentures at night if it is not possible to sleep without the dentures. These patients should be advised to remove the dentures for several hours every day to allow the supporting tissues to recover.
- *Cleaning*: A denture should be kept clean in order to avoid mouth odors and for attractive looking. The dentures should be taken out after meal and cleaned with a denture brush and soap or cleaner and water. Dentifrice should be avoided as they contains abrasives. It will cause wear of acrylic resin over time. If this fails to keep them clean the use of an effervescent denture cleaning power or solution is recommended. Commercial cleaners can be used and leaving the dentures overnight followed by brushing to remove plaques is usual. The dentures should be cleaned over half fill basin with water, this may prevent them breaking if dropped. The dentures should not be put in hot water or antiseptic solutions. If the patient has the calculus and cigarette and coffee stains or had *Candida* infection a solution of one part chlorine bleach to nine parts water is ideal for disinfecting the dentures. Undiluted bleach should be avoided as it may cause harm to the mucosa if not properly ringed. Dipping in bleach for prolonged time may cause the denture base to lose its color.

  The gentle brushing should be done with a soft rounded bristle toothbrush. It should follow by vigorous rinsing of oral cavity with water or mouthwash will help in maintaining oral hygiene and refreshing (Fig. 14.5).

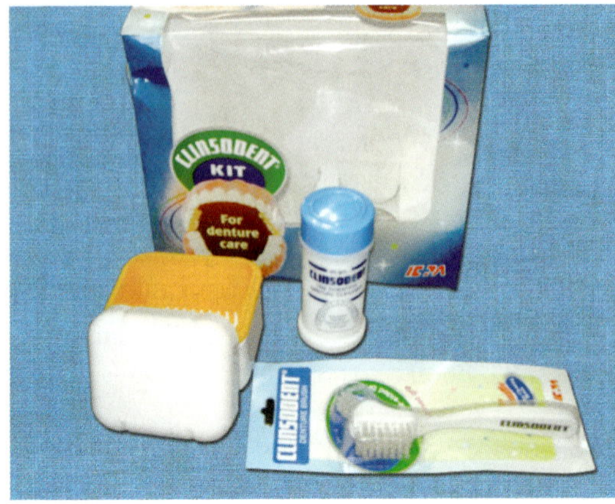

Fig. 14.5: Denture cleansing kit

  To remove calculus, overnight soaking with 114 ml of white vinegar is recommended. Only occasional soaking in white vinegar is necessary to control calculus formation. The sonic cleaners are effective in removing calculus.
- *Adhesives*: Some patients may need or want to use denture adhesives. This patient should be properly instructed about the proper use of denture adhesive particularly about the smallest amount to be used. Some adhesive are very tenacious, and complete removal from the denture is very difficult to remove from the mouth as well as from the denture and causes growth of harmful microorganism.

The following written instructions/suggestions are very helpful to patient during post-insertion period:

1. New dentures—mainly lower denture will feel strange and feeling of fullness of lips and cheeks.
2. Attempts should be made to rest the tongue forward so that the tongue rest on the inside (lingual) surfaces of the lower anterior teeth.
3. There may be excessive salivary secretion for the first few days.
4. Patients should make up his/her mind to master wearing of new dentures and to accept the new dentures in the mouth more than they are out of the mouth.
5. Difficulties to become accustomed with the new dentures are graded as follows:

First time denture wearers > Irregularly denture wearers > Regularly denture wearer

6. Spanning normally with dentures require several wears practice by various ways like speaking loudly in front of mirror, etc.
7. Learning of chewing normally requires 6–8 weeks minimum. Initially only chewing of soft nonsticky food cut into small pieces on both sides of the denture at the same time should be practiced. Front teeth should never be used for chewing.
8. Development of soreness in the mouth due to denture wearing is not uncommon and regular denture adjustment by operator according to the location of sore spots is essential.
9. Regular denture adjustment at various sites of the denture will be necessary. When the adjustment period has been completed there will be a charged (after 90 days) for future recall appointments.
10. Denture should be thoroughly brushed with soft toothbrushes and less abrasive agents at least twice daily and should be placed overnight in commercial denture cleansers once or twice weekly. Dentures never should be boiled or cleaned with hot water.
11. When cleaned the denture must be held over a water filled basin or wet washcloth to minimize chances of breaking of denture due to slipping from hands.
12. If at all possible leave your dentures out at night to give the tissues time to renew and refresh themselves. If it is not convenient the dentures must be kept out of mouth for some time during the day to rest your oral tissues and should be kept in water filled container covered with a lid. When not wearing them because dimensional change occur on drugging.
13. Periodic recall visits at least once yearly and regular medical checkups are essentially recommended.

Postinsertion Adjustment of Dentures

All new denture patients must be evaluated 24 hours of denture wearing because most tissue irritation will occur within the first 24 hours. The quick elimination of the cause of irritation will make the patient more comfortable and help him to adjust more rapidly to his dentures.

The second adjustment appointment should be 48 hours after the first adjustment and the third, 48 hours of the second adjustment or when problem arises. Some patients require two adjustments but some require many adjustment appointments. The sequence of clinical procedures for a 24 hours recall is as follows:

1. *Examination*: Thorough examination of the oral tissues are required for sore spot within the denture-bearing area or on the periphery. The area or on the periphery. The area is usually visible as an area of redness. If the injury is severe there will be ulceration. Tissues are dried with 2 × 2 inch gauze for inspection. The sore area is marked with indelible pencil wetting its tip. They dry denture is inserted in the mouth to transfer the marking to the denture. The denture is removed from the mouth examined to evaluate the sore areas. The sore areas are usually either due to (a) excessive displacement of the border tissues or (b) excessive pressure on the underlying mucosa beneath the denture base. The former is due to overextension of the denture borders and latter is produced due to occlusal error. Occlusal error is the main reason for soreness under the denture base so it should be corrected first by means of the check record procedure before adjusting the sore spots in basal seat area using pressure indicating paste.
2. *Detection of localized pressure areas in the denture base and adjustment*:
   i. The denture is dried. Using a disposable brush with course bristle a thin coat of

pressure indicating paste is painted over the whole fitting surface of the denture with the brush marking running in the same direction. The pressure relief paste is used to identify of areas of tissue displacement of the denture-bearing tissues. This is because the impression material used for denture construction does not differentiate between the different degrees of displacement in the denture supporting mucosa, e.g. thin soft tissue in the midline of the palate requires relief. All complete denture patients need a 12 month check up.

Each of the dentures is placed on the supporting tissue and firm pressure is applied on the occlusal surfaces of the teeth. The fitting surface is inspected for the disturbance of brush marks which indicates an area requiring adjustment. The denture base in the area is trimmed and a new application of paste is made and the dentures are placed in the mouth for testing.

ii. The recording and adjustment procedure is repeated until the paste exhibits a uniform pattern of contact when denture is seated with firm, even finger pressure.

3. *Detection of pressure areas in the denture border and adjustment*:
   i. The sore areas are located first.
   ii. A thin role of disclosing wax is adapted to the specific area of denture border. The denture is dipped in warm water and seated in the mouth carefully to avoid wiping off the wax. After the dentures are kept in the mouth and the patient is asked to swallow or border moulding movements are performed to determine the area of overextension.
   iii. The denture is removed and the base show through the wax is trimmed. The areas adjusted should be repolished with silicon wheel. The patient may still feel discomfort because the area remains irritated from sore. Usually there is some relief if the sore area is identified correctly and relief provided.

Table 14.1 Pain

Complaint	Causes	Remedy
a. Pain at periphery of the denture	Overextended periphery	Checking with disclosing wax, reduce and polish
b. Pain on residual ridge or palate	a. Faulty occlusion	a. Remounting and occlusal adjustment
	b. Bony spicules	b. Remove surgically
	c. Defect in impression or cast	c. Locating using pressure indicating paste and relieve
	d. Knife edge ridge	d. Relieve
	e. Pressure in mylohyoid ridge, mid-palatine raphe	e. Relieve
c. Pain on other areas	a. Check biting	a. Increase buccal overlap by rounding mandibular buccal cusps
	b. Pressure in retromylohyoid curtain due to overextension	b. Relieve
	c. Pain in temporomandibular joint due to incorrect vertical dimension of occlusion	c. Reset teeth at correct vertical dimension
d. Pain generalized over the ridge	Increased vertical dimension of occlusion	Reset teeth at correct vertical dimension

iv. The procedure is repeated until the base does not show through the wax.

Subsequent Adjustments

The second and third adjustments are similarly performed if required. If the patient complains of pain on lower ridge without localized sore spot the occlusal vertical dimension may be too much and must be corrected by taking a centric check record and mounting the dentures on an articulator and by selective grinding, or resetting the teeth and processing.

COMPLAINS OF DENTURES

It is impossible to discuss every complaint made by complete denture patients, but following are most common and will give a comprehensive outline to diagnose their causes and treatment.

1. Pain (Table 14.1)
2. Poor retention (Table 14.2)
3. Gagging (Table 14.3)
4. Chattering of teeth (Table 14.4)
5. Altered speech (Table 14.5)
6. Poor esthetics (Table 14.6).

Table 14.2 Loss of retention

Complaint	Causes	Remedy
a. Both the dentures all time	a. Overextension	Adjust periphery and polish
	b. Underextension	Border moulding with green stick compound and acrylic added.
	c. Ineffective post-palatal seal	Restored with green stick compound and acrylic added.
	d. Faulty occlusion	Remounting and occlusal adjustment
	e. Xerostomia	Sugar free lozenges to stimulate salivation or use artificial saliva
	f. Cramped tongue	Increase vertical dimension of occlsion
	g. Retruded tongue	Place a bleb on lower lingual flange to train patient
b. Maxillary denture on yawning	Excessive thickness of distobuccal flange	Reduce the denture and polish
c. Both dentures during eating	Unstable occlusion	Remounting and occlusal adjustment

Table 14.3 Gagging

Complaint	Causes	Remedy
a. On insertion	Lack of tissue adaptation	Reline
b. During the day	Cramped tongue	Increase VDO
c. While eating	Faulty occlusion	Remounting and occlusal adjustment

Table 14.4 Clicking of denture

Complaint	Causes	Remedy
Clicking	Excessive vertical dimension of occlusion	Reduce VDO
	Cramped tongue	Reset the teeth
	Overextension	Adjust denture border
	Underextension	Rebordering

Table 14.5 Inadequate speech

Complaint	Causes	Remedy
Inadequate speech	Faulty tooth arrangement	Reset the teeth
	Faulty palatal contours	Reduce thickness

Table 14.6 Poor esthetics

Complaint	Causes	Remedy
a. Denture teeth un-natural	a. Too dark	Mixing shades
	b. Too light	Reset teeth
	c. Too much or too little tooth visibility	
b. Denture base un-natural	a. Too thick	Reduce bulk
	b. Un-natural color	Use characterized denture base material
	c. Un-natural contour	Duplicate natural contour
c. Nose and chin approximation	VDO decreased	Remake with proper VDO

CONCLUSION

Tissues changes continuously and the rate of changes are depended on local and general conditions. A well fitted denture become ill fitting with time and can damage the oral tissues without the knowledge of patient. So, all edentulous patient wearing dentures should be examined by the dentist at least yearly. A list of patient should be maintained by the dentist for a recall visit for that purpose.

BIBLIOGRAPHY

1. Kouats JT. Clinical evaluation of the gogging denture patient. JDP. 1971;25:613.
2. Kubker. Denture problems. Quint Int. 1984;15:1035.
3. Lawson NA. Information and Advice for Denture Wearing. Dent Rec. 1965;15:402.
4. Murrel GA. The management of difficult lower dentures. JPD. 1974;32:243.
5. Nagle RJ. Postinsertion problem in complete denture prosthesis. JADA. 1958;57;187.
6. Robinson HBG. Diagnosis of lesions associated with dentures. JPD. 1957;7:338.
7. Sharry JJ. Denture failures related to occlusion. Dent Clin N Amer. 1972;16:119.
8. Silverman MM. The hustle and swish sound in denture patients. JPD. 1967;17:144.
9. Welker WA. Prosthodontic treatment of abused oral tissues. JPD. 1977;37:259.
10. Woods V. Management of post-insertion problems. Dent Clin N Amer. 1964. p. 742.

Chapter 15

Sequelae of Wearing Complete Dentures

EFFECTS OF COMPLETE DENTURES ON ORAL TISSUES

The wearing of complete denture may have some adverse effects on the oral environment particularly to the denture-bearing tissues. These effects can be divided into two types of sequelae:

a. Direct
b. Indirect.

Direct Sequelae

1. **Residual ridge reduction.**
2. **Mucosal reactions:**
   a. *Denture stomatitis:* The pathological reactions of the denture-bearing palatal mucosa.
   b. Angular cheilitis.
3. **Soft tissue hyperplasia:**
   a. *Flabby ridges*: It is mobile and extremely resilience alveolar ridge due to replacement of bone by fibrous tissue. It is often seen in long-term denture wearers due to residual ridge resorption. It has been observed in 24% of edentulous maxilla and 5% of edentulous mandible and most frequently in anterior region. It is seen most commonly in the anterior part of the maxilla, when anterior teeth remain in the mandible causing excessive loading.
   Treatment: Surgical removal is the common mode of treatment.
   b. Denture irritation hyperplasia.
   c. *Traumatic ulcers*: The small painful ulcers or sore spots commonly develop within 1 to 2 days after placement of dentures due to overextended borders or deflective occlusal contacts.
   d. A sequelae of wearing ill-fitting dentures causing tissue hyperplasia in denture border due to chronic injury by unstable dentures, thin or overextended borders.
   e. *Oral cancer*: It may develop in wearing ill-fitting dentures in alcoholic or tobacco use with uneducated and low socioeconomic groups of people.
4. **Burning mouth syndrome:** It is a burning sensation in one or several oral structures in contact with the denture with a feeling of dry mouth. It may be due to instability in denture, Vitamin deficiencies, and iron deficiency anemia, xerostomia induced by radiation or drugs or psychologic factors.
5. **Gagging:** It is triggered by tactile stimulation of the soft plate, the posterior part of tongue, and tonsils and psychologic factors.
6. **Altered taste perception.**

Indirect Sequelae

1. **Atrophy of masticatory muscles:** Atrophy of masseter and the medial pterygoid muscle occur in complete denture wearers particularly women with lessoning of bite forces progressively. The

reduced biting force and chewing efficiency is sequel of wearing complete dentures, resulting in impaired masticatory function. The placement of new denture will not cause improvement in masticatory efficiency. The old denture wearer gradually changes their food habit to softer food.

2. **Nutritional deficiencies:** In healthy adults there is no evidence that the nutritional intake is impaired in denture wearers of complete dentures so replacement of ill-fitting dentures with well-fitted new dentures will not improve the nutritional status. However, nutritional deficiencies occur, in patient with poor general health, poor absorption, intestinal, metabolic, and catabolic disturbances, anorexia and salivary gland hypofunction, or altered taste perception.
3. **Temporomandibular disorders:** Complete denture patients and patient with other types of dentition can be affected by temporomandibular disorders in a similar way. But as the severe signs and symptoms are rare there is relatively less number of complete denture wearer with temporomandibular disorders. Treatment with new complete dentures relieves the patient of signs and symptoms of the diseases.
4. **Masticatory ability:** A study shows that the great majority (70 to 85%) of edentulous patients was satisfied with the masticatory ability of their complete dentures. Older patients have been more satisfied with poorly fitting dentures and will not seek new denture. Measurements of masticatory force and ability to comminute a test food are drastically reduced in complete denture wearers in comparison to the people with natural teeth, as well as with implant supported dentures. Only 8% of totally edentulous patient would prepare to accept dental implants if available. The main reason for declining implant prosthesis was that they were satisfied with their present dentures.

RESIDUAL RIDGE REDUCTION (RRR)

Definition

Residual ridge reduction is a chronic, progressive, irreversible and cumulative disease.

Etiology

1. *Anatomic factors*
   a. Size and shape of ridge
   b. Type of bone
   c. Type of mucoperiosteum
   d. Ridge relation
2. *Metabolic factors*
   a. *Age*: The older the patient more the resorption of bone.
   b. *Sex*: The female at menopause are more prone to osteoporosis which increases bone resorption.
   c. *Hormonal balance*: Higher amount of parathyroid hormone causes more bone resorption.
   d. *Vitamins*: Deficiency of vitamin D can cause bone resorption deficiency of vitamin A and C affects bone growth.
3. *Mechanical factors*
   a. *Functional factors*: Cancellous bone can withstand compressive forces better than any other type of bone.
   b. *Prosthetic factors*: Form of teeth, arrangement of teeth, interocclusal distance.

Pathology

Longitudinal cephalometric studies by Atwood showed that there is continuous reduction of residual bone tissue after tooth extraction in complete denture wearers. It was considered by Atwood as "a major oral disease entity". It appears to be a process occurs in all patients. There is considerable individual variation in the rate of bone loss after tooth extraction and the wearing of complete dentures. The reduction of the residual ridge height is about 2 to 3 mm for the maxilla and

4 to 5 mm for the mandible during the first year of extraction. In mandible the annual reduction is 0.1 to 0.2 mm and it is four time less in the maxilla. The residual bone resorption may proceed throughout the lifetime of the denture wearer. The resorption is a consequence of bone remodeling due to altered functional stimulus on the jaw bone due to anatomic, metabolic, psychosocial and mechanical factors. The mechanical factors (masticatory or non-masticatory forces) transmitted by the denture or tongue to the residual ridge are assumed to be important factors in the remodeling process. However, the causes of the variations are not well understood. The pathogenesis of ridge resorption is also not known. It is assumed that ridge resorption results from combination of a number of factors, anatomical, metabolic psychological, and mechanical. Women are more affected than men. To provide simplified method for ridge resorption, a six order form has been described by Atwood (Fig. 15.1).

Treatment

Many prosthodontic and surgical treatments are performed in case of several residual ridge resorptions but without much success. The best treatment is preventive, i.e. avoiding total extraction, preservation teeth, and treatment with over dentures which cause much less bone resorption. In edentulous cases the placement of implants and the insertion of an implant-supported prosthesis reduce bone loss.

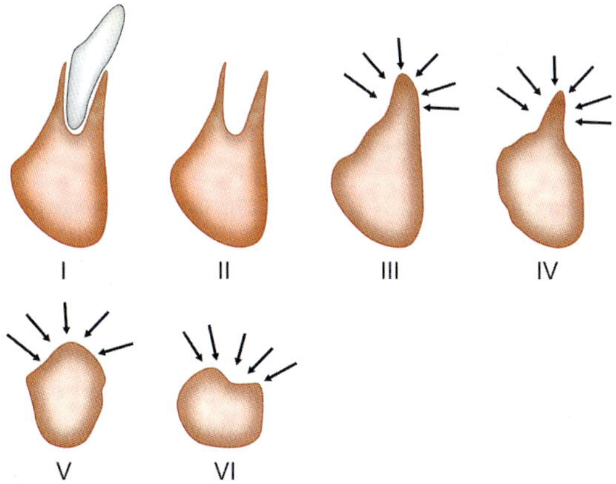

Fig. 15.1: Six orders of mandibular anterior residual ridge form (I) Preextraction; (II) Postextraction; (III) High, well-rounded; (IV) Knife edge; (V) Low, well-rounded; (VI) Depressed

DENTURE STOMATITIS

Etiology

1. Candida infection results in microbial plaque on the fitting surface of the denture.
2. Traumatic factors, e.g. mechanical, thermal, and chemical irritations.
3. Allergic reactions to denture base material.
4. Immunological disorders.

Treatment

The complete prevention of the causes by maintaining good oral hygiene, through cleaning of the dentures and increasing the period of rest of the denture bearing tissues combined with antifungal agents is the method of treatment.

ANGULAR CHEILITIS

Etiology

1. Candida infection.
2. Reduced vertical dimension of occlusion.
3. Nutritional deficiencies.
4. Immune dysfunction

FLABBY RIDGE

Etiology

It is most commonly seen in the anterior maxillary ridge when the natural mandibular anterior teeth are present.

BURNING MOUTH SYNDROME

The burning sensations of structures of mouth in contact with the dentures it occurs most frequently in tongue. It is more frequent in middle aged men and women.

Etiology

Local Factors

1. Mechanical irritation.
2. Tongue habits.
3. *Allergy:* True allergies to acrylic are rare. Allergy can be confirmed by a patch test on denture-bearing tissues or skin. If positive result is obtained the denture can be remade using another resin such as polystyrene, nylon, or polycarbonate, or cast chrome-cobalt. Free monomer present in incompletely cured denture may be the cause.
4. Pressure on nerve. A burning sensation in anterior part of palate may be due to excessive pressure from the denture on incisive papilla. Proper relief will cause immediate relief.
5. *Candida albicans* and bacterial infections.
6. Unstable dentures.
7. Smoking, tobacco chewing, mouth breathing, chronic alcoholism.
8. Intake of excessively seasoned foods.
9. Use of denture adhesives, cleansers, etc.
10. The patients with reduced tongue space, incorrect level of occlusal plane and increased vertical dimension of denture are more susceptible to BMS.

Systemic Factors

1. Vitamin deficiency anemia.
2. Menopause.
3. Xerostomia.
4. Systemic diseases.
5. Drugs.
6. Psychological and/or psychosocial disturbances like depression, anxiety.
7. Metabolic and circulatory disturbances, pernicious and iron deficiency anemia, gastrointestinal disorders, and hormonal imbalance.

Treatment

1. Optimization of deficient dentures.
2. If there is no denture deficiencies the psychological evaluation is essential in collaboration with psychologist.
3. An implant supported denture fabrication may be carried out along with psychotherapy.

GAGGING

It is a normal reflex to prevent foreign bodies from entering the trachea.

Etiology

1. The tactile stimulation of the soft palate, posterior part of tongue, and tonsil.
2. The sight, taste, noise, as well as psychological factors or combination of all these factors.
3. Persistent complaints of gagging may be due to overextended borders particularly at the posterior part.
4. The unstable occlusions or increased vertical dimension of occlusion may trigger gagging reflex.

Treatment

1. Correction of overextended dentures by proper trimming.
2. Correction of occlusal vertical dimension and occlusal prematurities.
3. Psychological: The patient who is wearers of old dentures, gagging may be due to some systemic diseases of the gastrointestinal tract, tonsil, and alcoholism.

CONTROL OF SEQUELAE OF WEARING COMPLETE DENTURES

The consequences of complete denture wearing are reduction of the residual ridges, and oral pathological changes. This results in discomfort, insufficient mastication and poor esthetic problems. The patient may be unable to wear the denture completely and will be leveled as prosthodontically maladaptive. These sequelae cannot be prevented but can be delayed as followed:

1. The treatment with complete denture by total removal of teeth should be avoided except in poor periodontal health. Instead partial denture should be planed. Some teeth or at least roots

should be preserved to act as a abutment for the over denture.

2. The complete denture patients should be placed on routine yearly recall and checkup plan so as to maintain the fit and occlusion.
3. The complete denture patients should be aware of benefit of implant-supported dentures.
4. The patient should be advice not to wear the dentures during the night.
5. The patient should be properly advised to clean and maintain the denture regularly and if necessary patient may be seen every three monthly intervals.

CONCLUSION

A complete denture use in the mouth invites various changes in oral tissues causing damage to them. It is important to inform the patient that the complete denture treatment is not a definitive treatment and requires regular check-up visits in preventing the long-term risks associated with the consequences of wearing complete dentures. This is required for prolong optimum use of the dentures.

BIBLIOGRAPHY

1. Atwood DA. A reduction of residual ridges a major disease entity. J Prosth Dent. 1972;26:266.
2. Gunnar E Carlsson. Clincal Morbidity and sequelae of treatment with complete dentures. J Prosth Dent. 1998;79:17.
3. Tallgren A. The continuing reduction of the residual alveolar ridges in complete denture wearer: A Mixed Longitudinal Study Covering 25 years. J Prosth Dent. 1972;27:120-32.

Chapter 16

Repair, Rebasing and Relining

REPAIR

Introduction

Aftercare of denture requires repair of a denture or repair of tooth of a denture. The cause of a fracture should be determined and failure to correct any underlying cause will result in repeated fracture.

Definition

It is the procedure by which the fractured parts of a denture are assembled and joined together using denture-base material of same type.

Cause of Fracture

1. *Intraoral causes*: Resorption of alveolar bone, causing denture rocking and fracture.
2. *Faulty construction*: These may be due to incorrect setting of teeth, inadequate polymerization time, denture base too thin or large labial frenum relief.
3. Accident of drop, during cleaning.

Treatment

1. Repair
2. Relining.

Materials

Broken acrylic resin complete denture can be repaired using heat curing or cold curing materials. The use of heat cured resin with flasking often results in dimensional change of the base material at the curing temperature. Nowadays self-curing resin is used to make fast, easy and very satisfactory repair. A broken tooth can be replaced with self-cure resin without flasking. A light cure resin may be used.

Types of Fracture

Simple

Single or several tooth facture or dislodgement.

Complex

Fracture of denture based in two or more pieces.

Techniques

Replacing Broken Teeth/Tooth

1. A reduction is made in the denture base material on lingual/palatal surface of the denture base where the tooth/teeth are broken or missing.
2. Tooth/teeth of correct mould and shade are placed or ground in position and held with sticky wax at the incisal edge. The denture may be articulated against opposing cast and teeth set up to ensure that no occlusal interferences occur.
3. Separating medium is applied to the labial surface and adjacent teeth, and an index is made of plaster or silicone putty.
4. The area of repair is moistened with cold-cure monomer with the help of a small glass dropper two or three times to make the area tacky.
5. The polymer is spread over the area from a small plastic bottle. This is followed by alternate

applications of monomer and polymer until the area is slightly over-filed. Always slight excess of monomer should be present there to assure complete polymerization.

6. A wet sheet of cellophane is placed on the acrylic and pressure is applied with the index for few minutes.
7. The denture is bench cured for about 20 minutes and polishing and finishing is done in the usual way (Figs 16.1A and B).

Repair of Midline Fractured Dentures

- Repair is not advisable if the fractured fragments cannot be accurately approximated. The technique for maxillary or mandibular denture is similar. The fracture parts are assembled together with sticky wax in correct position and the fragments are held together with one or more wooden match sticks to the occlusal surfaces of the teeth (Figs 16.2 and 16.3).
- The denture is tried in the mouth if possible for accuracy of reassembly. Any undercuts on fitting surface is blocked out with moist cotton wool and a plaster cast is poured into the denture and allowed to set.
- The pieces of denture are removed. The pieces are prepared by removing 3 mm of acrylic from the fracture line.
- A long rounded bevel (4–5 mm) is used to produce a bond of acceptable strength.
- Tin foil substitute is applied on cast to the area beneath the fracture. When dried the pieces are placed on the casts. The edges of the bevel are wetted with monomer. Monomer and polymer powder is placed in the areas of bevel incrementally.
- The plaster matrix is placed in position and held there for 10 minutes. It is allowed to stand for another 10 minutes for bench curing.
- In case of pressure curing unit is used to quicken curing and preventing porosity, the repair job is placed in the pressure unit and covered with water at 100° F. Compressed air is introduced

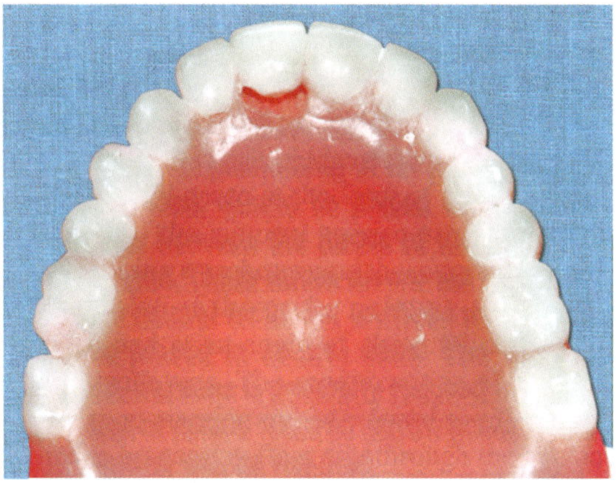

Fig. 16.1A: The acrylic is removed from the lingual side of the tooth and sticky wax maintain the new tooth in position when acrylic is added

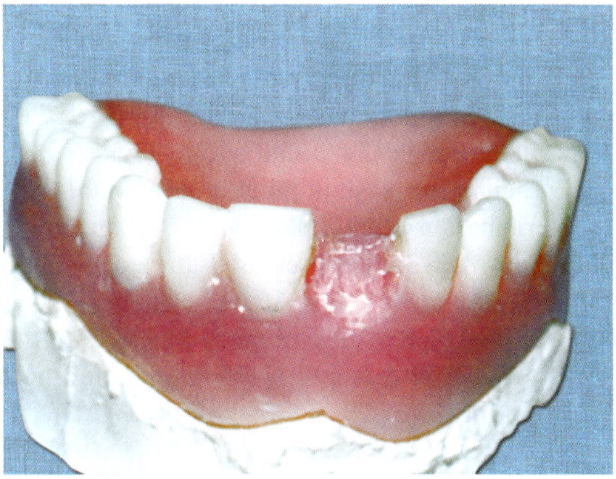

Fig. 16.1B: The buccal contour is not reduced

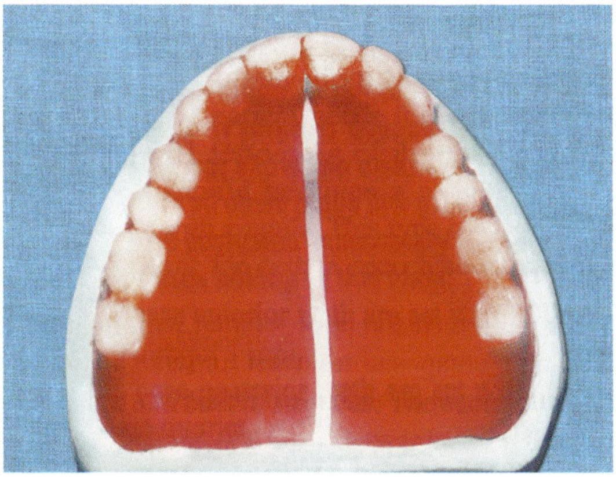

Fig. 16.2: Repair of midline fracture maxillary denture

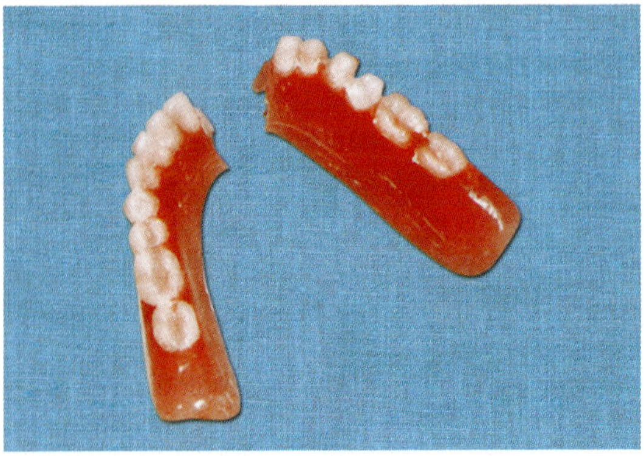

Fig. 16.3A: Fractures after occur at or near the midline of lower dentures

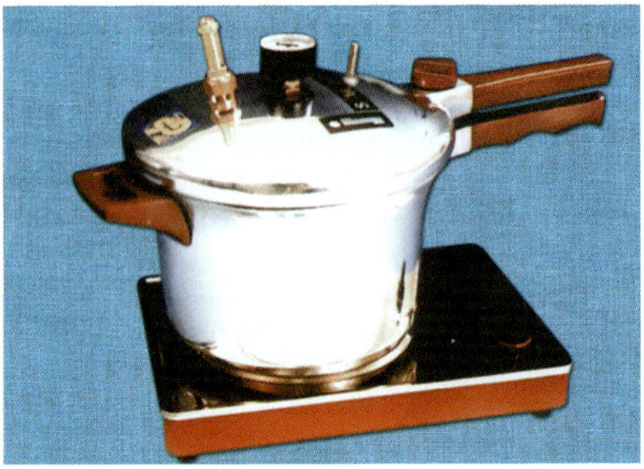

Fig. 16.4: The repaired denture placed in a pressure chamber at 20 to 30 lb of pressure for 30 minutes to prevent porosity

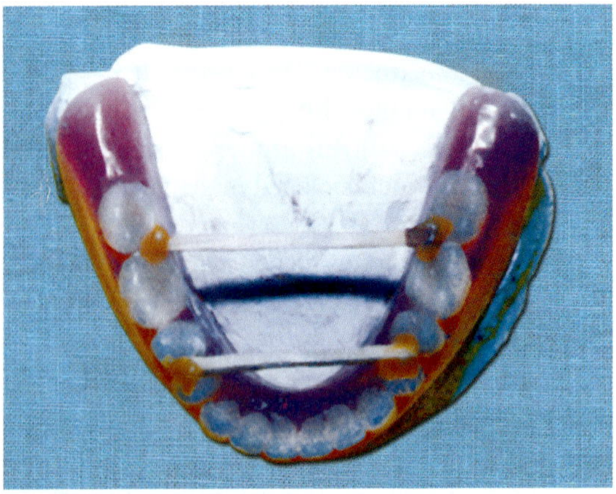

Fig. 16.3B: Repair of midline fracture mandibular denture. The fragments can be maintained in proper position by means of sticky wax and sticks. A cast is prepared

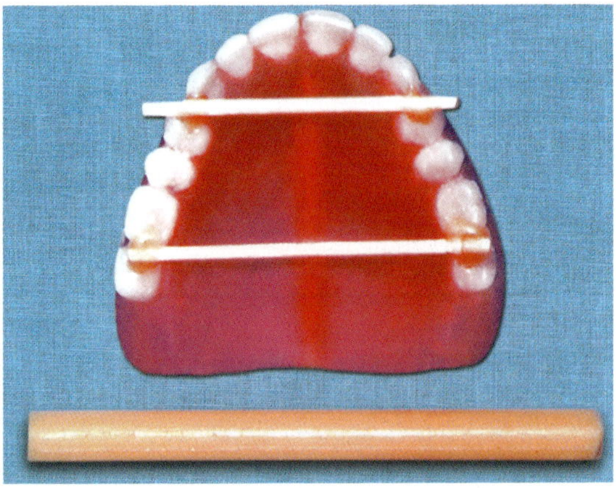

Fig. 16.5: A midline fracture of the upper denture held in proper relation by means of sticky wax and sticks

in curing unit at 30 lbs/sq for 10 minutes (Fig. 16.4).

- After curing the excess material is trimmed and polishing of denture is done.

Light-Cure Repair

Fiber reinforced composites along with light-cure flow able composite resin will provide a stronger and durable repair than resin repair.

1. First two fractured parts of the denture are rejoined with cyanoacrylate and stabilized with sticky wax and wooden sticks (Fig. 16.5).
2. Then stone cast is poured to maintain the orientation of two parts.
3. Gap of 2–3 mm is created and edges were beveled to 45° (Fig. 16.6).
4. Then space for fibers is made and the fracture site is prepared with monomer/bonding agent.

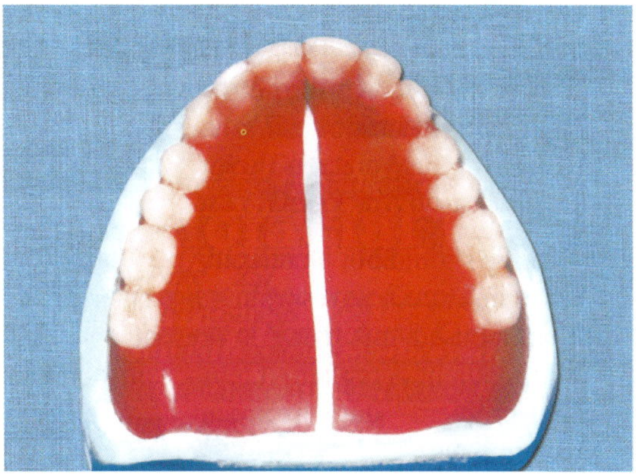

Fig. 16.6: The fracture line is enlarged with a No. 558 fissures bur and placed back on the cast for application of cold-cured acrylic resin

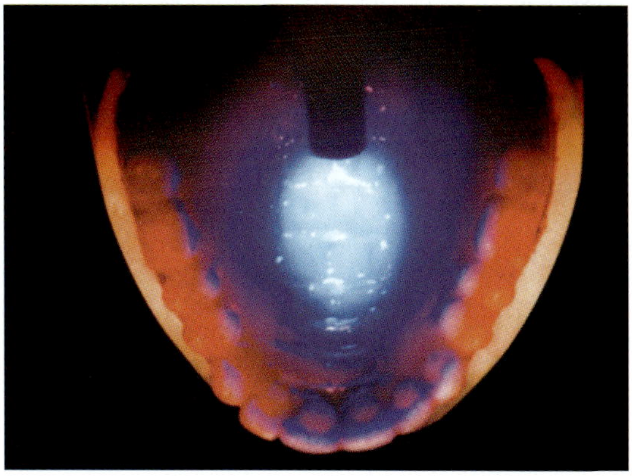

Fig. 16.8: FRC polymerized

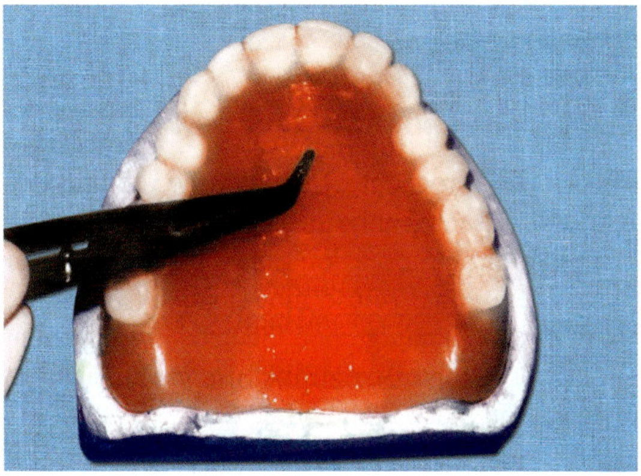

Fig. 16.7: FRC applied on fracture line

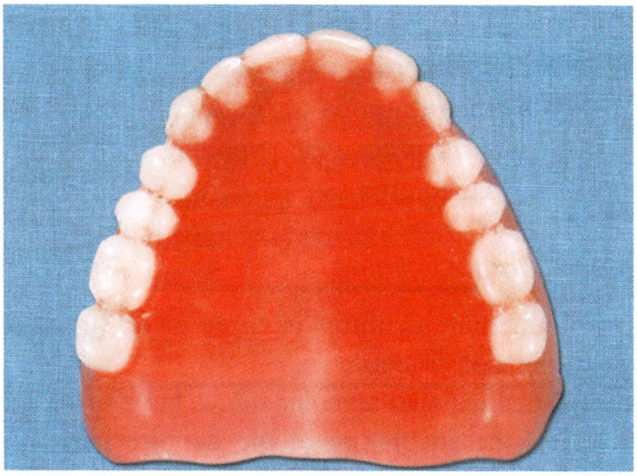

Fig. 16.9: The midline fracture of maxillary denture repaired with cold-cure acrylic resin

5. A thin layer of flow able composite resin was applied. It is not polymerized as it creates an adhesive surface that allows for the FRC to be tacked down.
6. Multiple strips of FRC are cut, tacked across the fracture site and light cured (Figs 16.7 and 16.8).
7. FRC repair is then covered with cold cure resin to mask the color of FRC. It is slightly overfilled to compensate the polymerization shrinkage (Fig. 16.9).
8. Then prosthesis was placed is warm water and allowed to polymerize in a pressure pot at 20 psi. After 15 minutes, the prosthesis is removed, pumiced and polished.

Advantages

1. Long lasting service due to enhance of strength of repaired denture.
2. Frequency of fracture of maxillary complete denture opening a natural dentition is reduced.
3. It is a simple straightforward procedure and can be easily done in dental office.
4. Esthetic is not compromised.
5. There is no increase in weight and bulk.

Relining

Relining is the process of resurfacing by adding base material in a quantity to fill the space between the tissue and the denture base created by the resorption of the supporting ridges.

Rebasing

Definition

Rebasing is the process of refitting a denture by replacing all the old denture base material with new material, without changing the occlusal relations of the teeth.

Objectives

The purpose of such process is to close contact between the supporting tissue and the denture base created by the resorption of tissues. If the change in the oral tissue is not great, "relining" rather than "rebasing" is required.

Indications for Relining

1. Immediate dentures at three or six months after construction.
2. When residual alveolar ridges have resorbed and the adaptation of the denture bases to the ridges is poor.
3. When the patient cannot afford the cost of having new denture construction.
4. When the construction of new dentures with series of appointments can cause physical or mental stress in geriatric or chronically ill patients.
5. When the occlusal vertical dimension is satisfactory.
6. When centric occlusion coincide with centric relation.
7. Patient's appearance is acceptable to the patient and the dentist.
8. The oral tissue is in optimum health.
9. The posterior limit of the maxillary denture is correct.
10. The denture base extensions are adequate.
11. Speech is satisfactory with the existing tooth arrangements.
12. There should be no severe bony undercuts or flabby tissues.

Contraindications for Relining

The denture should not be relined:
1. When an excessive resorption has taken place.
2. When abused soft tissue is present.
3. When patient complain of temporomandibular joint problem—until treatment of problem is accomplished.
4. If the denture have poor esthetics or unsatisfactory jaw relationships.
5. If the denture creates speech problem.
6. When severe bony undercut present.
7. Absence of freeway space.

Clinical and Laboratory Procedures

The clinical procedures for both the relining and rebasing is same, only the laboratory procedures are different. Impressions may be made either by the functional (close mouth) or by the static technique, depending upon the need of the patient and the decision of the dentist. Before impression is made, the mucosa should be free from irritation and it should be in healthy state. The denture should be left out the mouth for a minimum 2 to 3 days.

Functional Impressions

Tissue treatment material may be used for making a functional impression. This type of impression is indicated in dentures which require no modification of the vertical dimension of occlusion. The denture is prepared by removing all undercut areas so that the denture may be removed from the cast without damaging the latter. The denture border, in specific location such as frena, need to be relived, it is not necessary to cut away a portion of the entire border because the impression material should record the original relation of the border with the muscular borders. The vertical dimension may be altered by more or less than this relation.

The dentures are first relined with tissue treatment material (using a percentage of 1:1 powder liquid ratio) and placed in the mouth, and the patient is allowed to close lightly with teeth in centric occlusion. Care must be taken to prevent the displacement of the maxillary denture anteriorly. Border molding is accomplished by functional movements. The denture is removed from the mouth after 5 minutes for evaluation of the impression. It should have a smooth rounded border and surface free from imperfections, and accurate reproduction of the patient oral tissue. After removing the excess material from the facial surface of the denture, the patient is allowed to wear for 24 hours. The patient should return for evaluation of the denture. If the dentures have develop adequate stability and retention and stability and tissues do not show any sign of irritation, the dentures are relined with the same ratio of powder liquid (1:1). The upper and lower are loaded with the material at the same time inserted in the mouth and closed without much pressure on the teeth, and make open and close for 2 minutes. The dentures are kept in the mouth for 45 minutes. If they are removed earlier the material is not properly set and sticks to the tissues and gets distorted.

The maxillary denture is removed by asking the patient to blow with his mouth closed to preserve the peripheral border. The excess material which has flowed on the denture base 4 mm beyond the peripheral border is removed.

The occlusion is recorded with a plaster buccal key for remounting.

The dentures are removed from the mouth, and stone cast is poured by carefully covering the borders.

The buccal keys are secured to the dentures for remounting on an articulator.

The keys are removed, the dentures are cleaned and occlusion examined. The dentures are invested usually without removing the dentures from the casts.

To avoid distortion of the old denture base during processing, all the acrylic resin should be removed from the maxillary denture and rebasing is done, whereas relining is done in a mandibular denture.

Static Impressions

Separate impressions are made without utilizing the existing centric occlusion. The dentures should be left out of the mouth for at least 24 hours before impressions are made. All the undercuts are eliminated.

The denture borders are checked. Any overextension must be removed by grinding away the denture periphery in that area until they are at least 1 mm short of tissue reflection point. Any area of the denture base that impinged on soft tissue should be relieved before the entire fitting surface is reduced from 0.5 to 1.0 mm, depending upon the impression material used.

Four composition stops are placed in the alveolar groove area of the denture, one each in each canine and one each in the molar areas. The dentures are placed in the patient's mouth and addition or subtractions from the stops are made until the desired vertical dimension is obtained.

The dentures are border molded with green stick composition as a new denture impression.

If close mouth method is used, patient is closed the mouth each time border molding is done.

After the border molding is completed, the dentures should be retentive. All borders except the posterior palatal seal area on the maxillary denture and buccal shelves on the mandibular denture should be reduced 1.0 mm. Awash impression is made with zinc oxide paste or light body rubber base. The denture will now be retentive and stable. The vertical dimension and centric relation and appearance are rechecked. If correct the denture is boxed and cast is poured.

RELINING

The denture may be relined either with autopolymerizing acrylic resin or heat cure resin in laboratory. This is performed using any of the two methods:

a. Hooper duplicator method.
b. Jectron jig method (Figs 16.10 to 16.13).

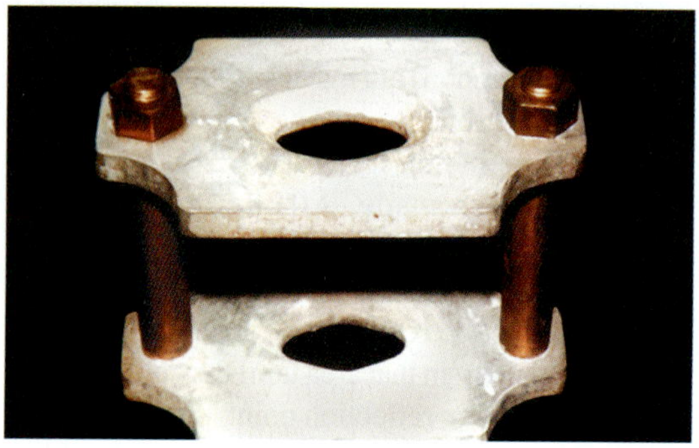

Fig. 16.10: The Jectron jig

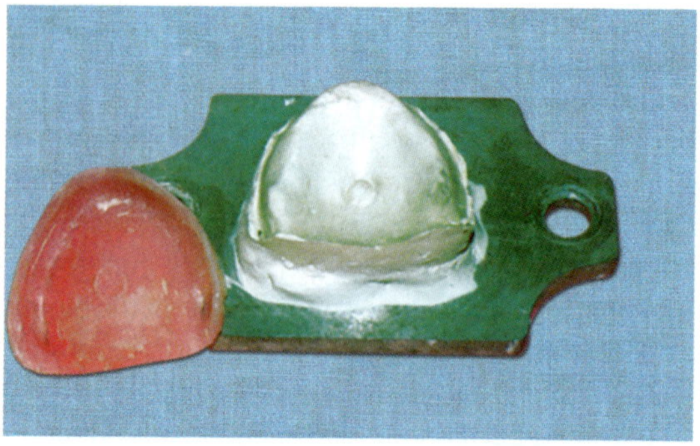

Fig. 16.11: The Jectron jig ready for mounting denture

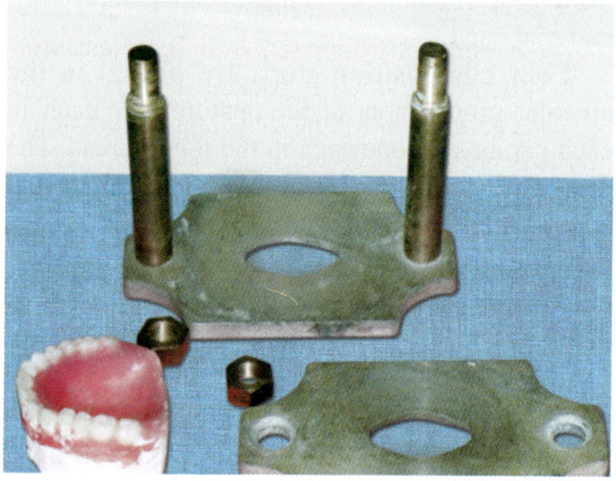

Fig. 16.12: The new cast has been mounted on the upper member of the jig

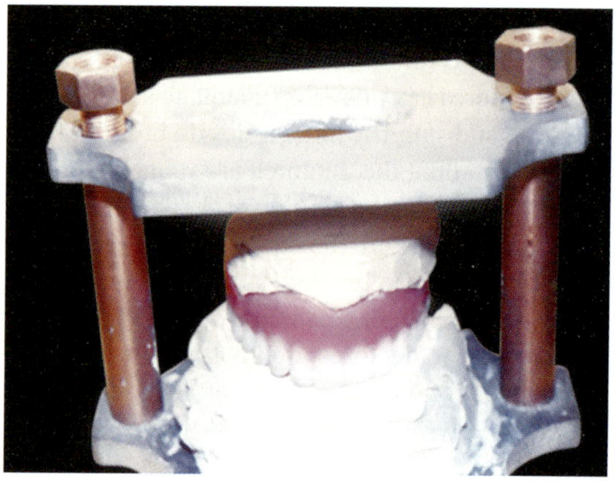

Fig. 16.13: The denture mounted in the jig with teeth set into a plaster plate form

The maxillary and/or mandibular casts are not separated and mounted in the top of jig or duplicator. A layer of plaster is placed in the lower member of the jig, and the upper member with the attached to it denture is closed into the soft plaster. So that the teeth penetrate the plaster surface to a depth of 3 mm approximately. The set plaster formed a key into which the teeth can be set repeatedly. The denture is now removed from the cast by dipping in hot water to soften the impression material. Now it should be decided whether to reline or rebase the denture.

The post dam groove is cut in the maxillary cast. Self-curing resin is mixed up as per manufacturers direction and poured in the space created by removal of the impression material. The gig or duplicator is closed to its original position.

The denture is finished and polished as usual. The intraoral checking of occlusal contacts and relationship should be performed during delivery.

Chairside Relining

Research continues to develop some material that can be added to the denture base and allowed to set in the mouth. Two types of material available temporary soft liner and permanent soft liner. The former is used to treat abuse tissue developed from wearing faulty denture without leaving the denture out of the mouth.

Procedure

Before t he placement of the tissue conditioner all occlusal adjustments and correction of underextension or overextension of denture borders should be performed. The material is placed as follows:

1. The tissue fitting surface (except the posterior palatal seal area) and the denture borders are reduced about 2 mm. Two anterior steps may be placed in canine region without relieving two (3 × 3 mm) areas.
2. The material is mixed (powder and liquid) according to the manufacturer's directions.
3. The material is evenly spread on the fitting surface of the dentures including the borders.
4. The dentures are placed in patient's mouth and the patient is advised to tap his teeth lightly together without putting excessive pressure.
5. Border-moulding is done functionally.
6. The denture is removed from the mouth and checked for voids if found and new material is to place over them and dentures returned to the mouth to correct these areas.
7. The pressure spots are relieved with round bur or carbide burs.
8. The centric relation must coincides centric occlusion at correct vertical dimension.
9. The patient is dismissed for 72 hours and asked not to brush the fitting surface and avoid hard food.
10. Additional treatment may be needed after 72 hours and the material is replaced by new material till tissues become normal.

REBASING

Indications

1. In case of excessive resorption of ridge.
2. When a denture has been repaired many times.
3. When a denture has been fractured into many pieces.

Procedures

1. When the denture is intact an impression is taken in the denture. When the denture is fractured, an impression is obtained from mouth in a stock tray.
2. A cast is poured into the impression and the polished surface is cleaned.
3. The denture and the cast are flasked in the shallow section of a flask.
4. When the plaster have set the denture is removed from the flask and cleaned of impression material along with the cast.
5. Denture base material is removed with a grinding wheel mounted on lathe until only teeth remain on a 5 mm of wide acrylic giving a horseshoe appearance. The denture base from interpoximal areas are removed with a No. 3 flat fissure bur.
6. A post dam is cut on the maxillary cast. The teeth one firmly seated into the flask and acrylic resin dough is packed.
7. The curving, deflasking, finishing and polishing done before delivery.

CONCLUSION

Relining should be carried out when the vertical dimension and centric relation of the dentures are correct and the patient is satisfied with the esthetics. In case the vertical dimension is reduced by 3 mm or more as a result of tissue changes and error in centric relation relining is not being successful. It is usually occur when the patient fails to come back for routine periodic check-up. Relining in this case will improve the adaptation but fails to eliminate the occlusal errors. Rebasing is needed in this case.

BIBLIOGRAPHY

1. Christensen FT. Relining techniques for complete denture. J Prosthet Dent. 1971;26:373.
2. Freilich MA, et al. Fibre reinforcements repaired acrylic resin removable dentures. Quintessence 1977;28:39-44.
3. Goel H, Das S. A simplified and innovative technique of denture repair by fibre-reinforced composite. Journal of Indian Prosthodontic Society. 2004;40:43-5.
4. Heartwell CM, Rahn AO. Syllabus of complete dentures, 2nd edn; 1874.
5. Tucker MT. Relining complete dentures with the use of a functional impression. J Prosth Dent. 1966;16:1054.

Chapter 17

Immediate Complete Dentures

INTRODUCTION

The patients excepting a few are willing to lose their anterior teeth without any form of immediate replacement. The best method is to make immediate denture. This method is convenient when large number of teeth becomes unserviceable and a complete denture is mandatory in near future. The posterior teeth are first extracted and after the healing a complete denture is made and inserted immediately after extraction of the remaining front teeth. The dentists are making immediate dentures at least for last 80 years. The construction of an immediate denture is one of the most challenging problems for the dentist. The most important single factor requires producing a natural appearance is the position of the teeth. Nowadays, with improvement of oral hygiene standard and good restorative procedure there is decrease in patient with large number of neglecting unsavable teeth. So, now transitional dentures are often become more appropriate method of easing a patient into edentulous state through the successive loss of natural teeth. The teeth lost are added to an existing partial denture and thus prolonged surgical trauma is avoided.

DEFINITION

A complete or removable partial denture constructed for insertion immediately following the removal of natural teeth (GPT).

TYPES OF IMMEDIATE DENTURE

Payne has classified immediate dentures as follows:

1. *Conventional or traditional immediate denture*: An immediate complete denture that usually constructed before all the remaining teeth have been removed and inserted immediately after the removal of the remaining teeth. This is advocated when only anterior teeth remain and the patient wants to extract the posterior teeth before immediate complete denture is provided. The posterior teeth are extracted and the posterior ridges are allowed to heal before impressions are made.
2. *Additive or convertible immediate denture*: A partial denture which the patient is already wearing is converted to an immediate denture by adding tooth or teeth to it for extracted areas after healing.
3. *Transitional or interim immediate denture*: An interim denture is denture prosthesis which replaces the remaining teeth without any preliminary extraction. These are designed to enhance esthetics, stabilization and/or function for a limited period of time, after which it is to be replaced by a definitive prosthesis. Often such prosthesis are used to assist in determination of the therapeutic effectiveness of a specific treatment plan or form and function of the planned for definitive prosthesis.

REQUIREMENTS OF IMMEDIATE DENTURES

A denture is a part of system composed of living tissues. It must be physiological and well-tolerated by the patient. To achieve the maximum success the immediate complete denture should have the following requirements:

1. Restoration of masticatory efficiency.
2. Restoration of the function of speech, respiration, and deglutition.
3. Restoration of acceptable esthetics.
4. Should be compatible with the surrounding tissues.
5. Preservation of the remaining oral tissues.

ADVANTAGES OF IMMEDIATE DENTURES

1. The patient does not suffer the edentulous period without artificial replacement. The patient's social and business activities are not hampered. The appearance and well-being of the patient can be maintained and sometimes improved, e.g. carious or grossly hyperplastic, or markedly proclination of teeth.
2. The form, size, color, and arrangement of natural teeth can be correctly reproduced in dentures easily when some of the natural teeth remain in the mouth. If require a change in position can be done. The most natural looking dentures are immediate dentures. The dentists have the opportunity to copy the size, shape and color and arrangement of the natural teeth.
3. *Speech impairment prevented:* Immediately following total extractions, speech becomes indistinct. Speech is not affected to such a marked degree as the placement of immediate denture preserve a clear speech, particularly labiolingual dental sounds. The necessity of two speech adaptations, one after the teeth extraction and another after the dentures delivery is thus avoided.
4. The remaining natural teeth help in maintenance of correct vertical dimension of occlusion that is essential for acceptability of any dentures. It is due to prevention of shortening of the muscles of mastication and ligaments, therefore, adapting a changed posture.
5. *Mastication not impaired*: The patient is no time remains without teeth, so mastication of food and digestion is not impaired and the nutrition is maintained. It helps to maintain the patient health.
6. It acts as a protective surgical splint to control bleeding after extraction with organization of clot and it reduces loss of blood and promotes healing.
7. *It prevents collapse of facial musculature*: The incisal third of the anterior teeth provide the lip support and normal lip contour. When the lips have not altered positions because of lack of tooth support, it is easier to obtain esthetic harmony with complete support is obtained and maintain neutral zone. A long edentulous period causes a decreased neutral zone—a space between the tongue in one side and the cheeks and lips on the other. A decreased neutral zone reduced the space for the lower denture and hampered the retention and the stability of the lower dentures. The insertion of immediate dentures preserved the proper neutral zone.
8. It prevents development of abnormal mandibular movement's pattern in absence of natural teeth.
9. It helps in preservation of ridge according some authorities. But the placement of immediate dentures does not helps to preserve the bony ridge.
10. It shorten learning period. As remaining toothless for a long period, patient develops habits specially tongue habits that cause difficulty in the use of dentures.

11. It removes the patient's fear of edentulous state and help to tide over it smoothly.
12. The change of tongue shape is prevented.

DISADVANTAGES OF IMMEDIATE DENTURES

Immediate denture possesses so many advantages mentioned above though it has very few disadvantages which are negligible. These are as follows:

1. Strain to the patient too much due to extraction of large number of teeth at a time. So, physical and mental condition of the patient is to be considered as a deciding factor.
2. *Additional cost of treatment*: There is an increased expense due to need for relining and remaking.
3. *Additional complex clinical procedures*: The final impression with border moulding is more difficult in presence of natural teeth.
4. Try-in with natural teeth in place not possible and patient got no opportunity to see the denture in mouth before it is processed.

INDICATIONS

1. Patients with a concern for appearance due to their professions.
2. Patients desire to follow the dentist's instructions.
3. Patients with little surgical risk.
4. Patients not requiring gross recontouring of bone.

CONTRAINDICATIONS

Local Conditions

1. Ankylosed teeth.
2. Embedded or impacted teeth.
3. Hypercementosis.
4. When excessive surgical correction of malrelated jaws is required.
5. When malposition of teeth requires extensive surgical reduction.
6. Excessive mobile teeth, large cysts or abscess requiring post-surgical drainage.

Systemic Conditions

1. Patient undergone recent radiation therapy.
2. Patients with systemic condition affecting blood coagulation and healing.
3. Fibrous dysplasia.
4. Aged or medically compromised patients who cannot withstand multiple extraction.
5. Patient with psychological disorders.
6. Patients with gross oral sepsis.

TREATMENT PLANNING FOR IMMEDIATE DENTURES

1. *Two-stage extraction technique:* It is technically possible to replace all 32 teeth at one time. However, a two stage technique of tooth removal is preferred. The first stage is to extract all the posterior teeth except the opposing premolars which are act as an occlusal stop to preserve the interarch distance during healing period. After the healing for several months a stable posterior ridge will have formed on which the second stage of treatment of immediate dentures fabrication can be started. The upper and lower anterior teeth maintain the appearance and are used in chewing during this healing period. The incisors and canines are extracted after the immediate dentures are made, and are replaced by the prosthesis. The two stage technique simplifies clinical procedures, reduces post-insertion care, and provides denture with improved stability and retention. This technique was first advocated by Swenson.
2. *Single stage extraction technique*: It is usually advised for patient with poor oral hygiene. Total extraction is done in one appointment.

The dentures are constructed from the casts of complete maxillary and mandibular impressions.

IMMEDIATE DENTURE TECHNIQUES

There are many methods of preparing the mouth for immediate denture. They can be divided into two groups:

1. *Without alveolectomy*: The artificial teeth are placed over the tooth sockets without alveolectomy.
2. *With alveolectomy*: Alveolectomy is carried out simultaneously with extractions.

Immediate Denture without Alveolectomy

This method is most suitable for replacing the single rooted teeth and usually used for incisors and canines. If some posterior teeth have also to be extracted they should, if possible be removed three or four months before making the immediate denture.

There are two methods as follows:

1st Method—Two Stage Extraction Method

The patient is examined first for paying attention to the occlusal relationship of the upper and lower anterior teeth. If the occlusion of these teeth is such that they give an accurate guide to the jaw relationship only they need to be retained for immediate replacement.

a. Once it is decided which teeth are to be retained, the extraction of posterior teeth is done in first visit. These create a partial edentulous situation for a period of time.
b. After 6–8 weeks extraction of anterior teeth is followed by replacement with immediate denture at the same sitting of extraction.

2nd Method—Single Stage Extraction Method

The second method of preparation of mouth for immediate denture consists of the extraction of all the existing teeth, at the time of placement of the denture. This method is more accepted because of its several advantages as follows:

a. Uniform healing and resorption of the whole arch.
b. Patient does not loose the function of masticatory apparatus.
c. Jaw relation and occlusion is maintained.
d. Transition from natural to artificial teeth is accomplished quickly and the appearance is not altered.

Immediate Denture with Alveolectomy

This technique is same as the previous method but it will only require some modification before it is used where a part of alveolar ridge requires to be removed. Alveolectomy is required for the following reasons:

1 Prominent premaxilla.
2. In a very close bite situation.
3. In order to provide better retention and stability.
4. Preference of the operator.

Clinical and Laboratory Procedures

Mouth Preparation

To improve oral hygiene removal of calculus and decreased gingival tissue is to be done before impressions.

1. *Preliminary impressions:* A preliminary impression in alginate is made on a stock metal tray that will provide 6 mm clearance. Two steps of utility wax are placed over the molar areas, and a platform of wax is placed in the anterior ridge area of the tray. The tray is placed in the mouth in such a way that the incisal edges of the teeth will be forced into this platform to a depth sufficiently to place the peripheral border 6 mm from the mucobuccal fold. These indentations provides anterior stop. A wax bead should also provide at the posterior border of the upper tray to prevent the flow of impression material to the throat (Figs 17.1A and B).

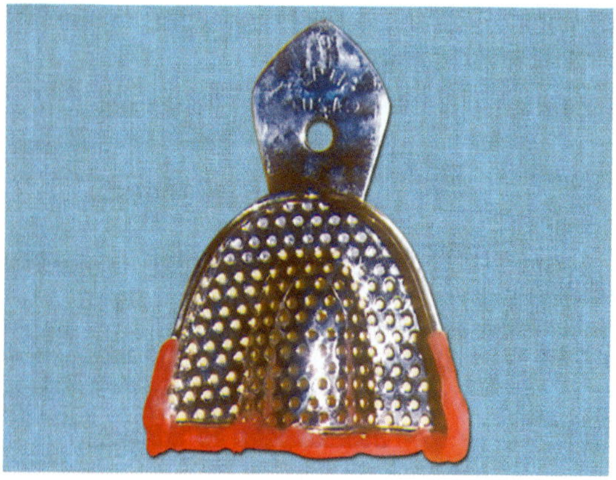

Fig. 17.1A: Addition of utility wax to the maxillary stock tray for preliminary impression

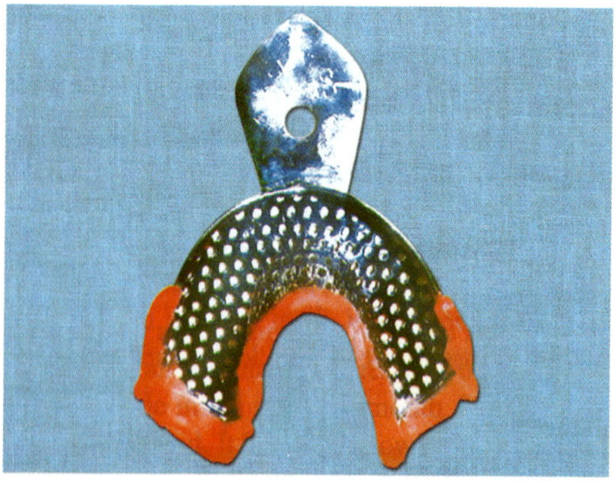

Fig. 17.1B: Addition of utility wax to the mandibular stock tray for preliminary impression

The upper try is loaded with alginate material and seated properly so that stops contacts the tissues. The patient is advised to move the upper lip downward, open wide, and move the lower jaw from side-to-side.

The impression is removed when set and examined for adequate tissue details, and stops just visible. The lower impression is recorded with tongue movement for proper border molding. Preliminary casts are secured.

2. *Fabrication of impression trays:* The border extension of the tray is drawn on the casts prepared from the preliminary impressions (study casts) as the line 2 mm from the mucobuccal fold. The undercuts are block out with wax and relief provided over displaceable tissues and bony prominences. Two layers of base plate wax are adapted to the upper preliminary cast so as to cover the basal seat and teeth. The wax is cut away from the incisal edges and the molar ridge to form stops. The cast is painted with alginate separating medium and allowed to dry. The tray is fabricated of cold cure acrylic resin (preferably sprinkled) fitted with a handle. The lower tray is made in the same way. After polymerization trays are trimmed smooth.
3. *Border molding and final impressions:* Border molding is performed with green stick compound to establish the correct peripheral extent. Movements of tongue, lips and cheeks should not displace the tray. Many 2 mm holes are drilled through the tray to provide retention for the alginate. The material is loaded into the tray and seated firmly in the mouth and held till sets.
   When set the impression is removed and inspected for the stops just visible. The cast is poured in a thick mix of stone and allowed to set.
4. *Jaw relation records:* The jaw relation is recorded with acrylic base with partial bite blocks (Fig. 17.2). The occlusal plane is determined on the lower bite block by cutting the bite rim posteriorly to follow the plane of the incisal edges of the standing anterior teeth. Unless it is decided to open the vertical dimension it is recorded by occluding the bite blocks at the first light contact of the opposing natural anterior teeth. The rims are sealed by softening the wax. If opening of bite has been decided, the space between upper and lower incisors serves as a guide. In case the upper and lower ridges are parallel, there is a tendency for anteroposterior movement of the bite blocks in the mouth. A denture adhesive, or wire clasps on abutment tooth should always be used to prevent the movement of bases during jaw

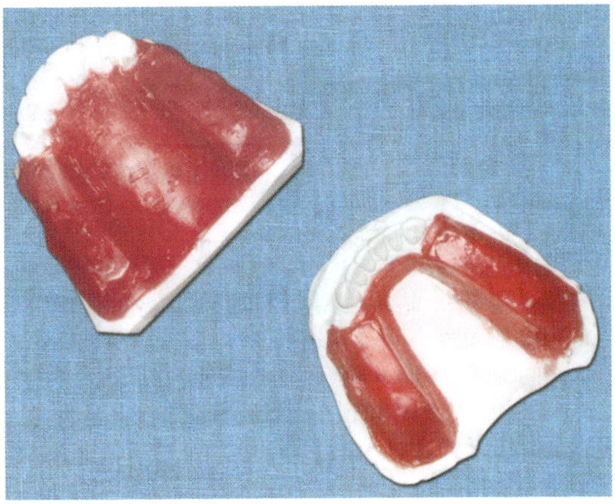

Fig. 17.2: Occlusion rims for upper and lower casts

relation record. Facebow record is obtained and casts are mounted on the articulator.

5. *Arrangement of posterior teeth:* Tooth selection is made at the jaw relation stage, acrylic teeth being preferred. Arrangement of the posterior tooth using stock tooth saves laboratory time.
6. *Try-in:* A modified try-in for patient mouth without the anterior tooth is advisable for verification of jaw relation. The patient is shown the wax-up dentures on the articulator for comments on color or arrangement of the teeth. The protrusive relation record is obtained by asking the patient to protrude the lower jaw until the incisal edges of the upper anterior teeth meets the lower anteriors and close. The lateral condylar guides are adjusted using Hanau's formula:

   $$L= H/8 +12$$
7. *Selection and arrangement of anterior teeth*: If positions of natural teeth are to be reproduced, arrangement of the anterior teeth is very much simplified because of the guidance of the remaining natural teeth. One stone tooth is removed by cutting down and flush with the gum, and replaced by a denture tooth. If they are not to be reproduced, the anterior teeth of one side of the arch is removed the teeth are arranged by scraping the cast.
8. Denture processing, finishing and polishing is done as in conventional dentures.
9. *Delivery:* The dentures should be ready before any surgical procedure is started. The patient is prepared and the condemned teeth are removed. A surgical transparent template may be used if contouring of ridge is done. The dentures are set in the mouth, overextensions and the pressure spots located and adjusted. The patient is given to bite on cotton rolls for 5 minutes and intraoral occlusal contacts verified and gross occlusal disharmonies are removed. The patient is advised not to remove the dentures for 24 hours.
10. *24 hours adjustment:* The dentures are removed carefully and intraoral examination is done for sore spots and necessary adjustments are done. If no alveolectomy was done remounting and occlusal adjustments can be done at that time. If alveolectomy was performed at delivery occlusal adjustments on articulator should be delayed. Intraoral adjustment should be done on first recall visit and occlusal adjustment on remounting should be done in subsequent visits. The sequence of recall appointments are 1, 2, 4, and 7 days post-delivery. The remounting and occlusal adjustment may be done at any of the visits.
11. *Relining:* The immediate dentures require relining for 5–6 months post-extraction or a new denture is fabricated after 8–12 months.

CONCLUSION

Teeth should be removed with minimum trauma and without surgical bone removal. Lan observed that after teeth have been removed, the maxillary anterior alveolar bone resorbs rapidly for one month. Then moderate resorption continue for 5 months after extraction. Wictorin observed that the residual ridge requires 8–12 months before reaching a stable form. Therefore, immediate dentures require continuous adjustments and temporary relines for 5–6 months. After 8–12 months a heat cure relining or new dentures should be made.

BIBLIOGRAPHY

1. Academy of prosthodontics, Glossary of prosthodontic terms: 7th edn, J Prosthet Dent. 1999;81:76-8.
2. Bruce RW. Immediate denture service designed to preserve oral structures. J Prosthet Dent. 1966; 16:811.
3. Chierici G, et al. Influence of immediate dentures on oral motor skill and speech. J Prosthet Dent. 1978;39:21.
4. Cho GC, Chee WW. Custom characterization of the provisional restoration. J Prosthet Dent. 1993;69(5): 529-32.
5. De Van MM. The transition from natural to artificial teeth. J Prosthet dent. 1961;11:677.
6. Demer WJ. Minimizing problems in placement of immediate dentures. J Prosthet Dent. 1972;27:275.
7. Javid N, Tanaka H. Split tray impression technique for immediate upper dentures. J Prosthet Dent. 1974;32:348.
8. Khan Z, Zaeberele CB. One appointment construction of an immediate transitional complete denture using visible light cured resin. J Prosthet Dent. 1992; 68(3):500-2.
9. Mc Cartney JW. The transitional immediate complete denture. J Prosthet Dent. 1978;40:593.
10. Payne SH. A transitional denture. J Prosthet Dent. 1964;14:221.
11. Payne H. A transitional denture. J Prosthet Dent. 1062;14:22.
12. Pound E. An all-inclusive immediate denture technique. JADA. 1963;67:16.
13. Wakh JF, Walsh T, Eriffiths R. An immediate denture technique to reproduce labial alveolar contour. J Prosthet Dent. 1977;37:222.
14. Waltz ME. Considerate Postoperative care for immediate denture patients. J Prosthet Dent. 1966;16:822.

Chapter 18

Dental Implants

INTRODUCTION

There was a long felt need to replace missing teeth without causing any damage or loading on the adjacent teeth and mucosa. The conventional dentures could only partly perform the masticatory function though perform the esthetic function very well. Dental profession in his attempt to find artificial substitutes for lost tooth conducted research in the use of metals for dental implants and established the basic ideas of using tolerable metals in the jaw bones. It was found that the main cause of failure of implant is due to the electrolytic action of metals in the presence of saliva. Vitallium—one metal alloy was found to produce no electrolytic action in the oral cavity. It is formulated from cobalt (65%), chromium (30%), molybdenum (5%) and minor elements including carbon, silica and manganese.

Implantology is the study of the placement of a foreign material into or onto the jaw bone to replace or support artificial denture. It consists of surgery, prosthetic, and biomechanical principles.

Implant is a graft or insert of alloplastic material set firmly or deeply, into or onto the alveolar process that may be prepared for its insertion; so as to support a prosthetic superstructure.

DENTAL IMPLANTS

A denture which receives its stability and retention from a substructure which is partially or wholly under the soft tissues of the denture basal seat.

Parts of Dental Implant

1. *Substructure*: The metal framework which is embedded beneath the soft tissues in contact with the bone for the purpose of supporting an implant denture superstructure.
2. *Superstructure*: The metal framework which is retained and stabilized by the implant denture substructure.

Indications for Implant Supported Prosthesis

1. It is to satisfy the edentulous patient who cannot tolerate conventional dentures because it would float on a movable muscle base.
2. It is well suited for sharp, spiny, uneven, ridges.
3. It is for case of a dehiscence of the mandibular canals, in which bone loss continues until the roof or covering of the mandibular canal becomes very thin or is completely lacking. In such condition pressure causes pain when treated with conventional dentures.
4. In extreme resorbed mandible the migration of muscle attachments superficial on which conventional dentures ride and unstable.
5. In case of a malformed mental foramens located unfavorably on superior surface of the ridge.
6. In patients who psychologically cannot wear a removable denture even if adequate denture retention or stability is present.
7. Where extremely prominent mylohyoid and internal oblique ridges present that cannot be easily and surgically corrected.

8. In case of enlarged tongue.
9. In prominent genial tubercles.
10. In case of prominent mental eminence.
11. In case of absence or minimal attached mucosa with unfavorable frenum attachment.
12. In hypermobile ridge tissue.
13. In case of atrophic mucosa.

Contraindications for Implant Supported Prosthesis

General Conditions

1. Uncontrolled diabetic. But a patient with controlled diabetic under supervision of a physician can have implants.
2. Leukemia, immunosuppressive disease, hypoparathyroidism, chemotherapy patient.
3. *Pregnancy:* It is best to place an implant after delivery.
4. *Handicapped persons:* Handicapped persons and persons with severe arthritis will not be able to use the brush and floss properly to keep the implant clean.
5. Psychiatric disorders or senility where communication with patient is not possible.
6. Heavy smoking.
7. Patient comfortable with present conventional complete denture and its function.
8. Patient general health condition not permitting a minor surgery.
9. Local anesthesia containing a vasoconstrictor is contraindicated.
10. Liver and kidney disorders.
11. Unrealistic expectation or improper motivation.
12. Lack of operation expertise.
13. Patient sensitive components.
14. Unable to restore prosthodontically.

Local Conditions

1. Small oral opening.
2. Insufficient interarch space.
3. Implants should not be placed in healing bone or infected areas within the bone.
4. In adequate in height and/width of residual ridge.
5. Radiotherapy to the area.

Advantages of Implant Supported Prosthesis

1. Bone maintenance automatic.
2. Occlusal vertical dimension is restored and maintained.
3. Facial esthetics (muscle tone) is maintained.
4. Teeth are positioned with improved esthetic.
5. Improved phonetics.
6. Improved occlusion.
7. Improved mastication and maintenance of muscles of mastication and facial expression.
8. Improved oral proprioception.
9. Reduced prosthesis size (absence of palate and flanges)
10. Improved stability and retention of prosthesis.
11. Long life span of prosthesis.
12. No need for adjustment.
13. Improved psychology of patient.

Types of Implants

There are three types of implants depending upon their site of placement in relation to bone.

1. *Endosteal*: An endosteal implant is an alloplastic material surgically inserted into a residual bony ridge primarily as a prosthodontic foundation (endo-within, esteal-bone). The implant is partially submerged within the bone; achieve a direct attachment of the bone (Fig. 18.1) to the surface of a load-carrying titanium implant. Osseointigration occur and long-term attachment can be maintained indefinitely with minimal amounts of marginal bone loss. Endosseous implant has several advantages over other types. There are three forms of endosteal implant depending upon the shape:
   i. A screw (Figs 18.2A and B)
   ii. A cylinder (Fig. 18.3)
   iii. A blade
2. *Subperiosteal*: The implant is a metal framework inserted beneath the mucoperiosteum and rest directly over the bone of the jaws and is covered by the mucoperiosteum. Vertical posts attached to the framework protrude through

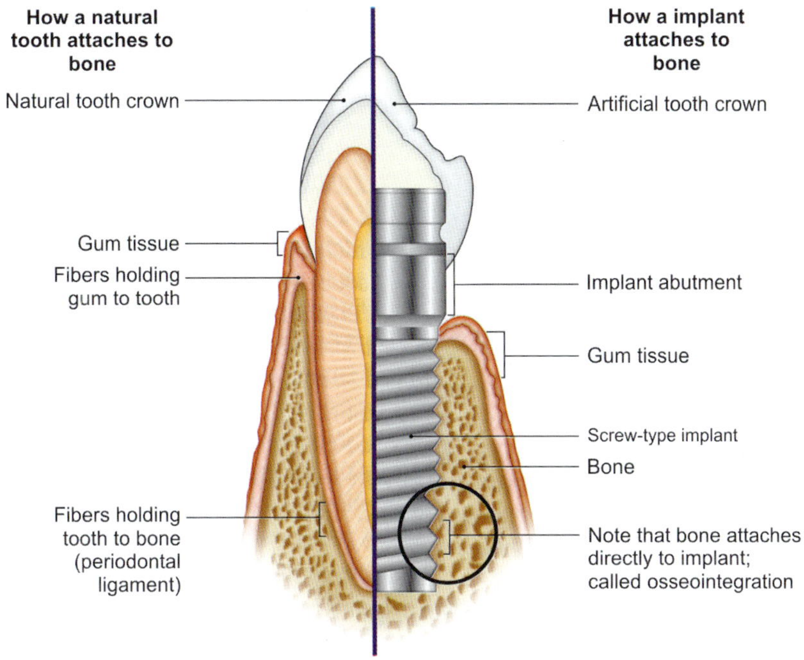

Fig. 18.1: Sketch of a natural teeth and an implant attaches to bone

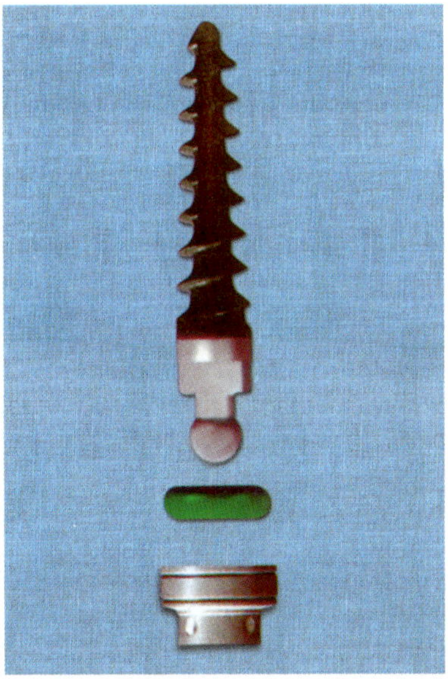

Fig. 18.2A: Endosseous root from screw threaded with cover

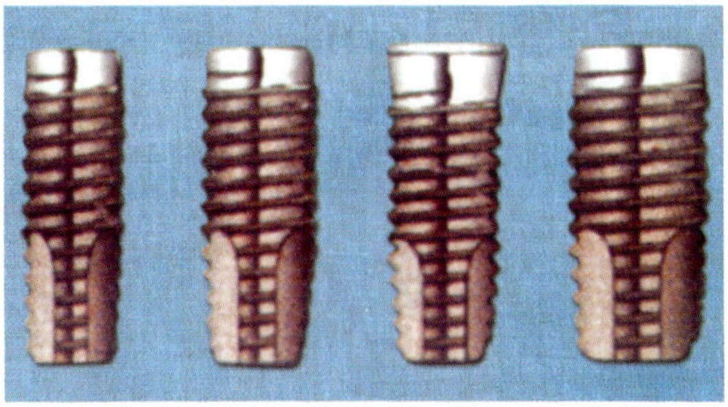

Fig. 18.2B: Endosseous implants screw and cylinders

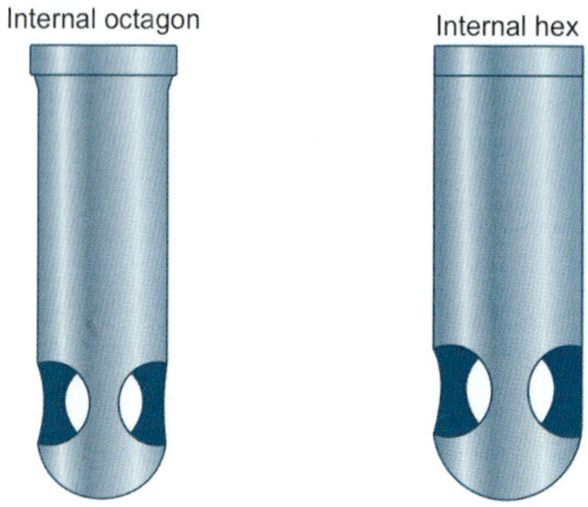

Fig. 18.3: Endosseous implants cylinder

the soft tissues support the dental prosthesis. Although varying degrees of success have been reported the loss of implant commonly occurs.

3. *Transosteal*: The implant passes through the bone of the lower jaw.

   This type of implant penetrates both cortical plates and passes through the full thickness of alveolar bone. It is of two types—staple bone plate or mandibular staple implant, and transmandibular implant.

Mandibular Staple

It consists of a metal plate with retentive pins that holds it against the inferior border of the mandible. The transosteal pins penetrates the full thickness of the mandible into the oral cavity through the ridge crest.

Transmandibular Implant

It is fixed to the jaw by five cortical screws. The prosthesis is fixed on to four threaded posts which penetrate the ridge crest. There are several types of implants.

- *Mucosal implants*: Mucosal implant consists of small metal studs, oval in cross-section, with a narrow neck and a wide base which is attached to the denture. The studs are placed at intervals in the fitting surface of the denture.

  Many attempts have been made to utilize nonendosseous types of implants. In some isolated cases these earlier forms of implant was successful, but fails in long run. Hence, there is growing popularity of separate endosseous implants with predictable results over decades.
- *Endodontic implants*: These are long pin implant inserted through the root canals of teeth into the bone of periapical region. They are usually used to stabilize mobile teeth.

  Osseointegration: It is defined as 'the apparent direct attachment or connection of osseous tissue to an inert, alloplastic material without intervening connective tissue'. It occurs when the bone growth within 100 Å space intervening.

  Biointegration: It is the interface where integration of ceramic implant with bone occur without having any intervening space.

Osseointegration Implant

An osseointegration implant is a cylinder or screw of biocompatible material that is precisely embedded into the jaw bone and allowed to integrate with the bone without any loading forces for certain period. This was devised by Branemark in 1970.

Parts of Branemark's implant consist of the following components:

1. *Fixture*: The part of implant embedded into the edentulous ridge. It is made up of titanium and may be coated with biocompatible, bone-regenerating material, e.g. hydroxyapatite.
2. *Abutment*: The transitional part that connects the prosthesis to the fixture.
3. *Dental prosthesis*: The visible part of the implant that is constructed and attached to the abutment after a few weeks of surgery.

Rate of Success of an Osseointegrated Implant

It depends upon many factors but long-term studies have predicted a success rate of 90%. The endosseous implants lasts for 10 years or more.

Osseointegration: It is defined as "the process whereby clinically asymptomatic rigid fixation of alloplastic materials is achieved and maintained in bone during functional and parafunctional loading". All forces applied to the prosthesis is transmitted through the implant abutment are absorbed and ultimately distributed throughout the surrounding viable bone and associated structures.

Usually dental implants are made up of titanium alloys.

IMPLANTS TREATMENT COURSE

There are one stage (non-submerged) and two stage (submerged osseointegrated implants (Figs 18.4A to C).

I. Two Stage Implant (Fig. 18.4C)

Examination and Diagnosis

Prior to surgery.

a. X-rays (Panoramic, occlusal, cephalometric films)
b. Investigation

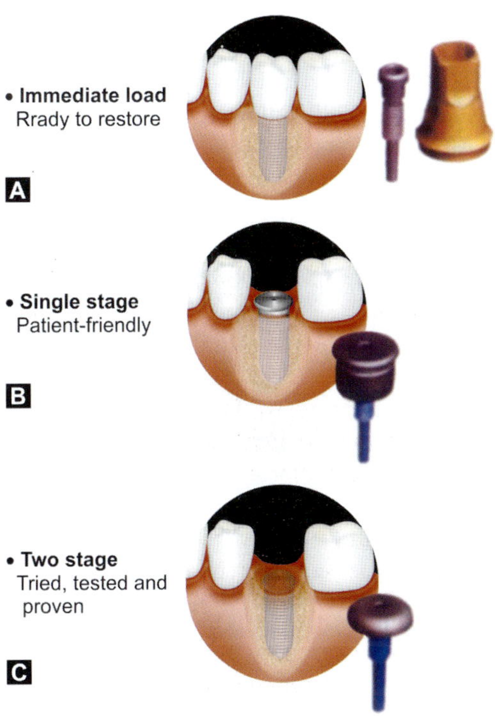

Figs 18.4A to C: Immediate load single stage implant

c. *Impressions*: The first step in the construction of the implant denture is to make correct impressions with alginate for custom tray fabrication as in conventional dentures. The casts are poured. Custom tray is prepared with opening over implant location. The selection of implant sites is limited in the edentulous mandible and the type of implant prosthesis is either fixed hybrid prosthesis or the removable overdenture. In the fixed-hybrid prosthesis the implant is located to the lingual of the anterior teeth or through the occlusal surfaces of the posterior teeth in the prosthesis. In the removable prosthesis, the abutment and its attachments should locate within the area of removal prosthesis. In maxilla, if the bone quality is in the A or B category, a fixed prosthesis is considerable. With the C, D, and E categories only removable prosthesis is considered and the implants are placed where bone or bone graft is present.
(**Note:** A—Abundant bone; B—Resorbed bone; C—Compromised bone; D—Deficient bone; E—Grafted bone)

Surgery—Stage I

Local anesthesia: Crestal incision and rising of flap to expose bone.

The surgical template is placed.

Preparation of implant sites with a series of drills (Fig. 18.5) which increase in width drilled at a speed of 500–2,000 rpm under copious saline irrigation. The atraumatic bone removal below 56 degree centigrade is recommended. The space between the implant and the wound should be less than 1 mm. There should be at least 2 mm space between the implant and the inferior dental canal. There should be at least 1 mm of bone on the buccal and lingual aspect of the implant. The guide drill is a small round bur used to pierce the outer cortex as indicated by the surgical stent. If self-tapping implant is used which have parallel sides appropriate size of drills are to select and used. It is necessary to flare the coronal third of the implant.

When inserting the self-tapping implant, it should be done in very low speeds using a high torque low speed handpiece or a hand ratchet instrument. For press fit implants gentle tapping with the instrument provided is used to push the implant into the bony socket. A covering screw is threaded into the upper part of implant body during healing period. The flap is sutured with a 3/0 reabsorbable material after proper irrigation of the area. The dentures may be provisionally fitted with soft liners at that time or 2 to 3 weeks later.

Surgery—Stage II

3 to 6 months after: This carried out stage I surgery.

a. Osseointegration checked by X-rays.
b. Implant uncovered by circular incision.

Removal of Screw and Abutment Placed

A surgical pack is kept over the abutment by means of a disposable healing cap.

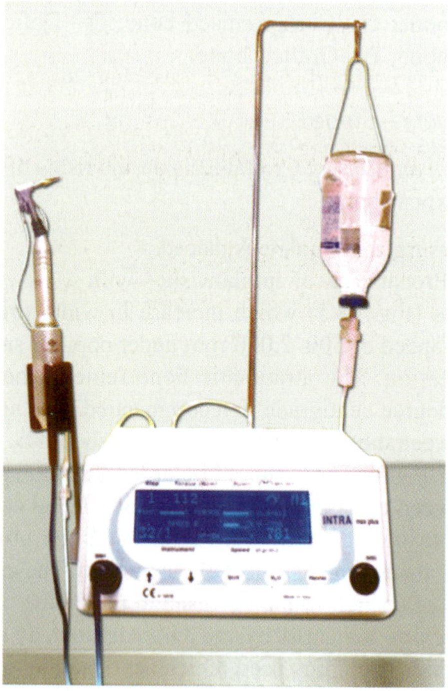

Fig. 18.5: Implant drill motor accessories

Follow Case

One month, three months and six months after restorative treatment and yearly thereafter.

II. Immediate Load Single Stage Implant

Modern one stage non-submerged implant are the dental implant specially designed to be placed as a single unit from gingival margin towards the apex. All abutments and restorations are then placed directly without lifting a mucoperiosteal flap. So, no second surgery is necessary to recover the implant. Designs of implants used in different situations:

1. Single tooth replacement (Fig. 18.6)
2. Three teeth prosthesis (Fig. 18.7)
3. Bar clip over denture (Fig. 18.8)
4. O-ring retained over denture.

Criteria for Implant Success

1. An unattached implant is immobile when tested clinically.
2. A radiograph shows no evidence of peri-implant radiolucency.
3. The mean vertical bone loss is less than 0.2 mm annually following first year of service.
4. Absence of persistence of sign and symptoms as pain, infections, neuropathies, paresthesia.

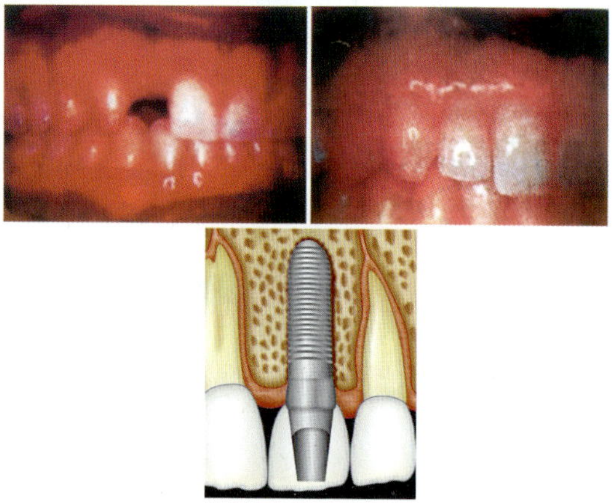

Fig. 18.6: Single tooth replacement

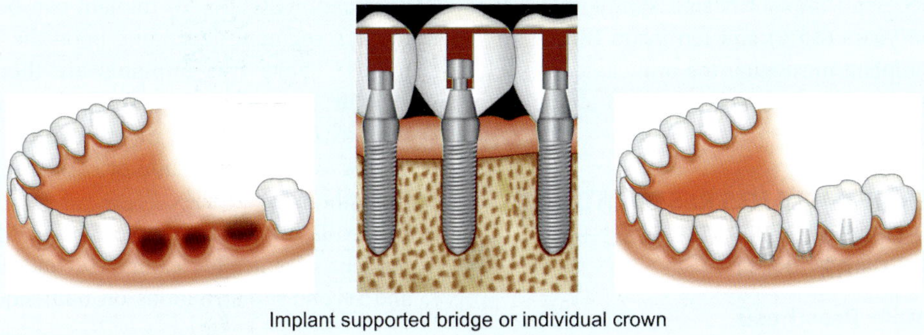

Fig. 18.7: Three teeth replacement prostheses

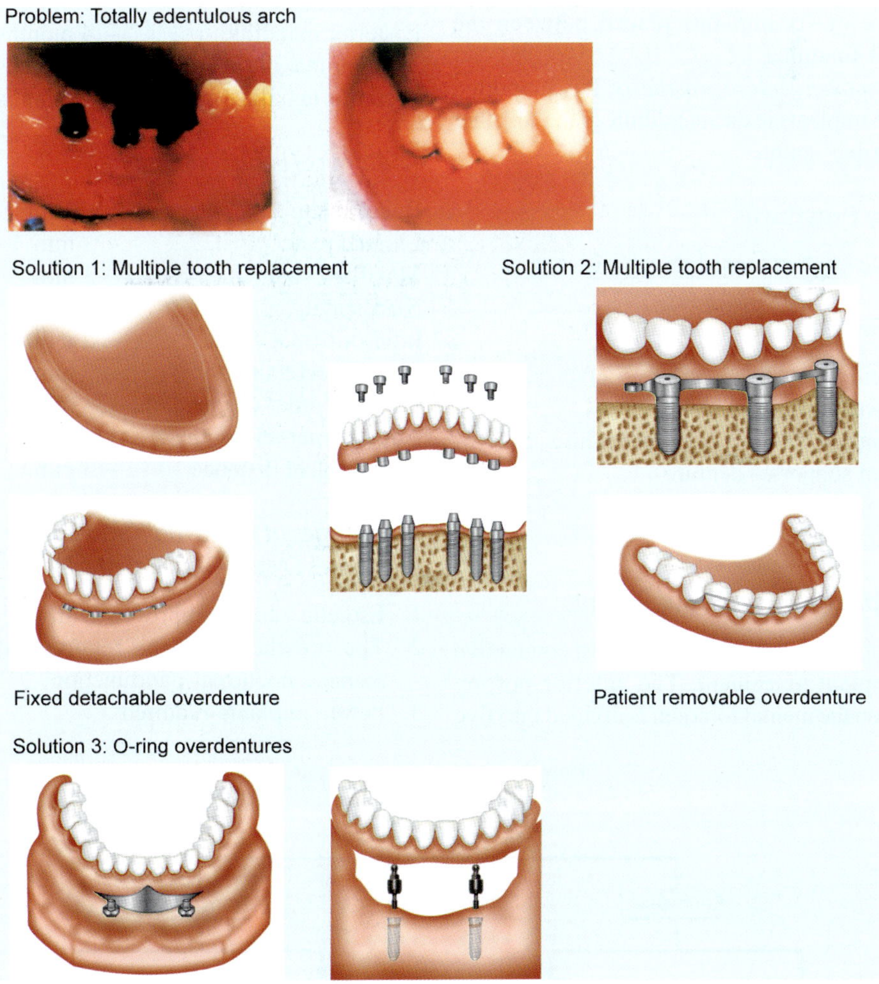

Fig. 18.8: Bar clip over denture

5. A successful implant is sign symptomless for a five years (85%) and ten years (80%).
6. The implant must enter the oral cavity in such a position that it can be used to support or retain prosthesis.

TYPES OF IMPLANTS RESTORATION FOR EDENTULOUS PATIENTS (FLOW CHART 18.1)

Mandibular Prosthesis

1. *Fixed hybrid prosthesis*: It is most commonly used prosthesis in the mandibule. It is supported by five or six implants placed between the mental foramina.
2. *Implant over denture prosthesis*: It is supported by two implants in the mandibule going together with a bar splint.

Maxillary Prosthesis

Removable implant loaded prosthesis.

Patients Benefit Scale

0—No teeth
2—Removable dentures
4—Implant and tissue supported denture
6—Implant supported denture
8—Fixed implant
20—Natural teeth.

Site of Implant for Edentulous Patients

a. In mandible the anterior part is most conductive for implant placement. The anterior portion between the mental foramen is divided into five segments ABCDE. An implant can be placed in each segment depending upon the requirements. Those five implants are themselves capable of supporting a full arch prosthesis, the posterior portions of the denture can be cantilevered up to 15 mm or can be supported from the ridge tissues.
b. In maxilla, implant requirement is rare. Maxillary implant sites are the canine, second premolar and second molar regions on both sides.

Minimum Integration

Anterior mandible – 3 months
Posterior mandible – 4 months
Anterior maxilla – 6 months
Posterior maxilla – 6 months

Anatomical Limit for Implant

Buccal plate – 0.5 mm
Lingual plate – 1 mm
Maxillary sinus – 1 mm
Nasal cavity – 1 mm
Inferior dental canal – 2 mm
Mental nerve anterior – 5 mm
Inferior border of mandible – 1 mm
Adjacent natural tooth – 0.5 mm
Inter-implant distance – 3 mm

Advantages of Removable Implant Supported Prostheses Over a Fixed Prosthesis

1. Esthetic can be improved with labial flange.
2. The prosthesis can be removed at night to manage nocturnal parafunction
3. Fewer implants required

Flow chart 18.1: Types of implants

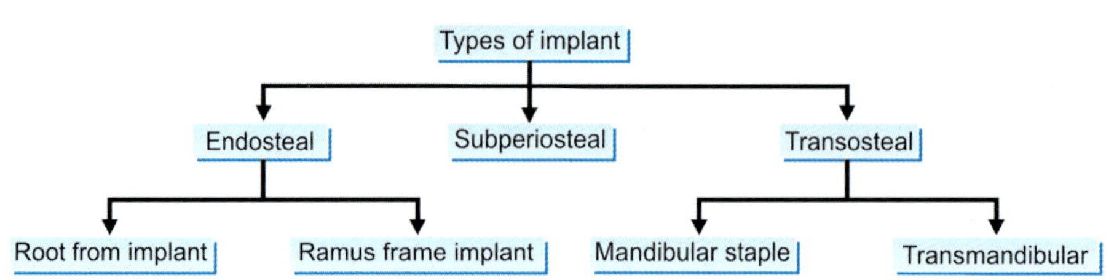

4. Less expensive
5. Daily home case in easier.

Advantages of Fixed Implant Supported Prostheses Over Removal Implant Supported Prosthesis

1. Psychologically better.
2. Less food entrapment.
3. Less maintenance.
4. Longevity in more.
5. Similar in cost as removal implant supported prostheses.

Disadvantages of Fixed Implant Supported Prostheses

1. Complications may be more difficult to treat.
2. Removal at night not possible to prevent nocturnal parafunction.
3. Lack of labial flange support.
4. Oral hygiene is difficult to maintain.

CLINICAL SUCCESS FOR ENDOSSEOUS IMPLANT

The clinical success is defined as an osseointegrated or biointegrated interface, no measurable mobility of the implant in any direction and ability to withstand the required occlusal forces over time. In most clinical cases 95% success rate is obtained if initial interference and occlusal load are not too great. The endosseous implants usually last 10 years or more. The bone support is essential around the implant for its longevity. The rate of success is low in case (a) the density or quality of bone is less, (b) one step technique is used, (c) immediate loading is done.

BIOMECHANICAL FACTORS IN LONG-TERM IMPLANT SUCCESS

The biomechanical factors responsible for implant success are:

1. Implant occlusion.
2. Implant and framework fit.
3. Shock absorbing element.

Implant Occlusion

a. Forces in long axis of the implants and minimum lateral force.
b. Minimum lateral force should be directed as per possible anteriorly.
c. Distribution of lateral force over as many as tooth as possible.

Implant and Framework Fit

Maximum fit of framework and the abutment.

Shock Absorbing Elements

The especially designed shock absorber in the implant system or use of acrylic teeth should be used.

CRITERIA FOR IMPLANT SUCCESS

1. An unattached endosseous implant had less than 0.5 mm of mobility in any direction when tested clinically. A radiograph shows no evidence of peri-implant radiolucency.
2. The mean vertical bone loss is less than 0.2 mm per year following first year of service.
3. Absence of persistence of sign and symptoms as pain, infections, neuropathies, paresthesia.
4. A successful implant is symptomless for a five years (85%) and ten years (80%).
5. The implant must enter the oral cavity in such a position that can be used to support or retain prosthesis.

Maintenance

Recall visits should be at least every 3 months during the first year. Implant mobility, framework and occlusion should be checked.

Removal of debris with plastic or wooden scalars if required as conventional metal scalars will scratch the implant.

Polishing of implant abutment using rubber cup with tin oxide polishing paste.

COMPLICATIONS OF IMPLANTS

Bone Loss

The longevity of implant depends upon the maintenance of bony support around it. The primary complication with dental implant treatment is bone loss. Some bone loss is usually seen around the implant but the rate of bone loss should not exceed 0.2 mm per year. The main causes of bone loss are inadequate number and sizes of implants, excessive occlusal loading, and smoking. If the loss occurs up to 25 to 30% repeat surgery should be considered.

Prosthetic Failure

The fracture of implant parts or the prosthesis due to overloading is due to faulty prosthetic design or procedures.

CONCLUSION

The implant prosthesis is not a substitute for a well-made conventional prosthesis. They are and should be constructed for those patients who are unable to wear conventional dentures successfully. It is the responsibility of the dentists to discuss all potential treatment options with the patient. The patient then can make the choice of the treatment that he or she wishes to undertake. The dentist should inform the patient about the pros and cons of the treatment with implant.

BIBLIOGRAPHY

1. Albrektsson T. A multicentre report on osseointegrated oral implants. J Prosthet Dent. 1988;60:75-84.
2. Branemark PI, Zarb GA, Albrektsson T, et al. Osseointegrated titanium fixtures in the treatment of edentulousness. Biomaterials. 1983;4(1):25-8.
3. Cune MS, de Putter C. Comparative evaluation of some outcome measures of implant systems and suprastructure types in mandibular implant overdenture treatment. Int J Oral Maxillofac Implant. 1994;9:548-55.
4. Jemt T. Implants treatment in resorbed edentulous upper jaw. Clinical Oral Implants Res. 1993;4:187-94.
5. Mish CE. Contemporary Implant Dentistry (2nd edn). St Louis: Mosby, Inc. 1999.
6. Zarb GA, Schmitt A. Osseointegration for elderly patients. The Toronto Study. J Prosthet Dent. 1994;72: 559-68.

Chapter 19

Overdentures

DEFINITIONS

Overdenture may be defined as a removable partial or complete denture that covers and rests on one or more remaining natural teeth or roots, and/or dental implant (GPT). Tooth supported complete overdentures are actually referred as overdentures or hybrid dentures. Overdentures were initially prescribed for patients with congenital or acquired defects where the need for maximum support is required.

OVERLAY DENTURE

An overlay or onlay denture is a denture used to alter the shape and height of the occlusal surfaces of the teeth over which it fits.

GOALS OF OVERDENTURES

1. An overdenture maintains teeth as an integral part of the residual ridge. This provides more support to the prosthesis than conventional denture.
2. It decreases the rate of bone resorption.
3. It increases the patient's manipulative skills in handling the dentures due to the presence of proprioceptive impulses in the periodontal membrane.

INDICATIONS

1. The overdentures are indicated for patient with badly mutilated teeth (Figs 19.1A and B).
2. They are indicated in patient with congenital or acquired intraoral defects.
3. They are indicated for patient with abnormal jaw relation and abnormal jaw size.

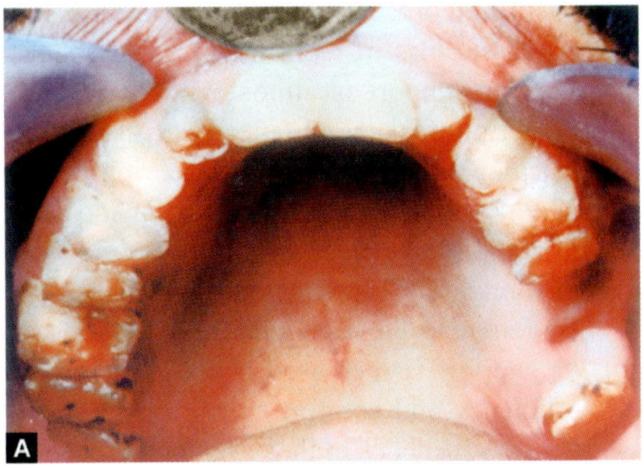
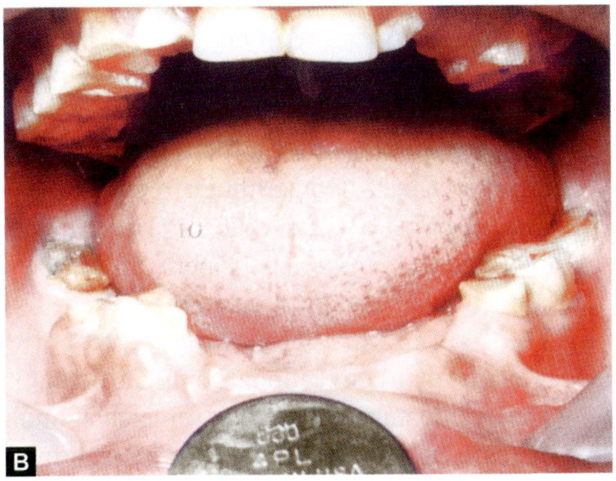

Figs 19.1A and B: Badly mutilated teeth require overdenture

CONTRAINDICATIONS

1. In high caries index and poor oral hygiene.
2. In abutments with poor periodontal conditions.
3. Bony undercuts adjacent to the supporting teeth.
4. In case of endodontic treatment produces poor prognosis.
5. Failure to establish a sufficient zone of attached gingiva.
6. Aged and uncooperative patients.

ADVANTAGES OF OVERDENTURE

1. Conservation of natural teeth and concomitant reduction of or slowing of residual ridge resorption.
2. Stability and support of overdenture is better than a conventional denture. In a patient with natural teeth the occlusal forces are sustained by the periodontal membrane. After the loss of teeth, the area of mucosa left for support is almost ¼th of the area of periodontal membrane. Watt (1961) has calculated the mean denture-bearing area as 22.96 centimeter square in maxilla and 22.25 in mandible whereas the area of periodontal membrane is 45 centimeter square in each jaw. By retaining the roots under the overdenture its support is increased. This gives greater efficiency and comfort.
3. Sensory feedback of the periodontal receptors is maintained and masticatory efficiency is better.
4. The procedures of overdenture are simple as conventional complete dentures. Moreover the presence of roots or teeth helps in registration of correct maxillomandibular records.
5. The repair, alterations or relining of overdenture can be easily performed as the conventional complete dentures.
6. The overdentures generally have better retention than conventional complete dentures.
7. The overdentures due to their same positioning of teeth as the natural teeth produces more esthetic results.
8. The maxillary overdentures without palate is possible if both anterior and posterior teeth are saved.
9. The time and cost of treatment is less than alternative fixed partial dentures.
10. The overdentures may be converted to transitional or treatment denture when patient lose the teeth or roots.
11. It is possible to produce a large vertical overlap of anterior teeth without displacing the denture during function.
12. Excellent patient acceptance.
13. Needs minimum adjustments.
14. Can be converted to complete denture.
15. The procedure is reversible.
16. Ease to clean than fixed partial denture.
17. Helps maintaining stability of existing oral structures.
18. It is particularly useful in patients with congenital defects, e.g. cleft palate, difficult class III occlusion, and cleidocranial dysostosis.

DISADVANTAGES OF OVERDENTURE

1. Maintenance of good oral hygiene is difficult and caries susceptibility and plaque accumulation is increased.
2. The additional time and cost due to additional preparation of copping.
3. Lack of the interocclusal distance leads to difficulty in tooth arrangement and weak dentures.
4. Maintenance of the abutments and dentures are time consuming.
5. Esthetics may have to be compromised.
6. It may be difficult to insert the denture flanges due to bony undercuts.

TYPES OF OVERDENTURES

Overdentures are of three basic types:

1. Immediate overdenture.
2. Transitional overdenture.
3. Remote overdenture.

Immediate Overdenture

It is the overdentures constructed for insertion immediately after the removal of hopeless natural teeth. The clinical and laboratory procedures are similar to the immediate denture except the selection, retention, and preparation of the abutment teeth. Most patient first receive an immediate overdenture.

Transitional Overdenture

It is an overdentures obtained by modifying an existing removal partial denture. It is worn for an interim period and is replaced if required later.

Remote Overdenture

A remote overdenture is constructed some time later, usually a year or more after the removal of the last hopeless teeth. It may be used for replacing an immediate or transitional overdenture following satisfactory use.

TECHNIQUES OF OVERDENTURE

There are several techniques in preparation of teeth to serve as abutments for overdentures:

1. *Simple tooth modification and reduction*: It is used in partially anodontic cases or in severe attrition cases. The remaining teeth are reshaped to eliminate undercuts and reduced in height if required to create interridge space for the overdenture (Fig. 19.2A).
2. *Tooth reduction and cast coping*: This is done because of sensitivity or prevention of caries. This is usually done with teeth with adequate bony support and good periodontal prognosis (Fig. 19.2B).
3. Endodontic therapy with amalgam filling (Fig. 19.2C).
4. Endodontic therapy with cast coping.
5. Endodontic therapy with cast coping using some attachment, e.g. stud attachments (Fig. 19.3).

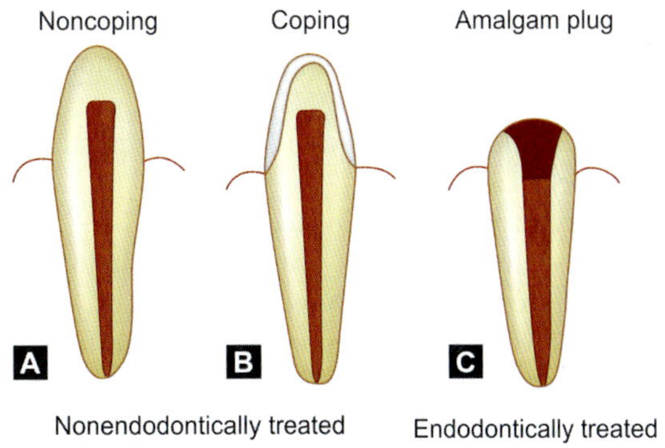

Figs 19.2A to C: Techniques of overdenture: (A) Simple tooth modification and reduction; (B) Tooth reduction and cast coping; (C) Endodontic therapy with amalgam filling

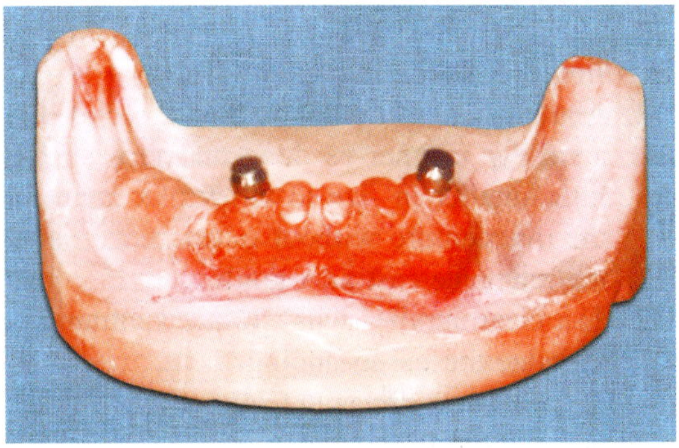

Fig. 19.3: Endodontic therapy with cast coping using some attachment

TREATMENT PROCEDURE FOR OVERDENTURE

The clinical procedure varies with the type of overdenture. It may be a tooth supported immediate complete denture, or tooth supported complete denture.

Immediate Overdenture

A typical procedure for immediate overdenture includes the following steps:

1. The hopeless posterior teeth are removed.
2. During the healing period prerequisite endodontic and periodontal treatment is completed.

3. Final impressions are made.
4. Recording of jaw relations and casts mounted on articulator.
5. Selection of acrylic anterior and posterior teeth is done.
6. Try-in with posterior teeth setting.
7. The anterior teeth are arranged using an adjacent stone tooth as guide.
8. The over-reduced abutment preparation is done on stone cast.
9. The acrylic abutment tooth is modified and set over the prepared stone abutment.
10. The denture is waxed, flasked, packed with high impact resin and cured in a conventional manner.
11. The denture is finished and polished and stored in water until insertion.
12. Abutment teeth in the mouth are reduced in a similar manner as done on the cast, but little smaller in size to allow placement of the overdenture without interference using the reference cast as a guide.
13. The clear acrylic stent is placed intraorally to judge the tissue impingement.
14. The abutment prepared teeth are treated with fluoride gel (APF) for 2 minutes, which is followed by application of 4% stannous fluoride gel.
15. The anterior hopeless teeth are removed and the overdenture is inserted. The peripheral extension and occlusion is checked.
16. The postinsertion instructions are provided and the patient is advised to report for 24 hours post-surgical appointment.
17. The 24 hours evaluation and necessary adjustments are made. The overdenture is adapted to abutments with tooth color autopolymerizing resin.
18. Follow-up care with application of fluoride on abutments.
19. Evaluation of oral hygiene, need for relining after six to eight weeks.
20. Yearly evaluation of oral hygiene and progress.

Tooth Supported Complete Denture

A typical procedure for tooth supported over dentures includes the following steps:

1. Preparation of abutments for copings.
2. The impression is made and dies are poured.
3. The waxing, investing, casting and polishing of copings.
4. Checking the fit of copings on teeth and cementation with glass ionomer cement.
5. The existing overdenture is relined with autopolymerizing resin to adapt the lubricated coping restored abutments.

Although a remote overdenture can be constructed in denture-base resin only, it is recommended to use metal-based overdenture in conjunction with abutment coping.

CONCLUSION

The overdenture is a special mode of treatment. The teeth used as abutments for support and retention are of critical importance for its maintenance. If control of caries by home care and periodontal disease by periodontal therapy and proper home care can be done success of the treatment outcome is assured for years together.

BIBLIOGRAPHY

1. Anderson JN, Storer R. Immediate and Replacement Dentures, 3rd edn, Blackwell, Oxford; 1981.
2. Boucher CO, Boucher's Prothodontic Treatment for Edentulous Patient. 8th edn, Hickey JC, Zarb GA (edn), Mosby, St Louis.
3. Brewer A, Morrow R. Overdentures, Saint Louis; Mosby; 1975.
4. Brewer AA. The tooth-supported dentures. J Prosthet Dent. 1973;20:703.
5. Craddock FW. Prosthetic Dentistry, London; Kimpton; 1951.
6. Crum R, Rooney G. Alveolar bone loss in overdentures. A five-year study. J Prosthet Dent. 1978;40:610.
7. Fish EW. Principles of full denture prosthesis, 5th edn, Staples Press, London; 1952.
8. Heartwell CM, Rahn AO. Syllabus of complete dentures, 5th edn, Macmillan, London; 1986.

9. Hobkirk JA. A colour atlas of complete dentures, Wolfe Medical, London; 1985.
10. Kotwal KR, Outline of standards for evaluating patients for overdentures. J Prosthet Dent. 1977;37:141.
11. Lamb DJ. Appearance and Aesthetics in Denture Practice, Wright, Bristol; 1987.
12. Lammie GA. Full Dentures, Oxford; Blackwell Scientific, 1956.
13. Lee JH. Dental Aesthetics, Wright, Bristol; 1962.
14. Mack A, Full Dentures, John Wright, Bristol; 1978.
15. Morrow RM, Rudd KD. Rhods JE. Dental Laboratory Procedures, Vol. I; Complete Dentures, 2nd edn, Mosby, St Louis; 1986.
16. Neil DJ, Naim, RI. Complete Denture Prosthetics, 2nd end, Wright, Bristol; 1983.
17. Sharry JJ, Complete Denture Prothodontics, 3rd edn, McGraw-Hill, New York; 1974.
18. Thayer HH, Caputo AA. Effects of overdentures upon remaining oral structures. J Prosthet Dent. 1977;37: 374.
19. Watt DM, Macgregor AR. Designing Complete Dentures, Saunders, Philadelphia; 1976.
20. Winkler S. Essentials of Complete Denture Prothodontics, 2nd edn, PSG Publishing, Massachusetts; 1987.

Chapter 20

Single Complete Denture

INTRODUCTION

A single complete denture is a conventional complete denture made against full complement of natural teeth, against a removable or fixed partial denture.

DEFINITION

The making of a maxillary or mandibular denture as distinguished from a set of complete denture. (GPT).

Since in single denture only one arch is involved it appears to be easy and require half as much work and time in comparison to a complete denture. It is not so easy to fabricate and it requires much skill and experience to produce a successful prosthesis.

INDICATIONS

Single complete denture may be indicated in the following situations:

1. Opposing the natural dentition only.
2. Opposing a combination of fixed and partial denture and natural teeth.
3. Opposing a removable partial denture and natural teeth.
4. Opposing an existing complete denture.

In the first three situations, the single maxillary denture opposing all or some of the mandibular teeth is the most common. This is because the maxillary denture is more stable and retentive than mandibular complete denture. The maxillary teeth are usually lost before the mandibular teeth.

CONTRAINDICATIONS

A mandibular single complete denture opposing maxillary natural teeth is usually contraindicated as less basal seat area to support the mandibular denture than a maxillary denture. The mucosa is thin and delicate, and a rapid loss of supporting bone. So, it may be necessary to extract healthy upper teeth looking after the long-term health of the mouth. The overdenture may be a better option to the problem of a mandibular denture opposing natural teeth. But mandibular denture opposing natural teeth may be considered in the following situations:

a. In class III jaw relationship mandibular complete denture against opposing upper natural teeth as the mandibular supporting tissues is able to resist the forces from upper natural teeth.
b. The patient with cleft palate the upper teeth are preserved as the prognosis of an upper complete denture is not good. A lower complete denture may be made against it.

PROBLEMS OF SINGLE COMPLETE DENTURE

1. The firmness and rigidity of the natural teeth are due to their anchorage in the bone. The force recorded on a single molar tooth is 198 lb where as a complete denture exerts a load of 26 lb. Therefore, the denture will be loose when natural teeth occlude against it.
2. The occlusal inclination and form of the remaining natural teeth which will guide the

occlusal form of the denture. The unfavorable occlusal form results in **shunting of denture**.

To overcome these problems, the following things are necessary:

1. Full use of every factor of retention and stability for success.
2. The forces applied on the denture must be reduced as far as possible by preparation or restoration of the remaining natural teeth so as to provide an acceptable occluding surface. The occlusal plane should exhibit no more than a gentle curve anteroposteriorly and mediolaterally.
3. The location of the occlusal plane in relation to the opposing supporting structures is below the middle of the interarch space, undesirable leverages may occur to either maxillary or mandibular complete dentures.
4. Teeth placed facial to the crest of the residual ridge induce torqueing and dislodging forces on denture during function.

FEES FOR SINGLE COMPLETE DENTURE

The construction of single denture is more difficult and time consuming than conventional dentures due to the several problems. But the fees for single complete denture is often underestimated with the assumption that the working and material cost is less for it in comparison to conventional complete denture. A single denture requires three quarter the time of fabrication and fitting of conventional complete dentures. The balancing of occlusion is more time-consuming in single dentures than in complete dentures. The fees must be set accordingly and the patient should be well-informed before the work is undertaken to prevent misunderstanding afterwards.

DIAGNOSIS AND TREATMENT PLANNING

The methods used the problems, the treatment plan, and the prognosis differ in all of these clinical situations. It is, therefore, convenient to consider the various clinical situations separately.

TOOTH MODIFICATION

In conventional complete dentures upper and lower teeth are be arranged to obtain occlusion and articulation. In case of a single complete denture the occlusal pattern of the natural teeth is already present. The natural teeth are modified by grinding or restoration to produce a more suitable occluding surface and grossly malpositioned teeth are extracted or orthdontically repositioned.

Three methods exist for tooth modification:

1. *Swenson's method*: The maxillary and mandibular casts are prepared. The recording of tentative jaw relation is done without making any adjustments to the natural dentition. These casts are mounted on an articulator and artificial teeth are set. The interferences in the natural occlusion is adjusted on the cast with a knife or bur and marked with pencil.

   The occlusal adjustments of natural teeth are carried out in the mouth, using the marked study cast and the trial dentures as guides.

   A new impression of the natural teeth is made and cast prepared and a definitive jaw relation record is made. The new cast is mounted on the articulator, and the artificial teeth are reset and adjusted for trial. The technique is accurate but time-consuming as several impressions and casts are to be made.
2. *Yurkstas method*: The mandibular study cast is evaluated with the help of U-shaped metal template with slight convex lower surface. The template is placed on the occlusal surface of mandibular teeth. The cusps high or low are observed. They are marked using articulating paper. The high cusps are judiciously equilibrated by removing a little of stone with knife on the study cast. This procedure is repeated by remarking and trimming until equalization is obtained. In most patient the natural teeth modifications requires enameloplasty only. The grinding should not be restricted to the tips of cusps but should extend on the buccal surface to prevent increase in occlusal table size.

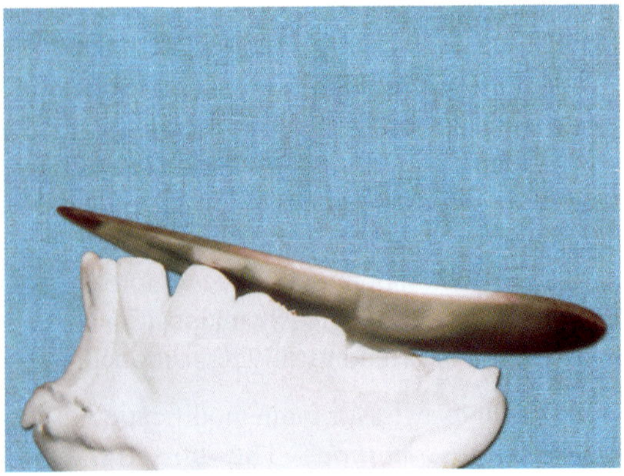

Fig. 20.1: The curved occlusal template used to identify the cusps which are too high or too low and which need modification to produce a suitable occlusal surface

3. *Bruce's method*: The method of tooth modification is done using same template but marking is done with the help of pressure indicating paste instead of articulating paper (Fig. 20.1).

METHODS USED TO OBTAIN BALANCED OCCLUSION

To achieve a harmonious balanced occlusion after tooth modification, there are two methods to do it.
1. Functional chew-in techniques (Stansbury, 1928)
2. Articulator-equilibration techniques.

Functional Chew-in Technique (Stansbury, 1928)

A compound maxillary rim is prepared against the mandibular natural teeth. It is trimmed buccally and lingually for freedom in lateral excursions. Soft carding wax is added on the compound rim and the patient is asked to perform lateral and protrusive chewing movements. The wax is abraded or reshaped to represent the functional paths of movement where as the compound preserve the vertical dimension. The paths are known as functionally generated path and occlusion developed by this method is known as functionally generated occlusion. The occlusion obtain is free from lateral and protrusive interferences. Stone is poured into the occlusal surfaces of the wax paths and without separation.

The mandibular cast mounted on the articulator is replaced by functionally generated cast. All interfering spots are ground until the incisal guide pin touches the incisal table and prevents further closure.

Articulator-Equilibration Techniques

This is the most common method indicated when the denture base lack stability or the patient is unable to perform eccentric movements to form a chew-in record.

The maxillary and mandibular casts are mounted on articulator with a tentative jaw relation without making any adjustments to the natural dentition. The relationship between the upper and lower posterior teeth are studied and following adjustments are done:

a. If the posterior denture teeth are to be placed too far lingually when articulated with the lower lingual cusps, they are reset to oppose the lower buccal cusps.
b. If the posterior denture teeth are to be placed too far lingually when articulated with the lower buccal cusps, they are reset to oppose the lower buccal cusps.

In this technique only the functional cusps are allowed to contact the central fossa. The inclines of the nonfunctional cusps are reduced.

If the lower buccal cusps are selected as the functional cusps, the lingual cusps are reduced.

If the lower lingual cusps are selected as the functional cusps, the buccal cusps are reduced.

At the wax try-in, eccentric records are made and the condylar inclinations are set on the articulator with the upper posterior teeth arranged in balanced occlusion.

The denture is processed. At the time of delivery a new centric record is made and balancing of occlusion is achieved on articulator.

OCCLUSAL MATERIALS FOR THE SINGLE COMPLETE DENTURE

The single denture is usually opposed to different types of teeth in the opposing arch so selection of occlusion forms for single denture should be done judiciously. The occlusal surface will be such so that it should not wear too fast or it should not cause wearing of the natural dentition. The following teeth may be considered with their relative advantages and disadvantages:

1. Vacuum fired porcelain.
2. Acrylic resin.
3. Gold occlusal.
4. Acrylic resin with amalgam stop.
5. Interpenetrating polymer network (IPN).

The use of maxillary porcelain teeth, will lead to rapid wear of the opposing natural teeth. Silver amalgam inserts or stops on occlusal surface wears out rapidly against the natural teeth. Gold occlusals are very effective against natural teeth to maintain vertical dimension without undergoing wear but very expensive and time consuming preparations are necessary. The use of acrylic resin or IPN teeth is the best alternative.

CLINICAL PROCEDURES FOR SINGLE COMPLETE DENTURE OPPOSING NATURAL TEETH

When a patient presents with a typical edentulous maxillary arch and a full complement of mandibular teeth (Fig. 20.2), a case history is taken and an oral examination is performed. Diagnostic casts are prepared and mounted on articulator in centric relation to study the existing interarch space, relationships plane of occlusion and other features and diagnosis, prognosis and treatment plan is formulated.

The mouth preparations are performed:

1. An impression of the natural mandibular teeth is made in alginate hydrocolloid, and cast is poured in stone.

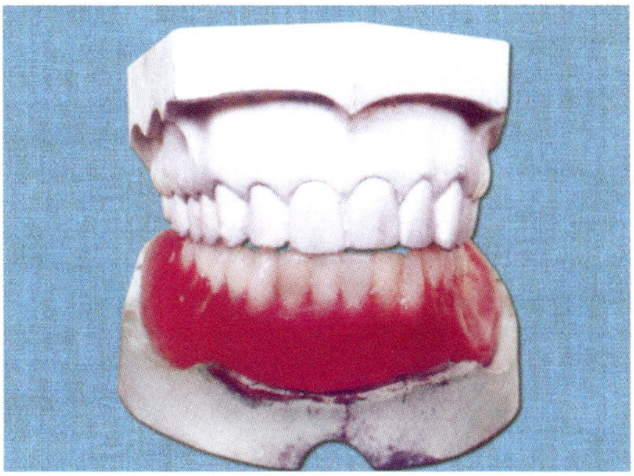

Fig. 20.2: Mandibular complete denture against maxillary natural

2. A preliminary impression of the maxillary arch is made with modeling compound. The special tray is fabricated on the preliminary cast. The final impression is made with zinc oxide paste. The master cast is poured in artificial stone.
3. A stabilized base plate with wax occlusal rim is constructed.
4. The occlusal rim is shaped to provide esthetic lip support; the preliminary vertical dimension of occlusion is established. The tentative centric relation is determined.
5. The facebow record is made and the maxillary cast is mounted on the articulator which is programmed with protrusive record.
6. The anterior artificial teeth are arranged to provide esthetic. The posterior teeth are arranged in centric occlusion.
7. The posterior teeth are rearranged to produce balanced occlusion. The occlusal surface of the mandibular cast is modified for balancing. The modified surfaces are marked with pencil to serve as a guide to accomplish the same in the patient mouth.
8. After modifications of the natural teeth a new impression of the mandibular ridge is obtained in alginate hydrocolloid and a stone cast is poured.

9. A new centric relation record is made, and the mandibular cast is remounted on the articulator.
10. The anterior teeth are reset to provide proper esthetic. The posterior teeth are reset in balanced occlusion.
11. The waxing and processing is done in usual manner and the facebow transfer is preserved.
12. The denture is processed, a new centric relation record is made by cheek-bite and the lower cast is remounted on the articulator and occlusion correction is done.
13. The denture is delivered with proper instructions.
14. The post-insertion cheek-up and adjustment are made as for conventional complete denture.

CONCLUSION

The single complete denture is sometimes required for patient who has all or some of the teeth in opposing arch. This single denture frequently creates some problems that interfere with the dentist ability to satisfy patients. All alternative methods should be chosen to give maximum patients satisfaction. Alteration of the occlusal plane of the opposing teeth to avoid unfavorable tooth contacts may be necessary and the consent of the patient for that is necessary. It is better to avoid mandibular single dentures in favor complete dentures if possible for better outcome.

BIBLIOGRAPHY

1. Bruce RW. Complete dentures opposing natural teeth. J Prosthet Dent. 1971;26:448.
2. Ellinger CW, Rayson JH, Henderson D. Single complete dentures. J Prosthet Dent. 1973:26:4.
3. Hansen CA, Clear K, Wright P. Simplified procedure for making gold occlusal surfaces on denture teeth. J Prosthet Dent. 1994;71:413-16.
4. Rudd KD, Morrow RM, Hall W. Occlusion and the single denture. J Prosthet Dent. 1973;30:4.
5. Scheider RL. Diagnosing functional complete denture fractures, J Prosthet Dent. 1985;54:809-14.
6. Sharry JJ. Textbook of Complete Denture Prosthodontics, 2nd edn, Englewood Cliffs. New Jersey, McGraw-Hill. 1968.p.299.
7. Stansbury GB. Single denture construction against a nonmodified natural dentition. J Prosthet Dent. 1960;10:37.
8. Vig RG. A modified chiew-in and functional impression technique. J Prosthet Dent. 1964;14:214.
9. Wallace DH. The use of gold occlusal surfaces in complete and partial dentures. J Prosthet Dent. 1964;14:326.

Chapter 21

Maxillofacial Prosthetics

DEFINITION

The branch of prosthodontics concerned with the restoration and/or replacement of the stomatognathic and craniofacial structures with prosthesis that may or may not be removed on a regular basis.

OBJECTIVES

The goal of maxillofacial prosthodontics is to restore the rudimentary functions of speech and swallowing, along with normal esthetics and mastication. These functions are disturbed because of congenital, traumatic and surgical procedures in oral cavity. Although normal function may not be achieved but optimum function should be restored.

The restoration of the rudimentary functions of speech and swallowing are made with various intraoral prostheses to compensate for loss of function.

CLASSIFICATION OF MAXILLOFACIAL DEFECTS

1. **Surgical:** The most common cause of maxillary defects are surgical removal of tumors. The removal of both maxillae is known as total maxillectomy. The resection of one or part of the maxilla is known as partial maxillectomy. Aramany developed a classification for partial maxillectomy defects resulting from resection content very different from Kennedy's classification for partially edentulous arch. The movement of the prostheses is more than normal partially edentulous arches, and increases with decrease in number of remaining natural teeth.
2. **Traumatic.**
3. **Congenital defects:** Congenital defects are craniofacial defect present from birth. The most common form includes cleft palate.
4. **Developmental anomalies:** These are defects that occur because of some genetic predisposition is expressed during growth and development.

TYPES OF SURGICAL DEFECTS IN MAXILLA

Aramany's Classification for Partially Edentulous Maxillectomy Defects (Fig. 21.1)

Class I – Midline resection.
Class II – Unilateral resection.
Class III – Central resection.
Class IV – Bilateral anteroposterior resection.
Class V – Posterior resection.
Class VI – Anterior resection.

TYPES OF SURGICAL DEFECTS IN MANDIBLE

Canter and Curtis classified the mandibular resections and their defects that provide a foundation for removable prosthesis design (Fig. 21.2).

Class I – Marginal resection (continuity defect)

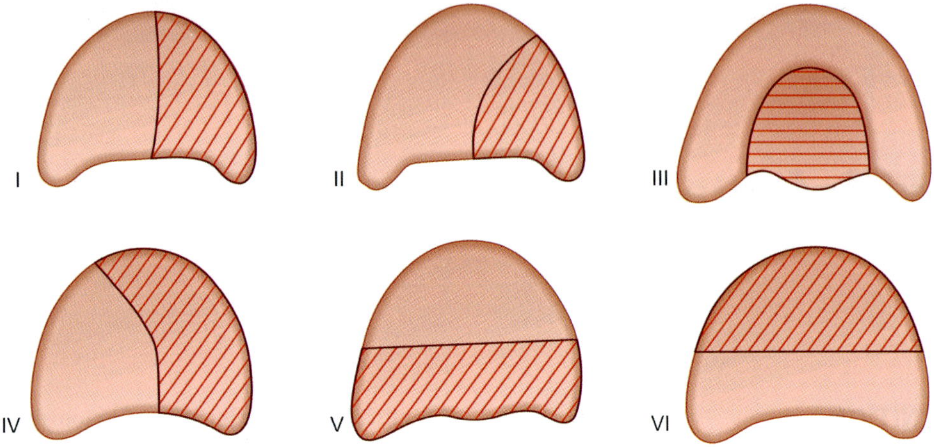

Fig. 21.1: Aramany's classification for partially edentulous maxillectomy dental arches: Class I—Midline resection; Class II—Unilateral resection; Class III—Central resection; Class IV—Bilateral anteroposterior resection; Class V—Posterior resection; Class VI—Anterior resection

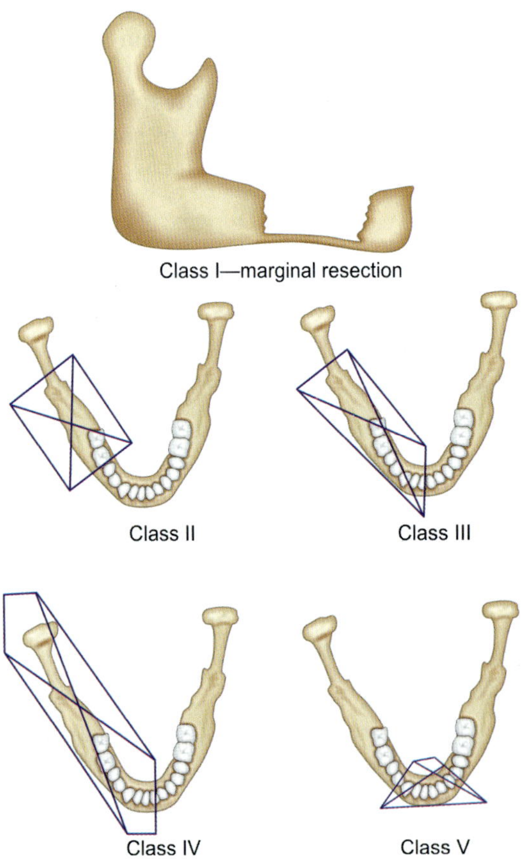

Fig. 21.2: Cantor and Curtis classification of partial mandibulectomy

Class II – Segmental free end resection (discontinuity defect)

Class III – Segmental free end resection up to or crosses the midline.

Class IV – Segmental free end resection up to or crosses the midline and resection of the temporomandibular joint

Class V – Anterior bounded resection

TYPES OF MAXILLOFACIAL PROSTHESIS

Extraoral Prosthesis

Extraoral prostheses are used to restore extraoral defects occur due to trauma, neoplasm or congenital malformation.

- Orbital and ocular prosthesis
- Nasal prosthesis
- Auricular prosthesis
- Combination prosthesis (Combination of one or more of above prosthesis).

Intraoral Prosthesis

Maxillary Prosthesis

- Obturators
- Speech aids
- Palatal lift prosthesis

- Palatal augmentation prosthesis
- Removable prosthesis for mandibulectomy
- Mandibular guide flange.

Treatment Prosthesis

- Stents
- Splints
- Carriers.

Extraoral Prosthesis

Orbital and Ocular Prosthesis

The ocular prosthesis is used to replace enucleated eyes. The lacrimal apparatus (eyelids and glands) is intact and the prosthesis only the eyeball. The orbital prosthesis is used when the entire orbit is removed, including the orbital bones and eyelids.

Nasal Prosthesis

It is fabricated for rhinectomy cases where tumors or cancers were present. The prosthesis may be a temporary or definite prosthesis.

Auricular Prosthesis

It is prosthesis for lost external ear as a results of surgery or from trauma or congenital abnormality. The prosthesis is constructed with silicone rubber with color matching.

Intraoral Prosthesis

Speech Aids Prosthesis

It is prosthesis aid in speech extending into the defect and functionally shaped to the palatopharyngeal musculature. It is done in defects in soft palate due to surgery or congenital anomaly.

Palatal Lift Prosthesis

It is a special type of obturator, to restore narrow palatopharyngeal opening for improving oral air pressure and help in speech.

Palatal Augmentation of Prosthesis

It is a prosthesis for speech and deglutition when surgical resection of tongue or flour of the mouth is done. The contour of palate is augmented by it to modify space of Donder.

CLEFT PALATE

Definition

A cleft palate may be defined as a lack of continuity of the palate either congenital or acquired as a result of injury or disease.

Classification

The failure of union of palate at any stage of development results in a congenital cleft palate which may be classified according to Veall as follows (Fig. 21.3):

- Class I – Cleft involving soft palate only
- Class II – Clefts involving soft and hard palates in the midline up to incisive foramen
- Class III – Clefts of soft and hard palate forward through the alveolar ridges and lip of one side
- Class IV – Clefts involve soft and hard palate forward through the alveolar ridge on both side of lip

Problems of Congenital Cleft Palate

1. Difficulty in ingestion of food and drinks.
2. *Speech*: The pronunciation of all oral sounds requires the air seal to nasal escape. In cleft

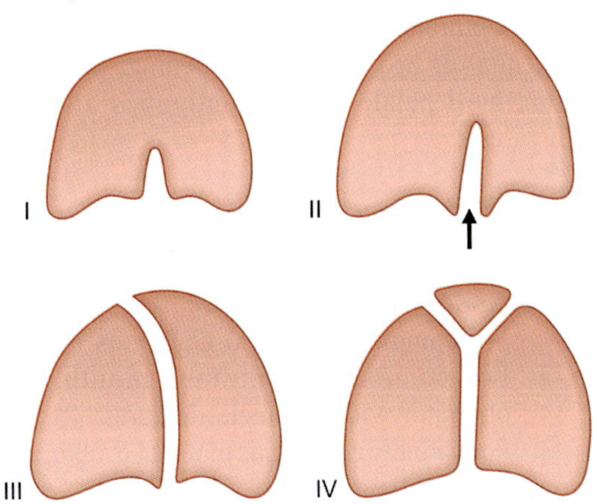

Fig. 21.3: Four types of cleft palate

palate cases this is not possible to control and the air escapes through the nose.

3. Esthetics is impaired when cleft is present.
4. Psychological effect on patient.

Treatment of Cleft Palate

The treatment of cleft palate is due to congenital defect. It should be dealt with by surgical and prosthetic treatment, i.e. by surgery and obturator. So, a team works between the plastic surgeon, prosthodontist and speech therapist is needed.

MAXILLARY PROSTHESIS

Obturator

The word obturator is originated from the Latin word "Obturarz" that means, "to stop up". So an obturator is a maxillofacial prosthesis that closes an opening between the nose and mouth preventing the passage of food and liquid. Obturator prosthesis is required for patient who undergoes maxillectomy due to tumors or has a cleft palate, or palatal injury from a trauma. The patient undergone maxillectomy is treated with obturator prosthesis in various stages of the surgical and post-surgical periods. These are surgical obturator, interim obturator and definitive obturator.

Definition

The "Glossary of prosthodontic terms" defines that an obturator as "A prosthesis used to close a congenital or acquired tissue opening, primarily of the hard palate and/or contiguous alveolar structures."

Types of Obturators

Obturators could be classified by various ways:

A. *Based on the area of restoration*:
   1. For complete or partial dentulous mouth
   2. For complete edentulous mouth, i.e. obturator with complete dentures.
   3. For partially edentulous mouth, i.e. obturator with partial denture.

B. *Based on function:*
   1. *Hinge type*: It moves up and down with the soft palate and formed in a piece of acrylic that is hinged to the base.
   2. *Fixed type*: It is directed towards or slightly above the Passavant's pad)
   3. *Meatus type*: It is directed upwards at approximately 90 degrees upward to the long axis of the palate to reach the roof of the nasopharynx.

C. *Based on phase of treatment*:
   1. *Immediate surgical obturator*: A temporary prosthesis used to restore the continuity of the hard palate immediately after surgery or traumatic loss of a portion or all of the hard palate and/or contiguous alveolar structures (i.e. gingival tissue, teeth). It restores the contours of the hard palate and if possible portion of the soft palate immediately after their loss by trauma or surgery—so has tremendous psychological benefit for the patients.
   2. *Interim surgical obturator*: A prosthesis that is made several weeks or months following the surgical resection of a portion or all of one or both the maxillae. It is frequently includes replacement of teeth and the defective area. This prosthesis, when used, replaces the surgical obturator that is placed immediately following the resection and may be subsequently replaced with a definitive obturator.
   3. *Definitive obturator*: "A prosthesis that artificially replaces part or all of the maxilla and associated teeth lost due to surgery or trauma" (GPT-7). It is for the patients whose healing after surgery or trauma is complete or patients having congenital palatal defects. All healing changes have stabilized and the patient has minimum discomfort. Patient may be dentulous or partial or complete edentulous and the defect can involve hard palate, soft palate, lip or all or any of the above. A hollow bulb

obturator is a definitive obturator modified to reduce the weight and increase patient's comfort. Hollow bulb may be of silicone bulb or acrylic bulb.

Immediate Surgical Obturator

The immediate surgical obturator may be placed immediately following surgery and will serve for 5 to 10 days approximately.

Goal

1. The obturator provides support to the surgical packing placed in the cavity.
2. It reduces the chances of infection contamination.
3. It restores the continuity of the hard palate.
4. It allows the patient to take food in immediate postoperative period if swallowing is not disturbed due to surgery.
5. The patient can speak normally after surgery.

Procedure

The obturator is made on a presurgical maxillary cast obtained during the examination.

The surgeon will plan the treatment to help in design the obturator. An existing well-fitted denture or a properly fitted base plate may be used. It is expected that when existing denture is used. It should be used as the interim prosthesis also. It is usually held by wires, sutures or bone screws

Interim Obturator

The interim obturator is required during the removal of immediate surgical obturator. It is made for wearing until healing occurs approximately 2 to 6 months.

The immediate surgical obturator can be converted to interim obturator by relining with soft resilient liner.

Definitive Obturator

The definitive obturator is fabricated when tissue healing and contraction are complete. The tissue must be stable before it is constructed 6 months after the radiation therapy is completed.

Procedure

1. The preliminary impressions are made in alginate hydrocolloid after block out of the surgical defect with vaseline gauze piece. The limited oral opening makes the impression little difficult. The maxillary custom tray should cover the defect will be helpful in fabrication of final prosthesis.
2. The preliminary cast is blocked out with modeling clay before making the trays.

Definitive Type of Obturator in Edentulous Individual with Complete Denture (Fig. 21.4)

Some characteristics of obturator with complete denture:

1. It should be light in weight, stable and retentive.
2. It should be nonirritating to oral and nasal soft tissues, i.e. comfortable to the patient.
3. It should be simple in design.
4. Readily removable by the patient.
5. An obturator must be capable of restoring both contour and physiologic functions such as speech and swallowing.
6. It should also satisfy the patient esthetically.

Functions of Obturator with Complete Denture

1. Helps in or enables feeding.
2. Prevents aspiration of food and drinks.
3. Enables phonation.
4. Some form of obturator try to correct the defect by restoring the anatomy and some heal the

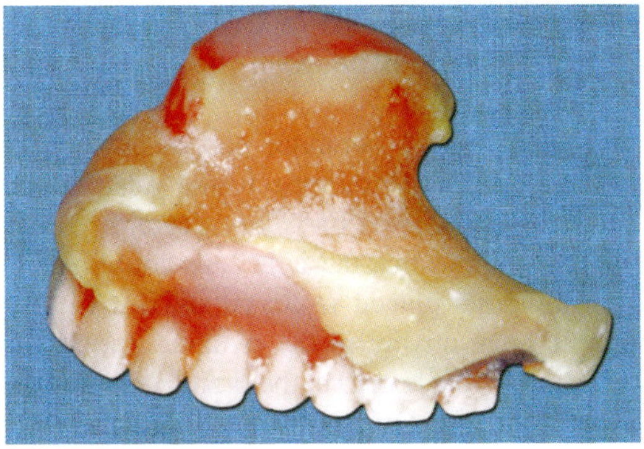

Fig. 21.4: Definitive obturator in edentulous patient with complete denture

defect with scar tissue by stimulating tissues around the void to granulate and scar.

5. Ultimately adds psychological benefit to the patient.
6. When with complete denture the total restoration fulfills all the structural, functional and esthetic requirements of complete denture.

It is often necessary to fabricate an obturator in a complete edentulous mouth. Many of the common defects either congenital or acquired of head and neck surgery may involve most of the areas of maxillae involving full dental arch. Maxillectomy may cause complete edentulism of upper arch. Congenital cleft lip and cleft palate patients are often with congenital missing teeth and also show early teeth shedding due to poor periodontal and alveolar bone support of the remaining teeth. So, it is often needed to restore all upper teeth with obturator. This complete denture with obturator is a prosthesis restoring all teeth of upper arch with an extended part separating the nasal cavity or nasopharynx from oral cavity or oropharynx.

When restoring by complete denture with obturator the edentulous patient with palatal defects due to surgery, congenital anomaly or trauma, the obturator portion of the prosthesis must add stability and retention by extending for enough into the defect to seal it and engage some small undercuts to help in holding the prosthesis in position. The complete denture portion should be constructed using accepted prosthodontic techniques. Modification of the posterior palatal seal and additional beading are often necessary for the denture portion.

The edentulous obturator patient has greater problem in retention, speech and mastication than the conventional maxillary denture patient. It seems obvious that these patients could benefit from implants placed in maxillae. But lack of suitable bone quality in the remaining arch and within the residual bones of the skull on the surgical site precludes widespread use of implants. Bone grafts and sinus lifts are usually needed in the remaining arch but patients are often reluctant to undergo more surgery. Adjunct radiotherapy leads to increased implant failure in the maxilla and implants placed within the surgical cavity are often not accessible through the oral opening for prosthetic restoration. In addition implant cost is still prohibitive. Consequently, few patients have been able to benefit from implants. If clinicians have an option to maintain one or two maxillary teeth, these teeth should be maintained rather than rendering the patient edentulous. Although some teeth may not be adequately positioned to retain conventional partial denture obturator prosthesis, they can become suitable over-denture abutments to be used in a coping/magnet system.

Finally, no matter what additional retentive elements may be employed, sound prosthodontic principles of using bony undercuts, achieving maximum tissue coverage without overextension and placing the dentition in harmony with the functional tissues are paramount for prosthetic success when treating the edentulous patients with palatal defects.

CLINICAL AND LABORATORY STEP BY STEP PROCEDURES OF FABRICATION OF COMPLETE DENTURE WITH OBTURATOR

1. Preliminary impression
2. Final impression
3. Jaw relation records
4. Mounting
5. Flasking
6. Insertion
7. Post-insertion instructions

Preliminary Impression

The preliminary impression should offer maximum extension within the surgical/defective site. In case of large maxillary cavity it is not necessary to block the cavity with gauge. Recent opinion is that blocking causes time loss, patient's discomfort and under-extension of impression due to material shifting during impression taking. In case of small defects, i.e. palatal fistula, the fistula can be blocked with a piece of gauge or cotton wedge tightly into the fistula and tied with floss extending out of mouth. It will prevent the impression material, e.g. alginate, etc. to mushroom into the small cavity that may tear from impression during removal of the tray.

A stock edentulous tray with fluid alginate or a stock edentulous with high viscosity alginate may be used for taking preliminary impression. In case of fluid alginate it is necessary to support the surgical side of the material by adding compound or wax and also necessary to inject the material into the cavity before seating the loaded tray. In case of high viscosity alginate the surgical side of the tray is loaded with more material and adding of compound or wax to the tray or injecting the material into the defect/cavity is not needed. So high viscosity alginate is mostly used. The preliminary impression should capture the periphery and carry into the defect 3–4 cm.

Final Impression

The custom acrylic resin tray should extend 2–3 mm into the cavity beyond the scar band and superior to the cut edge of the hard and soft palates, leaving space for 5–8 mm of compound to add to defective side. Within the cavity the cast undercuts must be blocked out or reduced from the tray before the impression taking. It is possible to make the tray hollow in the bulb area to reduce weight thus to prevent dislodgement of tray due to gravity. The nondefective portion of the palate should be impressioned first. The borders and cut edges of the palate should be border moulded and then impressioned with a definitive impression material. Performing this initial step creates a stable tray for addition of the cavity impression. Compound should be added incrementally to the periphery of the surgical side of the prosthesis. The tray should be supported diagonally against the residual palate or alveolus so as not to rotate the tray into the cavity. With each increment of compound the patient should go through swallowing and head movements. If any movement of tray occurs that area should be cut back and readapted before moving the next area. The defect cavity is convex from inferior to superior. At the height of the convexity the cavity walls begin to turn toward the center of the cavity. At this point the superior aspect of the prosthesis bulb should terminate. Superior extension beyond the greatest convexity aids weight of the prosthesis but adds no retention. An exception to this rule is at the junction of the oral cavity and surgical margin of the prosthesis. There the prosthesis should have more height to allow any liquid that express between the prosthesis and the tissue to travel along the same space by gravity back into the oral cavity. This height is 1–1.5 cm. Another exception involves contacting the remaining bony walls of the maxillary sinus. When the walls remain and have been resurfaced with the split thickness skin graft, there should be and attempt to capture those walls in the impression both peripherally and centrally. This lateral and posterior bony wall can offer support against superior displacement during swallowing and mastication. Following the use of compound, and impression wax can be placed over the compound surface. The surgical side of the impression can be dipped quickly into a hot water bath and then placed into the mouth. The area should be border moulded again. Thin area in the wax will denote the areas of pressure, which could be relieved in the compound impression and additional wax placed to repeat the procedure. A post-palatal seal can also be placed. Because of the large wax surface area the boxing can be done more easily with plaster and pumice.

Jaw Relation Records

Maxillectomy patients have loss of facial contour on the surgical side proportional to the amount of resected bone including alveolus. Infrastructural maxillectomies have minimal facial disfigurement. As the surgical defect includes the middle and superior portions of the maxillary bone at its junction with the zygomatic arch, the middle third of the face contracts. Finally if the floor of the orbit is resected the globe is also displaced. Often the maxillary resection crosses the midline, and if the nasal spine is resected, the nose is unsupported. There is a desire to use the obturator prosthesis to support the facial tissues. Unfortunately these tissues are fibrotic and can only be minimally displaced by prosthesis border. Trying to push the contracted tissues into their preoperative position can cause overextension of prosthesis border. This creates considerable prosthetic support of the face is limited by the amount of retention that can be achieved from the residual palate and undercuts within the defect cavity. When an individual had an infrastructure maxillectomy (alveolus and sinus floor only) that does not cross the anterior midline, the lip and cheek can be easily supported by the dentition of the obturator prosthesis. As more of the maxillary bones are resected, however, tooth position and the flange of prosthesis must be placed palatally due to tissue collapse. Attempting to maintain the dentition in its normal position will cause dislodging forces. There may be some scarring of the lip at the suture line that disrupts the normal drop of the lip, often requiring accommodation by changes in the occlusal plane and tooth position. Normal prosthetic landmarks cannot be used to position the dentition. Processed record bases are ideal for jaw relationship records for maxillofacial prosthetic patient. Because of the missing structures and unusual reconstruction, prosthetic retention and stability are gradually compromised. Blocking out of routine undercuts and the undercuts within the surgical area adds to instability of conventional record base. In the obturator cast the blocking out of undercuts within the surgical area adds to instability of conventional record base. In the obturator cast the blocking out of undercuts at the periphery will result in a trial base that does not extend to the periphery of the defect. After these block out it is possible to have trial base that makes no contact with the defective side. There will be no retention of prosthesis except for the adhesive on the hard palate. The prosthesis will fall into the oral cavity when attempting to establish the occlusal plane and locate into the defect when attempting the centric relation record. Without maximum extension of record base, one cannot determine the optimal position of the teeth to support the lip and cheek. A processed base will reveal the optimal retention of the obturator prosthesis before addition of teeth. It is quite common to find that retention become worse as the wax rim is added in its preoperative position. If retention is decreased as the wax rim is added, the position of the rim must be modified to establish retention. A compromise must be reached between tissue support and prosthesis retention. Often the lip is scarred and contracted creating too much or too little tooth display. Having the processed base allows the clinician to try different tooth position to optimize speech, esthetics and retention at the try-in appointment. It is important that the patient and clinician understand what can be accomplished prior to the insertion appointment.

The waxing of the processed obturator base can be solid in the area of the bulb and hollowed before jaw relationship records. When waxing the prosthesis on should recreate the palate contours on the surgical side to be identical to the contours on the remaining hard palate. The bulb can be processed hollow by waxing the external periphery of the bulb portion several millimeters thick and pouring a stone core through the back of the master cast or creating a stone core in the cope of the flask, in which case there will be a hole in the palate after processing primarily in the prosthesis this hole could be opened but opening must be wide enough to place a cleaning brush but later the hole in the prosthesis should be closed with a lid on the palate.

The jaw relationship appointment should progress as a routine denture appointment. Remount casts will be required for the processed bases. The usual parameter of speaking space and appearance should be considered for establishing vertical dimension of occlusion. The maxillary anterior rim should be placed at the wet dry line of the lower lip. There should be an attempt to displace the contracted lip to achieve appropriate position of the rim.

However, if the prosthesis begins to loose retention, the wax rim will require reduction on the facial aspect. Compensation of the contracted lip and cheek is often necessary on the defect side, and it may be necessary to gradually create a negative horizontal overlap or end-to-end occlusion extending from the midline to the posterior dentition. Lip closure may be a problem due to contracture and shortening of the upper lip. One may elect to decrease the vertical dimension of occlusion slightly to compensate for poor lip closure, but the decrease may result in tongue or lip biting on the nonsurgical side of the mouth. Therefore, one should attempt to improve lip closure by buccolingual tooth position rather than a severe decrease in vertical dimension.

The centric relation recording material should be selected by clinician's preference. As more of the maxillary arch and palate are resected, greater the instability of maxillary base. A processed should also be considered for edentulous mandible. When making the centric relation record, the clinician must manually stabilize the maxillary prosthesis but cannot do the same in case of mandibular prosthesis. In case of mandibular prosthesis this instability during jaw relationship record can be compensated to some extent by using a processed base. Both upper and lower prosthesis should be retained with adhesive during jaw relationship records and try-in. If the mandibular arch is partially dentate it should be restored to allow full arch occlusion. This will assist in reseating the maxillary obturator under function and maintaining the correct vertical dimension. At the try-in all records are verified. The patient and clinician will get an appreciation for the tooth position and tooth display. For the patients, edentulous in both the arches, a cuspless tooth allows freedom to create a negative horizontal overlap on the surgical side of the arch without having to create it on the nonsurgical side. Because these are processed bases the clinical remount is not needed at insertion but a laboratory remount can be performed after processing to correct errors.

The final palatal contour should be evaluated at the try-in appointment. It is likely that the contours are not symmetric because they were created arbitrarily on the surgical side of the palate with few visible landmarks at the initial wax up of the base. The vault may be of too high or too flat. It is often easy to detect the asymmetry by sweeping the thumb across the palate from cusps on one side of the arch to cusp tip of other side.

Place wax or reduce resin until the palate is symmetric. Finally pressure-indicating paste can be streaked across the palate from right to left. Seat the prosthesis and have the patient swallow and count. Where the tongue makes contact with the palate, the contact can be read in the pressure indicating paste. Heavy areas should be reduced and the entire palate is checked again. Wax may need to be added in the palate where there is no contact. If the patient lisps, air is escaping laterally from the tongue. The patient may be given water to wet the mouth slightly and ask to count again. Water well likely express out from the side of the mouth where the tongue is not making contact, and the pressure indicating paste likely to be thicker in this area. Wax should be flowed along the premolar and canine areas on that side of the palate. With repeated adjustments and palatograms, more even contact will be observed on the entire palate after swallowing and speaking. Because the teeth are placed palatally due to facial contracture, they may impinge on the tongue. Sometime, it is necessary to reduce the width of the occlusal table on the defective/surgical side to allow for tongue space. If the palatograms reveal a heavy contact against the palatal surface of the teeth, the occlusal table should be reduced. This palatal refinement should be incorporated in the final prosthesis when the teeth are processed to the baseplate. The prosthesis can be processed at a lower temperature than that used to process the base.

After deflasking the processed dentures can be replaced on the remount casts and a laboratory remount is performed. The clinician may place a lid on the obturator prosthesis or may insert the prosthesis with the bulb left open for several days after delivery. The patient then can make the choice between the closed or open obturator. Patients exhibiting problems during interim phase may need more adjustment to satisfy speech and swallowing. Too soon placement of lid may preclude adjustments without perforating the bulb.

Mounting

During mounting of casts for obturator with complete denture the articulator modification is done to increase the vertical space so that the articulator can accommodate casts. Both arcon and non-arcon Hanau articulator can be modified:

- For arcon articulator it is seen in the figures. When the recessed end is secured to the lower member of the articulator, the protruding stud permits attachment of the upper member. The upper member is thereby raised but the condylar elements remain in the original position.
- For non-arcon Hanau articulator, attachment of the studded end to the lower member also permits elevation of the upper member without altering the position of the condylar elements.
- Any rigid non-corrosive material can be selected and machined to the dimensions as seen in the figures. With the upper member of the articulator at an elevator position, machined incisal pins of proper length are required for both modified articulator.

Flasking

For flasking of obturator with complete denture the special maxillofacial flask that is oversized in all dimensions (especially in vertical dimension) should be used.

Insertion

At insertion the prosthesis should be evaluated for pressure areas using pressure indicating paste for residual palate. The bulb portion should be checked for functional pressure areas with a tissue conditioning material of contrasting color.

Post-insertion Instructions

Patient should be instructed to wear continuous even at night to manage sinus secretion and saliva at night. If removed at night the soft tissue periphery of the defect will change due to tissue edema and cause improper seat for about an hour of wearing the prosthesis in the morning. Mainly the teeth of the nondefective side of the arch should accomplish mastication. Denture adhesives also may be required.

Post-insertion Problems or Complains of Complete Denture with Obturator

Many patients eventually complain of: (a) Nasal reflux, i.e. fluid leakage due to inadequate seal and (b) Hypernasal speech due to escape of air for several months or even a few years after insertion of prosthesis. In most cases continued fibrosis in the tissues bordering the prosthesis is the cause. Use of tissue conditioning materials primarily and relining later on, use of silicone bulb obturator could be solution of the problems. Beside this loss of posterior and lateral extension, improper fit, fracture of acrylic, loss of labial tooth form and perforation of hollow bulb after adjustment may be there due to processing errors.

TREATMENT PROSTHESIS

Definition

A treatment prosthesis is "A prosthetic appliance used for the purpose of treating or conditioning the tissues that are called on to support and retain it."

Types of Treatment Prosthesis

- Surgical obturator
- Mandibular training flange
- Splints
- Stents

- Carriers
- Mouth protectors.

MANDIBULAR TRAINING FLANGE

It is prosthesis used by mandibulectomy patient to prevent the deviation of mandible towards the resected side because of the muscle pull results in derailment of occlusion. It helps to open and close in the normal occlusal relationship. It is a removable partial denture with a flange extended superior-laterally buccal to the maxillary posterior teeth on the normal side.

Procedures of Fabrication

1. The impressions of both the arches are obtained in alginate hydrocolloid and casts are poured.
2. The casts are mounted on articulator with normal cusp fossa relationship in the normal side.
3. A acrylic partial denture is fabricated with an acrylic extended flange for training to guide the mandible in normal occlusion.
4. A definitive prosthesis is fabricated and delivered to the patient after the deviation is corrected with regular use of the training flange.

SPLINTS

Definition

A splint is defined as "A rigid or flexible device that maintains in position a displaced or movable part; also used to keep in place and protect an injured part" (GPT-7).

Types of Splints

Gunning Splint (Figs 21.5A and B)

It is an acrylic device used to immobilize the jaws in occlusion and to hold together fractured segments of mandibular or maxillary bones. An external bandage helps immobilization of splint. It was first devised by Thomas Brian Gunning an American dentist. There are two types of gunning splints: (a) one piece gunning splint and (b) two piece gunning splint.

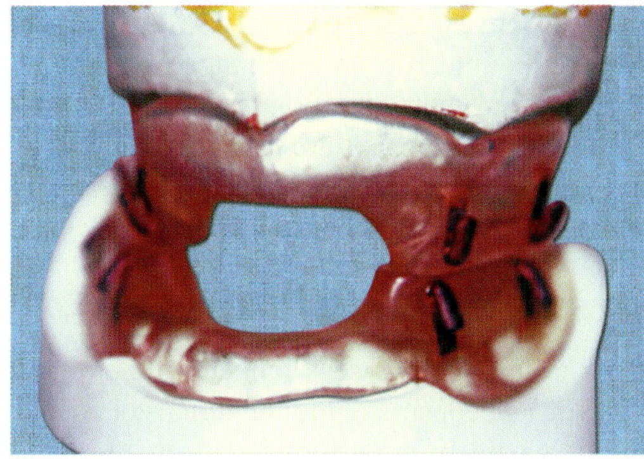

Fig. 21.5A: Two piece gunning splint assembled on casts

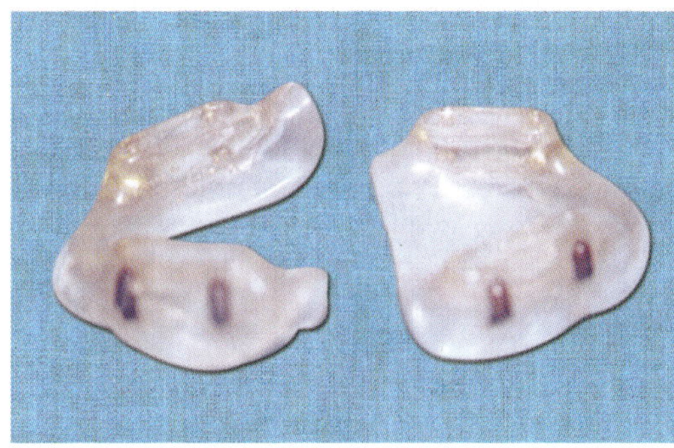

Fig. 21.5B: Two piece gunning splint separate

One piece gunning splint joins upper and lower bases in correct vertical dimension of occlusion. A space is created in incisor regions in the rims to facilitate breathing, feeding and postanesthesia vomiting.

Two piece gunning splint is used in edentulous case with bilateral fractures. A pair of existing complete denture may be produced to two piece gunning splint by removing few anterior teeth and drilling holes for wiring together. Retention may be improved by reline with gutta purcha or soft tissue liner.

In absence of existing denture two impressions of alginate hydrocolloid impression is obtained and stone casts are prepared. Base plates with occlusal rims are construction for both the arches. The casts are mounted on an articulator with vertical dimension and centric relation registration. Two to four stainless wire hooks are inserted in the buccal flanges for fixation with elastic bands. The splints are processed with acrylic resin.

Split Splint/Labiolingual Splint (Fig. 21.6)

These are acrylic devisees hinged with stainless steel wire and constructed for dentulous or edentulous or partially edentulous patient requiring fixation of fracture. Two to four stainless wire hooks are incorporated in the buccal flanges for fixation.

Fenestrated Splint

This splint is prepared by fenestration in the occlusal surfaces. Two or four stainless wire loops or holes in buccal flange is fixed for fixation. It is useful for fixation of fracture in children with deciduous teeth.

Kingsley Splint

The Kingsley splint in its original form used by Dr Norman Kingsley was applicable to either jaw, and was used for treatment of fractures of the mandible in place of gunning splint and for depressed fractures of the maxilla where upward traction was required. Modern variety is only used in the maxilla for both dentulous and edentulous patients. It consists of a shallow tray (Fig. 21.7) which is fitted with impression compound for attaching it to the teeth. A handle is protruded through the lips and fixed to a vertical rod by means of an universal joint and clamp. The rod terminates in a flat plate which is embedded to a plaster or other type headgear.

Metal Cap Splits

It is constructed of either of cast silver copper alloy, cobalt chrome or aluminum alloy. The pattern is fabricated with thin sheet of casting wax covering the coronal portion of the cast. The pattern is invested with investing material in a casting rim of appropriate size. The casting is done after removal of wax.

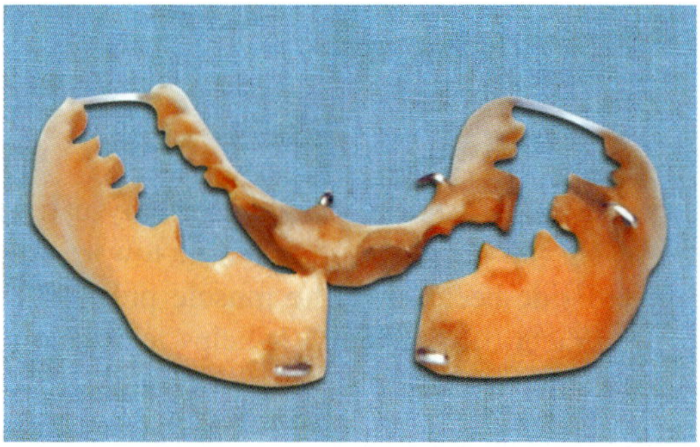

Fig. 21.6: Split splint for treatment of mandibular fracture

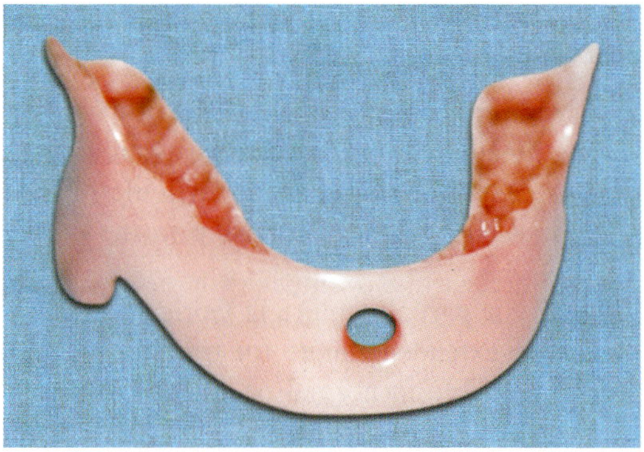

Fig. 21.7: Kingsley splint

Advantages of Cast Cap Splints

1. In presence of only two teeth on each fragment good anchorage and immobilization can be obtained.
2. These are comfortable to the patient and will cause little disturbance of oral function due to small mass.
3. They are not injurious to oral tissues.
4. There is less adjustment or attention is required.
5. The force is distributed on all remaining teeth attached to the splint.
6. The mastication is not impaired.

Disadvantages of Cast Cap Splint

1. Laboratory facility and the clinical assistance is required.
2. Time is required for construction.
3. Impression procedures are sometime difficult.
4. Decementation of splint may occur.
5. The splint is destroyed during removal.

STENTS

Charles R Stent, 1901.

Definition

A stent is an appliance to hold the tissue, i.e. graft in a predetermined position.

Antihemorrhagic Stent

This is a prosthesis used in hemophilic patient to control post-extraction bleeding. Pre-extraction casts are prepared and mounted on articulator in centric relation. The vertical dimension is increased by 1 mm. The teeth to be extracted are removed and sockets are prepared on the cast. An acrylic base plate is constructed and the stent is relined.

Drainage Stent

It is used to permit the drainage of pus, blood and exudates during healing period.

Paraplegic Stent

It is a device designed for feeding of paraplegic patient.

Periodontal Stent

It is a device designed to hold periodontal dressing in place after surgery.

Grafting Stent

It is a device designed to hold the graft during healing period. The most common stent is used in vestibuloplasty to prevent tissue attachment.

CARRIER

Definition

"A device used to administer radiation to confined areas by means of capsules, beads, or needles of radiation emitting materials such as radium or cesium. Its function is to hold the radiation source securely in the same position during the entire period of treatment (GPT-7).

Radiation carriers are of three types depends on their function as follows:

1. Protective carrier consisting of protective lead mask with a hole for passage of radiation. The lead mask protects the healthy tissue.
2. Positional carrier are used to recontour or reposition the tissues into or out of radiation target field.
3. Docking appliances are used to hold the radiation cone pointed to the target tissue.

MOUTH PROTECTORS

These are recommend to all players of contact sports like basketball, bax ball and so cure to protect orofacial structures from injury. Common trauma of teeth causes pupils, pulpal necrosis and resorption. Mouth protectors may be custom-made or mouth-formed or stock. The custom-made mouth protectors are formed from thermoplastic polymer sheets about 14 cm square. The common material is polyethylene or polyurethane. A vacum-forming machine is hold to produce it on an stone cast made from alginate impression.

CONCLUSION

The maxillofacial prosthodontics deals with the congenital, traumatic, or surgical abnormalities in the oral cavity and associated structures. The goal is to improve quality of life for the patient. Normal function of speech, swallowing may not be achieved but it is possible to obtain optimum functions.

BIBLIOGRAPHY

1. Bulbulian AH. Maxillofacial prosthetics: Evolution and practical application in patient rehabilitation. J Prosthet Dent. 1965;15:554.
2. Chalian VA, et al. Maxillofacial prosthetics.Wiilliams and Wilkins Co. Baltimore; 1977.
3. Laney WR, et al. Maxillofacial prosthetics, Littleton, Mass; 1979.
4. Murrow RM, Ruud KD, Rhoads JE. Dental laboratory procedures of complete denture; Vol 3 (2nd edn). Mosby, St Louis; 1986.
5. Rahn AO, Boucher LJ. Maxillofacial prosthetics, WB Saunders Co, Philadelphia; 1970.
6. Word RH, Carl W. Hollow silicone obturators for total maxillectomy: J Prosthet Dent. 1977;38:643.
7. Zarb, Bolender, Carlson. Boucher's prosthodontic treatment of edentulous patient (11th edn). Mosby; 1997.

Index

Page numbers followed by *f* refer to figure and *t* refer to table

A

Acrylic denture teeth chart 144*f*, 145*f*
Acrylic polishers 197*f*
Acrylic resin 103, 147, 253
Adhesion 50
Alveolar process 10
Alveolectomy 231
Angular cheilitis 217
Anterior teeth
  selection and arrangement of 233
  shade of 146
Antihemorrhagic stent 267
Anti-Monson curve 167*f*
Aramany's classification 255, 256*f*
Arch size 37
Articulators
  equilibration techniques 252
  parts of 107
  purpose of 108
  requirements of 108
  types of 111
  use of 108
Artificial teeth, number system of 146
Atmospheric pressure 51

B

Balanced articulation
  advantages of 172
  disadvantages of 172
Balanced occlusion, articulation of 169
Bases, types of 102
Bennett angle 24*f*, 170
Bennett movement 24, 24*f*
  types of 24, 24*f*
Biometer 125
Bone 10
  loss 244
Bonwill's circle 141*f*, 142*f*
  arch of 142*f*
Bonwill's triangle 141*f*
Bruce's method 252
Buccal frenum 63
Buccal shelf 11, 47, 48
Buccal vestibule 63
Buccinator 15
Buccolingual position 157
Buccolingual width 154
Burning mouth syndrome 215, 217

C

Camper's line 133*f*
Candida infection 210
Canine 152, 162
  lines 101, 135
  maxillary 161
Cantor and Curtis classification 256*f*
Capsular ligament 20
Cardiovascular diseases 35
Cast 92
  cap splint, disadvantages of 267
  guidelines, maxillary 150*f*
  pouring of 93, 98
  types of 92
Central incisor 151, 152, 160*f*, 162
  maxillary 161
Centric occlusion 25, 26, 126, 127*t*, 166
  selective grinding for 201
Christensen's phenomenon 166, 166*f*
Cleft palate 257
  treatment of 258
  types of 257*f*
Cold-cure acrylic resin 223*f*
Complete dentures 2, 3, 60, 62*f*, 177, 215, 228, 250
  complains of 264
  impression 60, 61
  indications of 4
  maxillary 46*t*
  occlusion, requirements of 167
  prosthesis 2, 4
  prosthodontics 1
  retention 49
  scope of 5
  selection of articulator for 113
  steps of insertion of 206
Composite resin 147
Compound impression 93
Condylar guidance 170
Condylar path, fixed 113
Congenital cleft palate 257
Congenital defects 255
Corner lines 101, 135
Cosmetic index 34
Cusp angle 171
Cusp height 171

D

Debris, removal of 19
Dental prosthesis 238
Dentures 2
  adhesives 53
  base
    adaptation of 55
    fitting surface of 58
    material 44, 193*f*
    maxillary 183*f*
    shade 44
  bearing areas 63
  borders 15
  checking retention of 178
  checking stability of 178
  cleansing kit 210*f*
  complains of 213
  finishing of 185
  flanges 18
  implant 235
  insertion of 178
  inspection of 206

maxillary 63, 183*f*, 188, 208
meniscus 50*f*
periphery 207
postinsertion adjustment of 211
press 193*f*
shunting of 251
stomatitis 215, 217
techniques 231
teeth 140
test for retention of 208
Depressor anguli oris 16
Depressor labii inferioris 16
Digestion, initiation of 19
Drainage stent 267

E

Edentulous mouth 43, 60
Electromyography 124
Endodontic implants 238
Endodontic therapy 247*f*
Endosseous implants 243
cylinder 237*f*, 238*f*
screw 237*f*
Esthetics 2, 62, 125
Extraction method, two stage 231
Extraction technique
single stage 230
two stage 230
Extraoral articulator method 179
Extraoral gothic arch tracer 128*f*

F

Fabrication 102
procedures of 265
rules for 104
Facebow 107, 113
arbitrary 116, 116*t*
kinematic 116*t*
necessity of 115
purpose of 114
record, preservation of 206
types of 116
use of 115
Facial expression, muscles of 14, 14*f*
Facial measurements 123
Facial musculature, collapse of 229
Fixed implant supported prostheses, disadvantages of 243
Flange method 190
Former denture, measurement of 123
Fovea palatine 63
Fracture, types of 220
Freeway space 125*t*

G

Gag reflex 41
Genial tubercles 12
Genioglossus muscle 17
Gothic arch tracing method, contraindications of 129
Grafting stent 267
Greater palatine foramen 10*f*
Groove indexing method 100
Gunning splint 265
Gysi simplex articulator 109*f*

H

Hanau arbitrary facebow 117*f*
Hanau kinematic facebow 117*f*
Hanau's formula 138, 170, 170*f*
Hanau's quints 169*f*
Hard palate 63
Hard tissues 57
Hard wax 103
Heat cure acrylic resin base 103
Hinge articulator 113
Hinge axis 114, 117
Hybrid prosthesis, fixed 242
Hydraulic denture press 193*f*
Hyoglossus muscle 18

I

Implants
complications of 244
denture, parts of 235
supported prostheses, advantages of 236
types of 236, 242
Impressions, types of 60
Incisal plane 179
Incisive fossa 11
Incisive muscles 16
Incisive papilla 63
Indexing cast 100
Infrahyoid muscles 21
Interarch distance 45
Interarch space 38
Intercommissural distance 141
Interim surgical obturator 258, 259
Interpenetrating polymer network acrylic resin 147
Intraborder movements 26
Intraoral gothic arch tracer 128*f*

J

Jaw closing reflexes 26
Jaw opening reflexes 26
Jectron jig 226*f*
Joint, diseases of 35

K

Keratinized mucosa 9*f*

L

Labial contour 101
Labial frenum 63
Labial sounds 180
Labial vestibule 63
Labiodental sounds 180
Labiolingual inclination 152
Lamina propria 10
Levator anguli oris 16
Lingual surface 190
Lingual tuberosity 13
Lingualized articulation 174, 175, 175*f*
Linguodental sounds 180
Lining mucosa 9
Lips 37
Local anesthesia 239
Lower anterior teeth, selection of 144

M

Mandible, gross anatomy of 11
Mandibular anterior teeth, arrangement of 161
Mandibular canine 100
Mandibular complete denture 47*t*, 253*f*
Mandibular denture 189, 208, 209*f*
Mandibular depression, muscles of 16
Mandibular impression, wax boxing of 99*f*
Mandibular movement 22
determinants of 26, 27
muscles of 21
regulation of 26
Mandibular posterior teeth, arrangement of 162
Mandibular ridge
prognosis 47
types of 47
Mandibular rim 105
Mandibular teeth, plane of 180
Mandibular training flange 265
Masseter muscle 16
Master cast 92
boxing and pouring of 97

Master impression 60
Mastication 2, 3, 229
Masticatory muscles 16, 20
atrophy of 215
Maxilla, gross anatomy of 10, 10*f*
Maxillary anterior teeth, arrangement of 160
Maxillary central incisor
arrangement of 161*f*
width of 141
Maxillary denture, midline fracture of 223*f*
Maxillary impression, wax boxing of 99*f*
Maxillary posterior teeth, arrangement of 162
Maxillary rim 105
width 106*f*
Maxillary supporting structures, anatomy of 63
Maxillary torus 47
Maxillofacial defects, classification of 255
Maxillofacial prosthesis, types of 256
Maximum mouth opening 25, 26
Maximum protrusion 25, 26
Menopause 35
Mental foramen 13
Mesiodistal inclination 152
Mesiodistal width 154
Midline fracture
mandibular denture, repair of 222*f*
maxillary denture, repair of 221*f*
Midpalatal suture 10*f*
Model former method 93
Molars and premolars, crossbite arrangement of 164*f*
Monoplane articulation 173, 174
Monson, curve of 167, 167*f*
Mould, classification of 146
Mouth protectors 267
Mucoperiosteum 10
Mucosa 8
masticatory 8
types of 8, 9
Mucosal implants 238
Mucosal reactions 215
Mucosal shade 34
Muscle tone 37, 47
Mylohyoid ridge 12

N

Natural teeth, removal of 228
Nonarcon articulators 111

O

Obturator
types of 258, 259
Occlusal plane 101
Occlusion
nomenclature and terminology of 166
preliminary vertical dimension of 130
rims 104, 233*f*
fabrication of 104
vertical dimension of 120
Oral cancer 215
Oral mucosa, types of 9*f*
Oral structures, preservation of 2
Orbicularis oris 15
Overdenture
techniques of 247, 247*f*
types of 246

P

Palatal glands, excessive salivation of 19
Palate, ulceration of 54*f*
Palatine bones 11
Palatoglossus muscle 18
Partial denture 2
fixed 2
prosthodontics 1
removable 2
Partial mandibulectomy 256*f*
Partially edentulous maxillectomy defects 255
Periodontal stent 267
Peripheral seal 52
Permanent base, advantages of 102
Pharyngeal muscles 17
Polishing wax 190
Posterior teeth
arrangement of 154, 156, 233
buccal cusps of 167*f*
normal arrangement of 164*f*
selection of 154
Post-extraction methods 123
Prosthesis 1, 256, 257, 264
auricular 256, 257
combination 256
extraoral 256, 257
intraoral 256, 257
mandibular 242
maxillary 242, 256, 258
nasal 256, 257
orbital and ocular 256, 257
palatal augmentation of 257
types of 2
Prosthetic dentistry 1
Prosthetic failure 244
Prosthodontics 1
branches of 1
care 44
fixed 1
implant 1
maxillofacial 1
Protrusive balance 173, 186*f*
selective grinding for 203
Protrusive interocclusal record 137
Protrusive occlusion 166
Pterygoid
external 21
hamulus 10*f*, 11
internal 21
lateral 16, 20
medial 16, 20
Pterygomaxillary notch 63

Q

Quadratus labii superioris 16

R

Remount cast 92
Removable prosthodontics 1
Residual ridge 63
Residual ridge
reduction 215, 216
relationship 14, 55
Retromolar pad 100, 159*f*
Retromylohyoid space 40
Ridge
parallelism 38, 123
shape of 37, 46, 53
size of 11, 46
tapering arch form of 12*f*
Rubber suction disk 54*f*
use of 54*f*

S

Sagittal axis 23
Salivary glands and saliva 19
Shock absorbing elements 243
Silverman's closest speaking space 124

Silverman's phonetic methods 124
Simple hinge articulator 110*f*, 111
Soft palate, muscles of 17
Soft tissue 57
  hyperplasia 215
Space envelope 26*f*
Spee, curve of 167, 167*f*
Splints 265
  types of 265
Split remounting indexing method 100
Sprinkle-on method 103
Square shaped maxillary arch 37*f*
Styloglossus muscle 18
Sublingual fold space, nature of 47
Submandibular and sublingual salivary glands, excessive salivation of 19
Suction chambers 54
Suction disks 54
Suprahyoid muscles 21
Surgical obturator 258, 259
Swenson's method 251

T

Tapering-shaped maxillary arch 38*f*
Teeth
  anatomic and nonanatomic 155*f*
  arrangement of 149, 157, 163, 164, 175, 186
  extraction of 35, 43
  final arrangement of 185
  mesiodistal inclination of 152*f*
  methods of selection of 139
  nonanatomic 155
Temporalis muscle 16
Temporomandibular disorders 216
Temporomandibular joint 20*f*, 21*f*, 26, 37, 109, 120
  anatomy of 19, 27
Three digit number system 146
Three teeth replacement prostheses 241*f*
Tissue
  health of 57
  tone 48
Tongue
  muscles of 17, 18
  position 41, 47
Tooth replacement 240*f*
Torus palatini 39*f*
Translation horizontal axis 25, 26
Transmandibular implant 238
Traumatic ulcers 215
Tuberosities 53
  size of 47

U

Upper anterior teeth, selection of 140
Upper denture, midline fracture of 222*f*

V

Vacuum fired porcelain 253
Valsalva maneuver 182*f*
Vertical dimension 101, 120
  significance of 121
Vitamins 216

W

Wax 103
  boxing 97
Whip-mix articulator 111*f*, 112
Willis gauge, use of 134*f*
Wilson, curve of 167, 167*f*
Wright's classification 48

X

Xerostomia 19

Y

Yurkstas method 251

Z

Zinc oxide eugenol impression paste 103
Zygomatic crest 63
Zygomatic process 63
Zygomaticoalveolar crest 10